Evidence-Based Public Health

Evidence-Based Public Health

SECOND EDITION

Ross C. Brownson
Elizabeth A. Baker
Terry L. Leet
Kathleen N. Gillespie
William R. True

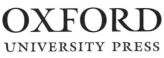

OXFORD
UNIVERSITY PRESS
2011

OXFORD
UNIVERSITY PRESS

Oxford University Press, Inc., publishes works that further
Oxford University's objective of excellence
in research, scholarship, and education.

Oxford New York
Auckland   Cape Town   Dar es Salaam   Hong Kong   Karachi
Kuala Lumpur   Madrid   Melbourne   Mexico City   Nairobi
New Delhi   Shanghai   Taipei   Toronto

With offices in
Argentina   Austria   Brazil   Chile   Czech Republic   France   Greece
Guatemala   Hungary   Italy   Japan Poland   Portugal   Singapore
South Korea   Switzerland   Thailand   Turkey   Ukraine   Vietnam

Published by Oxford University Press, Inc.
198 Madison Avenue, New York, New York 10016
www.oup.com

Oxford is a registered trademark of Oxford University Press

Library of Congress Cataloging-in-Publication Data

Evidence-based public health / Ross C. Brownson ... [et al.]. — 2nd ed.
p. ; cm.
Includes bibliographical references and index.
ISBN 978-0-19-539789-5 1. Public health. 2. Evidence-based medicine. I. Brownson, Ross C.
[DNLM: 1. Public Health. 2. Evidence-Based Practice. 3. Public Health Administration.
WA 100 E93 2010]
RA427.E954 2010
362.1—dc22
2010020134

9 8 7 6 5 4 3 2
Printed in the United States of America
on acid-free paper

We dedicate this book to our close colleague and friend, Terry Leet. We lost Terry in the spring of 2009 while this second edition was being developed. Terry was an outstanding scholar and teacher and we miss him every day.

Foreword

Evidence-based public health has become an often-used phrase by both practitioners and policymakers. However, its meaning and proper place in the development, conduct, and evaluation of public health programs and policies are often misunderstood. When we hear the word *evidence,* most of us conjure up the mental picture of a courtroom, with opposing lawyers presenting their evidence, or of law enforcement personnel sifting through a crime scene for evidence to be used in judicial proceedings.

Evidence, so central to our notion of justice, is equally central to public health. This is because it should inform all of our judgments about what interventions to implement, in what populations, and when and how to determine both positive and sometimes negative effects of those interventions. Our commitment to justice also comes with the responsibility to find effective ways to reduce the health disparities among groups that exist in virtually all geopolitical units.

In public health, there are four principal user groups for evidence. Public health practitioners with executive and managerial responsibilities and their many public and private partners want to know the evidence for alternative strategies, be they policies, programs, or other activities. Too infrequently do busy practitioners find the time to ask the fundamental question, "What are the most important things I can do to improve the public's health?" In pursuit of answers, population-based data are the first prerequisite, covering health status, health risks, and health problems for the overall population and sociodemographic subsegments. Also important are the population's attitudes and beliefs about various major health problems.

The second prerequisite is data on potential interventions. What is the range of alternatives? What do we know about each? What is their individual and conjoint effectiveness in improving health in the populations we are serving? This marriage of information can lead to a rational prioritization of opportunities, constrained only by resources and feasibility.

More often, public health practitioners and their partners have a more narrow set of options. Funds from national, state, or local governments are earmarked for a specific purpose, such as surveillance and treatment of sexually transmitted diseases, inspection of retail food establishments, or treatment for substance abusers. Still, practitioners have the opportunity, even the obligation, to survey the evidence carefully for alternative ways to achieve the desired health goals. Those on the frontlines share the responsibility to seek evidence on how they can be most effective and efficient overall and on their effects on health disparities in different groups.

The next user group includes policymakers at local, regional, state, national, and international levels. They are faced with macrolevel decisions on how to allocate the public resources for which they have been elected stewards. This group has the additional responsibility of making policies on controversial public issues. Under what conditions should private gun ownership be allowed? How much tax should be levied on cigarettes, and how should these tax revenues be used? Should needle exchange programs be legal for intravenous drug addicts? Should treatment be the required alternative for perpetrators of nonviolent offenses who committed crimes while abusing alcohol or other drugs? What are the best strategies to reverse the obesity epidemic? Good politicians want to know the evidence for the effects of options they are being asked to consider or may want to propose.

Key stakeholders are a third user group for evidence. This group includes many nongovernment organizations whose missions focus on or include improving health, directly or through enhancing the social and physical environments that are key population health determinants. Other stakeholders include the public, especially those who vote, as well as interest groups formed to support or oppose specific policies, such as the legality of abortion, what foods should be served at public schools, or whether home visiting for the families of neonates should be a routine health benefit. While passion on these issues can run high, evidence can temper views or suggest a feasible range for compromise among opposing views. Sometimes voters are asked to weigh in on proposed policies, such as clean indoor air ordinances or whether to legalize marijuana.

The final user group is composed of researchers on population health issues, who evaluate the impact of specific policies or programs. They both develop and use evidence to explore research hypotheses. Some are primarily interested in the methods used to determine the quality and implications of research on population-based interventions. They frequently ask, "Was the study design appropriate?"

and "What are the criteria for determining the adequacy of the study methods?" Others look at the factors that facilitate or retard progress in translating evidence into practice, or in what range of situations an evidence-based intervention can be applied with confidence as to its effectiveness. And an increasing number of researchers are looking at how to best extract evidence from common practices.

This volume should be sweet music to all of these groups. Anyone needing to be convinced of the benefit of systematic development and synthesis of evidence for various public health purposes will quickly be won over. A step-by-step approach to compiling and assessing evidence of what works and what does not is well explicated. In a logical sequence, the reader is guided in how to use the results of his or her search for evidence in developing program or policy options, including the weighing of benefits versus barriers, and then in developing an action plan. To complete the cycle of science, the book describes how to evaluate whatever action is taken. Using this volume does not require extensive formal training in the key disciplines of epidemiology, biostatistics, or behavioral science, but those with strong disciplinary skills will also find much to learn from and put to practical use here.

If every public health practitioner absorbed and applied the key lessons in this volume, public health would enjoy a higher health return on the taxpayer's investment, and public health practitioners would be more successful in competing for limited public dollars because they would have evidence of what works that is easy to support and difficult to refute. The same cannot be said for most of the competing requests for scarce public resources.

Jonathan E. Fielding, M.D., M.P.H., M.B.A.
Director of Public Health and Health Officer
County of Los Angeles
Professor of Health Services and Pediatrics
School of Public Health University of California, Los Angeles

Preface

As we complete this second edition of *Evidence-Based Public Health*, we return to the question: "How much of our work in public health is evidence based?" Although the precise answer to that question cannot be known, it is almost certainly "Not enough!" Public health has successfully addressed many challenges, yet nearly every success story is a two-edged sword. Programs and policies have been implemented and, in some cases, positive results have been reported that show improvements in population health. Yet some populations suffer health disparities and social inequalities. This leads us to questions such as, Are there ways to take the lessons learned from successful interventions and apply them to other issues and settings? Are we applying the evidence that is well established in scientific studies? How do we foster greater political will that supports evidence-based decision making? How do we develop incentives so practitioners will make better use of evidence? Here are a few examples showing the potential and work yet undone:

- The eradication of smallpox in 1980 demonstrated the powerful combination of vaccination, patient and worker education, and public health surveillance in disease reduction. Other vaccine-preventable diseases such as measles, hepatitis B, and rubella might also be eradicated with a global commitment.
- State-based programs to reduce tobacco use have demonstrated progress in California, Massachusetts, Florida, and elsewhere, yet declining rates of tobacco use appear to be plateauing for some population subgroups and many

states and communities are not implementing comprehensive, evidence-based interventions to control tobacco use.

• There are large health disparities (e.g., among racial/ethnic groups, across socioeconomic gradients) in the United States and many other countries. Although some promising behavioral interventions have been shown to address these disparities, new approaches are needed that include a focus on the "upstream" causes, such as income inequality, poor housing, racism, and lack of social cohesion.

As noted over two decades ago by the Institute of Medicine,[1] there are multiple reasons for the inefficiency and ineffectiveness of many public health efforts. There are at least four ways in which a public health program or policy may not reach stated goals for success:

1. Choosing an intervention approach whose effectiveness is not established in the scientific literature
2. Selecting a potentially effective program or policy yet achieving only weak, incomplete implementation or "reach," thereby failing to attain objectives (some call this Type III error)
3. Conducting an inadequate or incorrect evaluation that results in a lack of generalizable knowledge on the effectiveness of a program or policy
4. Paying inadequate attention to adapting an intervention to the population and context of interest

To enhance evidence-based practice, this book addresses all four possibilities and attempts to provide practical guidance on how to choose, carry out, and evaluate evidence-based programs and policies in public health settings. It also begins to address a fifth, overarching need for a highly trained public health workforce. Our book deals not only with *finding* and *using* existing scientific evidence but also with implementation and evaluation of interventions that *generate* new evidence on effectiveness. Because all these topics are broad and require multidisciplinary skills and perspectives, each chapter covers the basic issues and provides multiple examples to illustrate important concepts. In addition, each chapter provides linkages to diverse literature and selected websites for readers wanting more detailed information. Readers should note that websites are volatile, and when a link changes, a generic search engine may be useful in locating the new web address.

We began to see a need for this book through our experiences in public health practice, health care delivery, and teaching. Much of the book's new material originated from several courses that we have taught over the past 12 years. One that we offer with the Missouri Department of Health and Senior Services, "Evidence-Based Decision-Making in Public Health," is designed for midlevel managers in state health agencies and leaders of city and county health agencies. We developed a national version of this course with the National Association of Chronic Disease Directors and the Centers for Disease Control and Prevention (CDC). The same course has also been adapted for use in several other U.S. states. To conduct international trainings we have received support from the CDC, WHO/PAHO, the CINDI (Countrywide Integrated Non-communicable Diseases Intervention) Programme, and the CARMEN Initiatives (Conjunto de Acciones para la Reduccion Multifactorial de las Enfermedades No transmisibles, or Integrated Prevention of Non-communicable Diseases in the Americas).

The format for this second edition is very similar to the approach taken in the course and the first edition. Chapter 1 provides the rationale for evidence-based approaches to decision making in public health. Chapter 2 presents concepts of causality that help in determining when scientific evidence is sufficient for public health action. Chapter 3 describes a set of analytic tools that can be extremely useful in finding and evaluating evidence—these include economic evaluation, health impact assessment, meta-analysis, and expert guidelines. The next seven chapters lay out a sequential framework for

1. Conducting a community assessment
2. Developing an initial statement of the issue
3. Quantifying the issue
4. Searching the scientific literature and organizing information
5. Developing and prioritizing intervention options
6. Developing an action plan and implementing interventions
7. Evaluating the program or policy

The second edition includes a new chapter on emerging issues that are relevant to evidence-based public health. While an evidence-based process is far from linear, these seven steps are described in some detail to illustrate their importance in making scientifically based decisions about public health programs and policies.

This book has been written for public health professionals without extensive formal training in the public health sciences (behavioral science, biostatistics, environmental and occupational health, epidemiology, health management, and policy) and for students in public health and preventive medicine. We hope the book will be useful for state and local health agencies, nonprofit organizations, academic institutions, health care organizations, and national public health agencies. While the book is intended primarily for a North American audience, this second edition draws more heavily on examples from many parts of the world, and we believe that although contextual conditions will vary, the key principles and skills outlined are applicable in both developed and developing countries. The first edition of *Evidence-Based Public Health* was translated into Chinese and Japanese.

The future of public health holds enormous potential, and public health professionals have more tools at their fingertips than ever before to meet a wide range of challenges. We hope this book will be a useful resource for bridging research with policies and the practice of public health.

R. C. B.

E. A. B.

T. L. L.

K. N. G.

W. R. T.

REFERENCE

1. IOM. Committee for the Study of the Future of Public Health. *The Future of Public Health.* Washington, DC: National Academie Press, 1988.

Acknowledgments

We are grateful to numerous individuals who contributed to the development of the second edition of this book.

We particularly wish to thank Garland Land, who chaired the original work group that developed the concept for our course, "Evidence-Based Decision Making in Public Health." A number of outstanding graduate students have helped us with the course, including Laura Caisley, Mariah Dreisinger, Carolyn Harris, Lori Hattan, Julie Jacobs, Shannon Keating, and Leslie McIntosh. We are grateful for support from the Centers for Disease Control and Prevention: Ginny Bales, Wayne Giles, and Mike Waller; and to leaders in the CINDI and CARMEN networks: Gunter Diem, Vilius Grabauskas, Branka Legetic, and Aushra Shatchkute. Many other course instructors and collaborators contributed to this work: Claudia Campbell, Linda Dix, Ellen Jones, Aulikki Nissinen, Darcy Scharff, Paul Siegel, Eduardo Simoes, Sylvie Stachenko, Erkki Vartiainen, Fran Wheeler, and Jozica Zakotnik. This second edition benefitted by reviews and input from Laura Brennan, Carol Brownson, Jonathan Fielding, Larry Green, Julie Jacobs, Shannon Keating, Chris Maylahn, and Tracy Orleans. Perhaps most important, we thank the hundreds of dedicated public health practitioners who have taken our courses and have added many important ideas to the discourse on evidence-based decision making in public health.

Finally, we are indebted to Regan Hofmann, Oxford University Press, who provided valuable advice throughout the production of this second edition.

Contents

1. The Need for Evidence-Based Public Health   *3*

2. Assessing Scientific Evidence for Public Health Action   *35*

3. Understanding and Applying Analytic Tools   *60*

4. Community Assessment   *101*

5. Developing an Initial Statement of the Issue   *117*

6. Quantifying the Issue   *133*

7. Searching the Scientific Literature and Organizing Information   *158*

8. Developing and Prioritizing Intervention Options   *178*

9. Developing an Action Plan and Implementing Interventions   *206*

10. Evaluating the Program or Policy   *232*

11. Emerging Issues in Evidence-Based Public Health   *259*

Glossary   *273*

Index   *285*

Evidence-Based Public Health

1

The Need for Evidence-Based Public Health

> Public health workers ... deserve to get somewhere by design, not just by perseverance.
>
> —McKinlay and Marceau

Public health research and practice are credited with many notable achievements, including much of the 30-year gain in life expectancy in the United States that occurred during the twentieth century.[1] A large part of this increase can be attributed to the provision of safe water and food, sewage treatment and disposal, tobacco use prevention and cessation, injury prevention, control of infectious diseases through immunization and other means, and other population-based interventions.[2]

Despite these successes, many additional opportunities to improve the public's health remain. To achieve state and national objectives for improved population health, more widespread adoption of evidence-based strategies has been recommended.[3–7] An increased focus on evidence-based public health (EBPH) has numerous direct and indirect benefits, including access to more and higher-quality information on what has been shown to improve the public's health, a higher likelihood of successful programs and policies being implemented, greater workforce productivity, and more efficient use of public and private resources.[4,8,9]

Ideally, public health practitioners should always incorporate scientific evidence in selecting and implementing programs, developing policies, and evaluating progress.[10,11] Society pays a high opportunity cost when interventions that yield the highest health return on an investment are not implemented.[12] In practice, intervention decisions are often based on perceived short-term opportunities, lacking systematic planning and review of the best evidence regarding effective approaches. These concerns were noted two decades ago when the Institute of Medicine Committee for the Study of the Future of Public Health[13] determined that decision making in public health is often driven by "crises, hot issues, and concerns of organized interest groups" (p. 4). Barriers to implementing EBPH include the political environment (including lack of political will) and deficits in relevant and timely research, information systems, resources, leadership, and the required competencies.[10,14-17]

Several concepts are fundamental to achieving a more evidence-based approach to public health practice. First, scientific information is needed on the programs and policies that are most likely to be effective in promoting health (i.e., undertake evaluation research to generate sound evidence).[4,8,18,19] An array of effective interventions is now available from numerous sources, including *The Guide to Community Preventive Services*,[20,21] the *Guide to Clinical Preventive Services*,[22] Cancer Control PLANET,[23] and the National Registry of Evidence-based Programs and Practices, a service of the Substance Abuse and Mental Health Services Administration.[24] Second, to translate science into practice, we need to marry information on evidence-based interventions from the peer-reviewed literature with the realities of a specific real-world environment.[4,25,26] To do so, we need to better define processes that lead to evidence-based decision making. Finally, wide-scale dissemination of interventions of proven effectiveness must occur more consistently at state and local levels.[27]

It is difficult to estimate how widely evidence-based approaches are being applied. In a survey of 107 U.S. public health practitioners, an estimated 58% of programs in their agencies were deemed evidence-based (i.e., based on the most current evidence from peer-reviewed research).[28] This finding in public health settings appears to mirror the use of evidence-based approaches in clinical care. A random study of adults living in selected U.S. metropolitan areas found that 55% of overall medical care was based on what is recommended in the medical literature.[29] Thacker and colleagues found that the preventable proportion (i.e., how much of a reduction in the health burden is estimated to occur if an intervention is carried out) was known for only 4.4% of 702 population-based interventions.[30] Similarly, cost-effectiveness data are reported for a low proportion of public health interventions.[21]

This chapter includes five major sections: (1) relevant background issues, including definitions, an overview of evidence-based medicine, and other concepts underlying EBPH; (2) several key characteristics of an evidence-based process; (3) analytic tools to enhance the uptake of EBPH; (4) a brief sketch of a framework for EBPH in public health practice; and (5) a summary of barriers and opportunities for widespread implementation of evidence-based approaches. A major goal of this introductory chapter is to move the process of decision making toward a proactive approach that incorporates effective use of scientific evidence and data.

BACKGROUND

Formal discourse on the nature and scope of EBPH originated about a decade ago. Several authors have attempted to define EBPH. In 1997, Jenicek[31] defined EBPH as the "conscientious, explicit, and judicious use of current best evidence in making decisions about the care of communities and populations in the domain of health protection, disease prevention, health maintenance and improvement (health promotion)." In 1999, scholars and practitioners in Australia[5] and the United States[10] elaborated further on the concept of EBPH. Glasziou and colleagues posed a series of questions to enhance uptake of EBPH (e.g., "Does this intervention help alleviate this problem?") and identified 14 sources of high-quality evidence.[5] Brownson and colleagues[4,10] described a six-stage process by which practitioners are able to take a more evidence-based approach to decision making. Kohatsu and colleagues[25] broadened earlier definitions of EBPH to include the perspectives of community members, fostering a more population-centered approach. In 2004, Rychetnik and colleagues[32] summarized many key concepts in a glossary for EBPH. There appears to be a consensus that a combination of scientific evidence, as well as values, resources, and contexts, should enter into decision making[3,4,32,33] (Figure 1-1). A concise definition emerged from Kohatsu[25]: "Evidence-based public health is the process of integrating science-based interventions with community preferences to improve the health of populations" (p. 419).

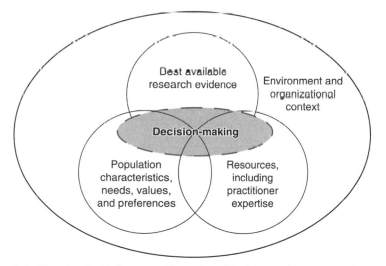

FIGURE 1-1. Domains that influence evidence-based decision making. (From Satterfeld et al.[35])

Defining Evidence

At the most basic level, *evidence* involves "the available body of facts or information indicating whether a belief or proposition is true or valid."[34] The idea of evidence often derives from legal settings in Western societies. In law, evidence comes in the form of stories, witness accounts, police testimony, expert opinions, and forensic science.[35] For a public health professional, evidence is some form of data—including epidemiologic (quantitative) data, results of program or policy evaluations, and qualitative data—to use in making judgments or decisions[36] (Figure 1-2). Public health evidence is usually the result of a complex cycle of observation, theory, and experiment.[37,38] However, the value of evidence is in the eye of the beholder (e.g., the usefulness of evidence may vary by stakeholder type).[39] Medical evidence includes not only research but also characteristics of the patient, a patient's readiness to undergo a therapy, and society's values.[40] Policy makers seek distributional consequences (i.e., who has to pay, how much, and who benefits),[41] and in practice settings, anecdotes sometimes trump empirical data.[42] Evidence is usually imperfect and, as noted by Muir Gray,[3] "The absence of excellent evidence does not make evidence-based decision making impossible; what is required is the best evidence available not the best evidence possible."

Several authors have defined types of scientific evidence for public health practice[4,10,32] (Table 1-1). Type 1 evidence defines the causes of diseases and the magnitude, severity, and preventability of risk factors and diseases. It suggests that "Something should be done" about a particular disease or risk factor. Type 2 evidence describes the relative impact of specific interventions that do or do not improve health, adding, "Specifically, this should be done."[4] It has been noted that adherence to a strict hierarchy of study designs may reinforce an "inverse

• Scientific literature in systematic reviews
• Scientific literature in one or more journal articles
• Public health surveillance data
• Program evaluations
• Qualitative data
  – Community members
  – Other stakeholders
• Media/marketing data
• Word of mouth
• Personal experience

Objective

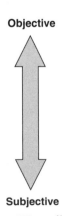

Subjective

FIGURE 1-2. Different forms of evidence. (From Chambers and Kerner[38])

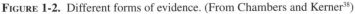

Table 1-1. Comparison of the Types of Scientific Evidence

Characteristic	Type 1	Type 2	Type 3
Typical data/ relationship	Size and strength of preventable risk—disease relationship (measures of burden, etiologic research)	Relative effectiveness of public health intervention	Information on the adaptation and translation of an effective intervention
Common setting	Clinic or controlled community setting	Socially intact groups or community-wide	Socially intact groups or community-wide
Example	Smoking causes lung cancer.	Price increases with a targeted media campaign reduce smoking rates.	Understanding the political challenges of price increases or targeting media messages to particular audience segments
Quantity	More	Less	Less
Action	Something should be done.	This particular intervention should be implemented.	How an intervention should be implemented

evidence law" by which interventions most likely to influence whole populations (e.g., policy change) are least valued in an evidence matrix emphasizing randomized designs.[43,44] A recent study from Sanson-Fisher and colleagues[45] showed the relative lack of intervention research (Type 2) compared with descriptive/ epidemiologic research (Type 1). In a random sample of published studies on tobacco use, alcohol use, and inadequate physical activity, their team found that in 2005–2006, 14.9% of studies reported on interventions, whereas 78.5% of articles were descriptive or epidemiologic research. There is likely to be even less published research on Type 3 evidence—which shows how and under what contextual conditions interventions were implemented and how they were received, thus informing "how something should be done."[37] Studies to date have tended to overemphasize internal validity (e.g., well-controlled efficacy trials) while giving sparse attention to external validity (e.g., the translation of science to the various circumstances of practice).[46,47]

Understanding the context for evidence. Type 3 evidence derives from the context of an intervention.[32] While numerous authors have written about the role of context in informing evidence-based practice,[8,32,39,48–52] there is little consensus on its definition. When moving from clinical interventions to population-level and policy interventions, context becomes more uncertain, variable, and complex.[53] One useful definition of context highlights information needed to adapt and implement an evidence-based intervention in a particular setting or population.[32] The context for Type 3 evidence specifies five overlapping domains (Table 1-2).

Table 1-2. Contextual Variables for Intervention Design, Implementation, and Adaptation

Category	Examples
Individual	Education level
	Basic human needs[a]
	Personal health history
Interpersonal	Family health history
	Support from peers
	Social capital
Organizational	Staff composition
	Staff expertise
	Physical infrastructure
	Organizational culture
Sociocultural	Social norms
	Values
	Cultural traditions
	History
Political and economic	Political will
	Political ideology
	Lobbying and special interests
	Costs and benefits

[a]Basic human needs include food, shelter, warmth, and safety.[55]

First, there are characteristics of the target population for an intervention such as education level and health history.[54] Next, interpersonal variables provide important context. For example, a person with a family history of cancer might be more likely to undergo cancer screening. Third, organizational variables should be considered. For example, whether an agency is successful in carrying out an evidence-based program will be influenced by its capacity (e.g., a trained workforce, agency leadership).[8,28] Fourth, social norms and culture are known to shape many health behaviors. Finally, larger political and economic forces affect context. For example, a high rate for a certain disease may influence a state's political will to address the issue in a meaningful and systematic way. Particularly for high-risk and understudied populations, there is a pressing need for evidence on contextual variables and ways of adapting programs and policies across settings and population subgroups. Contextual issues are being addressed more fully in the new "realist review," which is a systematic review process that seeks to examine not only whether an intervention works but also how interventions work in real-world settings[55]

Challenges related to public health evidence.   Evidence for public health has been described as underpopulated, dispersed, and different.[56,57] It is underpopulated because there are relatively few well-done evaluations of how the effects of public health interventions (Type 2 evidence) apply across different social groups (Type 3 evidence). Information for public health decision making is also more dispersed than is evidence for clinical interventions. For example, evidence on the health effects of the built environment might be found in transportation or planning journals. Finally, public health evidence is different, in part because much of the science base for interventions is derived from nonrandomized designs or "natural experiments" (i.e., generally takes the form of an observational study in which the researcher cannot control or withhold the allocation of an intervention to particular areas or communities but where natural or predetermined variation in allocation occurs[56]).

Triangulating evidence.   Triangulation involves the accumulation of evidence from a variety of sources to gain insight into a particular topic[59] and often combines quantitative and qualitative data.[4] It generally involves the use of multiple methods of data collection and/or analysis to determine points of commonality or disagreement.[60] Triangulation is often beneficial because of the complementary nature of information from different sources. Although quantitative data provide an excellent opportunity to determine how variables are related for large numbers of people, these data provide little in the way of understanding why these relationships exist. Qualitative data, on the other hand, can help provide information to explain quantitative findings, or what has been called "illuminating meaning."[60] There are many examples of the use of triangulation of qualitative and quantitative data to evaluate health programs and policies, including AIDS prevention programs,[61] occupational health programs and policies,[62] and chronic disease prevention programs in community settings.[63]

Cultural and geographic differences.   The tenets of EBPH have largely been developed in a Western, European American context.[64] The conceptual approach arises from the epistemologic underpinnings of logical positivism,[65] which finds meaning through rigorous observation and measurement. This is reflected in a professional preference among clinicians for research designs like the randomized controlled trial. In addition, most studies in the EBPH literature are academic research, usually with external funding for well-established investigators. In contrast, in developing countries and in impoverished areas of developed countries, the evidence base for how best to address common public health problems is often limited even though the scope of problem may be enormous. Cavill and colleagues[66] compared evidence-based interventions across countries in Europe, showing that much of the evidence base in several areas is limited to empirical observations. Even in more developed countries (including the United States), information published in peer-reviewed journals or data available through websites and official organizations may not adequately represent all populations of interest.

Audiences for Evidence-Based Public Health

There are four overlapping user groups for EBPH as defined by Fielding in Brownson et al.[67] The first includes public health practitioners with executive and managerial responsibilities who want to know the scope and quality of evidence for alternative strategies (e.g., programs, policies). In practice, however, public health practitioners frequently have a relatively narrow set of options. Funds from federal, state, or local sources are most often earmarked for a specific purpose (e.g., surveillance and treatment of sexually transmitted diseases, inspection of retail food establishments). Still, the public health practitioner has the opportunity, even the obligation, to carefully review the evidence for alternative ways to achieve the desired health goals. The next user group consists of policy makers at local, regional, state, national, and international levels. They are faced with macro-level decisions on how to allocate the public resources for which they are stewards. This group has the additional responsibility of making policies on controversial public issues. The third group is composed of stakeholders who will be affected by any intervention. This includes the public, especially those who vote, as well as interest groups formed to support or oppose specific policies, such as the legality of abortion, whether the community water supply should be fluoridated, or whether adults must be issued handgun licenses if they pass background checks. The final user group is composed of researchers on population health issues, such as those who evaluate the impact of a specific policy or programs. They both develop and use evidence to answer research questions.

Similarities and Differences between Evidence-Based Public Health and Evidence-Based Medicine

The concept of evidence-based practice is well established in numerous disciplines including psychology,[68] social work,[69,70] and nursing.[71] It is probably best established in medicine. The doctrine of evidence-based medicine (EBM) was formally introduced in 1992.[72] Its origins can be traced back to the seminal work of Cochrane, who noted that many medical treatments lacked scientific effectiveness.[73] A basic tenet of EBM is to deemphasize unsystematic clinical experience and place greater emphasis on evidence from clinical research. This approach requires new skills, such as efficient literature searching and an understanding of types of evidence in evaluating the clinical literature.[74] There has been a rapid growth in the literature on EBM, contributing to its formal recognition. Using the search term "evidence-based medicine," there were 254 citations in 1990, rising to 7331 citations in 2008 (Figure 1-3). Even though the formal terminology of EBM is relatively recent, its concepts are embedded in earlier efforts such as the Canadian Task Force on the Periodic Health Examination[75] and *The Guide to Clinical Preventive Services*.[76]

There are important distinctions between evidence-based approaches in medicine and public health. First, the type and volume of evidence differ. Medical studies of pharmaceuticals and procedures often rely on randomized controlled trials of individuals, the most scientifically rigorous of epidemiologic studies. In contrast, public health interventions usually rely on cross-sectional studies, quasi-experimental designs, and time-series analyses. These studies sometimes

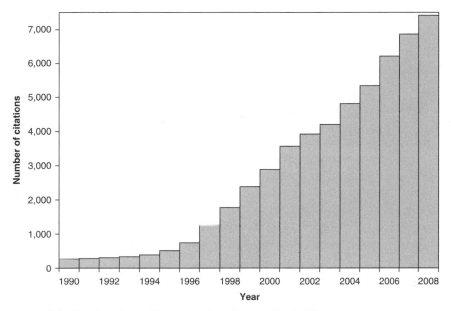

FIGURE 1-3. Citations for evidence-based medicine, 1990–2008.

lack a comparison group and require more caveats in interpretation of results. During the past 50 years, there have been more than 1 million randomized controlled trials of medical treatments.[77] There are many fewer studies of the effectiveness of public health interventions,[4,78] because the studies are difficult to design and often results are derived from natural experiments (e.g., a state adopting a new policy compared with other states). EBPH has borrowed the term "intervention" from clinical disciplines, insinuating specificity and discreteness. However, in public health, we seldom have a single "intervention" but rather a program that involves a blending of several interventions within a community. Large community-based trials can be more expensive to conduct than randomized experiments in a clinic. Population-based studies generally require a longer time period between intervention and outcome. For example, a study on the effects of smoking cessation on lung cancer mortality would require decades of data collection and analysis. Contrast that with treatment of a medical condition (e.g., an antibiotic for symptoms of pneumonia), which is likely to produce effects in days or weeks, or even a surgical trial for cancer with endpoints of mortality within a few years.

The formal training of persons working in public health is much more variable than that in medicine or other clinical disciplines.[79] Unlike medicine, public health relies on a variety of disciplines and there is not a single academic credential that "certifies" a public health practitioner, although efforts to establish credentials (via an examination) are under way. Fewer than half of public health workers have formal training in a public health discipline such as epidemiology or health education.[80]

This higher level of heterogeneity means that multiple perspectives are involved in a more complicated decision-making process. It also suggests that effective public health practice places a premium on routine, on-the-job training.

KEY CHARACTERISTICS OF EVIDENCE-BASED DECISION MAKING

It is useful to consider several overarching, common characteristics of an evidence-based approach to public health practice. These notions are expanded on in other chapters. Described next, key characteristics of these various attributes of EBPH include:

- Making decisions based on the best available peer-reviewed evidence (both quantitative and qualitative research)
- Using data and information systems systematically
- Applying program planning frameworks (which often have a foundation in behavioral science theory)
- Engaging the community in assessment and decision making
- Conducting sound evaluation
- Disseminating what is learned to key stakeholders and decision makers

Accomplishing these activities in EBPH is likely to require a synthesis of scientific skills, enhanced communication, common sense, and political acumen.

Decisions Are Based on the Best Possible Evidence

As one evaluates Type 2 evidence, it is useful to understand where to turn for the best possible scientific evidence. A starting point is the scientific literature and guidelines developed by expert panels. In addition, preliminary findings from researchers and practitioners are often presented at regional, national, and international professional meetings. In Box 1-1, the decision to address the lack of physical activity in youth was based on a large body of epidemiologic studies showing the causal associations between inactivity and numerous health outcomes. This large body of evidence has led to effective intervention strategies.[81]

Data and Information Systems Are Used

A tried and true public health adage is, "What gets measured, gets done."[83] This has typically been applied to long-term endpoints (e.g., rates of mortality) and

---

Box 1-1. Promoting Physical Activity in Youth

It is now well established that regular physical activity reduces the risk of premature death and disability from a variety of conditions including coronary heart disease, diabetes, colon cancer, osteoarthritis, and osteoporosis. In spite of these benefits, data from the 2007 Youth Risk Behavior Surveillance System report that nationwide only one third of high school students had met the recommended levels of physical activity. To address inactivity in youth, interventions have used modified curricula and policies to increase the amount of time students spend being active in physical education (PE) classes. This can be done in a variety of ways, including (1) adding new (or additional) PE classes, (2) lengthening existing PE classes, or (3) increasing moderate to vigorous physical activity of students during PE class without necessarily lengthening class time. A systematic review of these interventions showed strong evidence that school-based PE is effective in increasing levels of physical activity and improving fitness.[81] Despite convincing evidence of effectiveness, there are real world constraints to dissemination of these programs (i.e., key considerations in external validity). For example, schools often feel pressure for students to perform well on standardized reading and math tests which may in turn take time away from PE. However, recent longitudinal data suggest that increasing time spent in PE may benefit academic achievement in math and reading.[82]

---

data for many public health endpoints and populations are not readily available at one's fingertips. Data are being developed more for local level issues (e.g., SMART BRFSS) and a few early efforts are under way to develop public health policy surveillance systems. For example, a group of federal and voluntary agencies have developed policy surveillance systems for tobacco, alcohol, and, more recently, school-based nutrition and physical education.[84-87]

Systematic Program Planning Approaches Are Used

When an approach is decided on, a variety of planning frameworks and behavioral science theories can be applied. As an example, ecological, or systems, models are increasingly used in which "appropriate changes in the social environment will produce changes in individuals, and the support of individuals in a population is seen as essential for implementing environmental changes."[88] These models point to the importance of addressing problems at multiple levels and stress the interaction and integration of factors within and across all levels—individual, interpersonal, community, organizational, and governmental. The goal is to create a healthy community environment that provides health-promoting information and social support to enable people to live healthier lifestyles.[89] Effective interventions are most often grounded in health-behavior theory.[38,90]

Community Engagement Occurs

Community-based approaches involve community members in research and intervention projects and show progress in improving population health and addressing health disparities.[91,92] Practitioners, academicians, and community members collaboratively define issues of concern, develop strategies for intervention, and evaluate the outcomes. This approach relies on "stakeholder" input,[93] builds on existing resources, facilitates collaboration among all parties, and integrates knowledge and action that seek to lead to a fair distribution of the benefits of an intervention for all partners.[92,94]

Sound Evaluation Principles Are Followed

Too often in public health, programs and policies are implemented without much attention to systematic evaluation. In addition, even when programs are ineffective, they are sometimes continued because of historical or political considerations. Evaluation plans must be laid early in program development and should include both formative and outcome evaluation. For example, an injury control program was appropriately discontinued after its effectiveness was evaluated. This program evaluation also illustrates the use of both qualitative and quantitative data in framing an evaluation.[95]

Results Are Disseminated to Others Who Need to Know

When a program or policy has been implemented, or when final results are known, others in public health can rely on findings to enhance their own use of evidence in decision making. Dissemination may occur to health professionals via the scientific literature, to the general public via the media, to policy makers through personal meetings, and to public health professionals via training courses. Effective interventions are needed in a variety of settings, including schools, worksites, health care settings, and broader community environments.

ANALYTIC TOOLS AND APPROACHES TO ENHANCE THE UPTAKE OF EVIDENCE-BASED PUBLIC HEALTH

Several analytic tools and planning approaches can help practitioners in answering questions such as:

- What is the size of the public health problem?
- Are there effective interventions for addressing the problem?

- What information about the local context and this particular intervention is helpful in deciding its potential use in the situation at hand?
- Is a particular program worth doing or policy worth having (i.e., is it better than alternatives), and will it provide a satisfactory return on investment, measured in monetary terms or in health impacts?

Public Health Surveillance

Public health surveillance is a critical tool for those using EBPH. It involves the ongoing systematic collection, analysis, and interpretation of specific health data, closely integrated with the timely dissemination of these data to those responsible for preventing and controlling disease or injury.[96] Public health surveillance systems should have the capacity to collect and analyze data, disseminate data to public health programs, and regularly evaluate the effectiveness of the use of the disseminated data.[97] For example, documentation of the prevalence of elevated levels of lead (a known toxicant) in blood in the U.S. population was used as the justification for eliminating lead from paint and then gasoline and for documenting the effects of these actions.[98] In tobacco control, agreement on a common metric for tobacco use enabled comparisons across the states and an early recognition of the doubling and then tripling of the rates of decrease in smoking in California after passage of its Proposition 99,[99] and then a quadrupling of the rate of decline in Massachusetts compared with the other 48 states.[100]

Systematic Reviews and Evidence-Based Guidelines

Systematic reviews are syntheses of comprehensive collections of information on a particular topic. Reading a good review can be one of the most efficient ways to become familiar with state-of-the-art research and practice on many specific topics in public health.[101–103] The use of explicit, systematic methods (i.e., decision rules) in reviews limits bias and reduces chance effects, thus providing more reliable results on which to make decisions.[104] One of the most useful sets of reviews for public health interventions is *The Guide to Community Preventive Services* (the *Community Guide*),[21,105] which provides an overview of current scientific literature through a well-defined, rigorous method in which available studies themselves are the units of analysis. The *Community Guide* seeks to answer (1) What interventions have been evaluated and what have been their effects? (2) What aspects of interventions can help *Guide* users select from among the set of interventions of proved effectiveness? (3) What might this intervention cost, and how do these costs compare with the likely health impacts? A good systematic review should allow the practitioner to understand the local contextual conditions necessary for successful implementation.[106]

Economic Evaluation

Economic evaluation is an important component of evidence-based practice.[107] It can provide information to help assess the relative value of alternative expenditures on public health programs and policies. In cost-benefit analysis, all of the costs and consequences of the decision options are valued in monetary terms. More often, the economic investment associated with an intervention is compared with the health impacts, such as cases of disease prevented or years of life saved. This technique, cost-effectiveness analysis (CEA), can suggest the relative value of alternative interventions (i.e., health return on dollars invested).[107] CEA has become an increasingly important tool for researchers, practitioners, and policy makers. However, relevant data to support this type of analysis are not always available, especially for possible public policies designed to improve health.[42,108]

Health Impact Assessment

Health impact assessment (HIA) is a relatively new method that seeks to estimate the probable impact of a policy or intervention in nonhealth sectors, such as agriculture, transportation, and economic development, on the health of the population.[109] Some HIAs have focused on ensuring the involvement of relevant stakeholders in the development of a specific project. This latter approach, the basis of environmental impact assessment required by law for many large place-based projects, is similar to the nonregulatory approach that has been adopted for some HIAs. Overall, HIA, in both its forms, has been gaining acceptance as a tool because of mounting evidence that social and physical environments are important determinants of health and health disparities in populations. It is now being used to help assess the potential effects of many policies and programs on health status and outcomes.[110-112]

Participatory Approaches

Participatory approaches that actively involve community members in research and intervention projects[91,92,113] show promise in engaging communities in EBPH.[25] Practitioners, academicians, and community members collaboratively define issues of concern, develop strategies for intervention, and evaluate the outcomes. This approach relies on "stakeholder" input,[93] builds on existing resources, facilitates collaboration among all parties, and integrates knowledge and action that, it is hoped, will lead to a fair distribution of the benefits of an intervention or project for all partners.[92,94] Stakeholders, or key players, are individuals or agencies that have a vested interest in the issue at hand.[114] In the development of health policies, for example, policy makers are especially important stakeholders.[115] Stakeholders should include those who would potentially receive, use, and benefit from the program or policy being considered. As described in Chapter 5, three groups of stakeholders are relevant: people developing programs, people affected by interventions, and people who use results of program evaluations. Participatory approaches may also present challenges in adhering to EBPH principles, especially in reaching agreement on which approaches are most appropriate for addressing a particular health problem.[116]

AN APPROACH TO INCREASING THE USE OF EVIDENCE IN PUBLIC HEALTH PRACTICE

Strengthening EBPH competencies needs to take into account the diverse education and training backgrounds of the workforce. The emphasis on principles of EBPH is not uniformly taught in all the disciplines represented in the public health workforce. For example, a public health nurse is likely to have had less training in how to locate the most current evidence and interpret alternatives than has an epidemiologist. A recently graduated health educator with a master's in public health is more likely to have gained an understanding of the importance of EBPH than has an environmental health specialist holding a bachelor's degree. Probably fewer than half of public health workers have any formal training in a public health discipline such as epidemiology or health education.[80] An even smaller percentage of these professionals have formal graduate training from a school of public health or other public health program. Currently, it appears that few public health departments have made continuing education about EBPH mandatory.

While the formal concept of EBPH is relatively new, the underlying skills are not. For example, reviewing the scientific literature for evidence and evaluating a program intervention are skills often taught in graduate programs in public health or other academic disciplines, and they are the building blocks of public health practice. The most commonly applied framework in EBPH is probably that of Brownson and colleagues (Figure 1-4), which uses a seven-stage process.[4,28,117] The process used in applying this framework is nonlinear and entails numerous iterations.[118] Competencies for more effective public health practice are becoming clearer.[119–121] For example, to carry out the EBPH process, the skills needed to make evidence-based decisions require a specific set of competencies[122] (Table 1-3).

To address these and similar competencies, EBPH training programs have been developed in the United States for public health professionals in state health agencies,[28,123] local health departments, and community-based organizations,[124,125] and similar programs have been developed in other countries.[117,126,127] Some programs show evidence of effectiveness.[28,125] The most common format uses didactic sessions, computer labs, and scenario-based exercises, taught by a faculty team

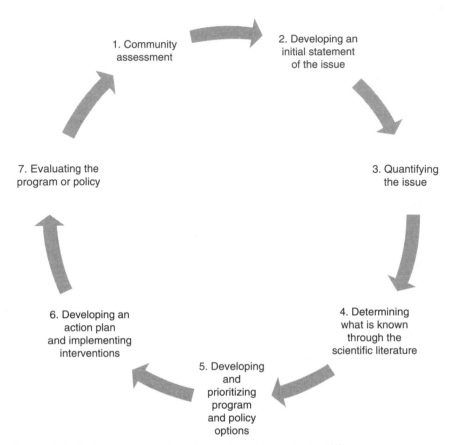

Figure 1-4. Training approach for evidence-based public health.[4,116]

with expertise in EBPH. The reach of these training programs can be increased by emphasizing a train-the-trainer approach.[117] Other formats have been used, including Internet-based self-study,[124,128] CD-ROMs,[129] distance and distributed learning networks, and targeted technical assistance. Training programs may have greater impact when delivered by "change agents" who are perceived as experts yet share common characteristics and goals with the trainees.[130] A commitment from leadership and staff to life-long learning is also an essential ingredient for success in training.[131]

Implementation of training to address EBPH competencies should take into account principles of adult learning. These issues were recently articulated by Bryan and colleagues,[132] who highlighted the need to (1) know why the audience is learning; (2) tap into an underlying motivation to learn by the need to solve problems; (3) respect and build on previous experience; (4) design learning

Table 1-3. Competencies in Evidence-Based Public Health[a]

Title	Domain[b]	Level[c]	Competency
1. Community input	C	B	Understand the importance of obtaining community input before planning and implementing evidence-based interventions.
2. Etiologic knowledge	E	B	Understand the relationship between risk factors and diseases.
3. Community assessment	C	B	Understand how to define the health issue according to the needs and assets of the population/community of interest.
4. Partnerships at multiple levels	P/C	B	Understand the importance of identifying and developing partnerships in order to address the issue with evidence-based strategies at multiple levels.
5. Developing a concise statement of the issue	EBP	B	Understand the importance of developing a concise statement of the issue in order to build support for it.
6. Grant writing need	T/T	B	Recognize the importance of grant writing skills including the steps involved in the application process.
7. Literature searching	EBP	B	Understand the process for searching the scientific literature and summarizing search-derived information on the health issue.
8. Leadership and evidence	L	B	Recognize the importance of strong leadership from public health professionals regarding the need and importance of evidence-based public health interventions.
9. Role of behavioral science theory	T/T	B	Understand the role of behavioral science theory in designing, implementing, and evaluating interventions.
10. Leadership at all levels	L	B	Understand the importance of commitment from all levels of public health leadership to increase the use of evidence-based interventions.
11. Evaluation in "plain English"	EV	I	Recognize the importance of translating the impacts of programs or policies in language that can be understood by communities, practice sectors, and policy makers.
12. Leadership and change	L	I	Recognize the importance of effective leadership from public health professionals when making decisions in the middle of ever-changing environments.
13. Translating evidence-based interventions	EBP	I	Recognize the importance of translating evidence-based interventions to unique "real-world" settings.
14. Quantifying the issue	T/T	I	Understand the importance of descriptive epidemiology (concepts of person, place, time) in quantifying the public health issue.

(continued)

Table 1-3. (Continued)

Title	Domain[b]	Level[c]	Competency
15. Developing an action plan for program or policy	EBP	I	Understand the importance of developing a plan of action that describes how the goals and objectives will be achieved, what resources are required, and how responsibility of achieving objectives will be assigned.
16. Prioritizing health issues	EBP	I	Understand how to choose and implement appropriate criteria and processes for prioritizing program and policy options.
17. Qualitative evaluation	EV	I	Recognize the value of qualitative evaluation approaches including the steps involved in conducting qualitative evaluations.
18. Collaborative partnerships	P/C	I	Understand the importance of collaborative partnerships between researchers and practitioners when designing, implementing, and evaluating evidence-based programs and policies.
19. Nontraditional partnerships	P/C	I	Understand the importance of traditional partnerships as well as those that have been considered nontraditional such as those with planners, department of transportation, and others.
20. Systematic reviews	T/T	I	Understand the rationale, uses, and usefulness of systematic reviews that document effective interventions.
21. Quantitative evaluation	EV	I	Recognize the importance of quantitative evaluation approaches including the concepts of measurement validity and reliability.
22. Grant writing skills	T/T	I	Demonstrate the ability to create a grant including an outline of the steps involved in the application process.
23. Role of economic evaluation	T/T	A	Recognize the importance of using economic data and strategies to evaluate costs and outcomes when making public health decisions.
24. Creating policy briefs	P	A	Understand the importance of writing concise policy briefs to address the issue using evidence-based interventions.
25. Evaluation designs	EV	A	Comprehend the various designs useful in program evaluation with a particular focus on quasi-experimental (nonrandomized) designs.
26. Transmitting evidence-based research to policy makers	P	A	Understand the importance of coming up with creative ways of transmitting what we know works (evidence-based interventions) to policy makers in order to gain interest, political support, and funding.

[a]Adapted from Brownson et al.[121]

[b]C, community-level planning; E, etiology; P/C, partnerships and collaboration; EBP, evidence-based process; T/T, theory and analytic tools; L, leadership; EV, evaluation; P, policy.

[c]B, beginner; I, intermediate; A, advanced.

approaches that match the background and diversity of recipients; and (5) actively involve the audience in the learning process.

In this section, a seven-stage, sequential framework to promote greater use of evidence in day-to-day decision making is briefly described[10] (Figure 1-4). It is important to note that this process is seldom a strictly prescriptive or linear one, but it should include numerous feedback "loops" and processes that are common in many program-planning models. Each of these stages is discussed in more detail in subsequent chapters.

Community Assessment

Community assessment typically occurs before the development of a program or policy and seeks to understand the public health issues and priorities in a given community. It also begins to identify current resources already in place to address the concern. Data are sometimes available through surveillance systems and national and local data sets. Other information that is useful at this stage is documentation of the context, or setting, within which the health concern is occurring, including an assessment of the social, economic, and physical environment factors. Community assessment data can be collected through quantitative (e.g., questionnaires) or qualitative (e.g., individual or group interviews) methods.

Developing an Initial Statement of the Issue

The practitioner should begin by developing a concise statement of the issue or problem being considered. To build support for any issue (with an organization, policy makers, or a funding agency), the issue must be clearly articulated. This problem definition stage has some similarities to the beginning steps in a strategic planning process, which often involves describing the mission, internal strengths and weaknesses, external opportunities and threats, and vision for the future. It is often helpful to describe gaps between the current status of a program or organization and the desired goals. The key components of an issue statement include the health condition or risk factor being considered, the population(s) affected, the size and scope of the problem, prevention opportunities, and potential stakeholders.

Quantifying the Issue

After developing a working description of the public health issue of interest, it is often useful to identify sources of existing data. Such descriptive data may be available from ongoing vital statistics data (birth/death records), surveillance systems, special surveys, or national studies.

Descriptive studies can take several forms. In public health, the most common type of descriptive study involves a survey of a scientifically valid sample (a representative cross section) of the population of interest. These cross-sectional studies are not intended to change health status (as would an intervention) but rather they serve to quantify the prevalence of behaviors, characteristics, exposures, and diseases at some point (or period) of time in a defined population. This information can be valuable for understanding the scope of the public health problem at hand. Descriptive studies commonly provide information on patterns of occurrence according to such attributes as person (e.g., age, gender, ethnicity), place (e.g., county of residence), and time (e.g., seasonal variation in disease patterns). Additionally, under certain circumstances, cross-sectional data can provide information for use in the design of analytic studies (e.g., baseline data to evaluate the effectiveness of a public health intervention).

Determining What Is Known through the Scientific Literature

Once the issue to be considered has been clearly defined, the practitioner needs to become knowledgeable about previous or ongoing efforts to address the issue. This should include a systematic approach to identify, retrieve, and evaluate relevant reports on scientific studies, panels, and conferences related to the topic of interest. The most common method for initiating this investigation is a formal literature review. There are many databases available to facilitate such a review; most common among them for public health purposes are MEDLARS, MEDLINE, PubMed, PsycInfo, Current Contents, HealthSTAR, and CancerLit. These databases can be subscribed to by an organization, can selectively be found on the Internet, or sometimes can be accessed by the public through institutions (such as the National Library of Medicine [http://www.nlm.nih.gov], universities, and public libraries). There also are many organizations that maintain Internet sites that can be useful for identifying relevant information, including many state health departments, the Centers for Disease Control and Prevention, and the National Institutes of Health. It is important to remember that not all intervention (Type 2) studies will be found in the published literature.

Developing and Prioritizing Program Options

Based largely on the first three steps, a variety of health program or policy options are examined. The list of options can be developed from a variety of sources. The initial review of the scientific literature can sometimes highlight various intervention options. More often, expert panels provide program or policy recommendations on a variety of issues. Summaries of available evidence are often available in systematic reviews and practice guidelines. There are several assumptions or contexts underlying any development of options. These considerations focus in five main areas: political/regulatory, economic, social values, demographic, and technological.[133]

In particular, it is important to assess and monitor the political process when developing health policy options. To do so, "stakeholder" input may be useful. The stakeholder for a policy might be the health policy maker, whereas the stakeholder for a coalition-based community intervention might be a community member. In the case of health policies, supportive policy makers can frequently provide advice regarding timing of policy initiatives, methods for framing the issues, strategies for identifying sponsors, and ways to develop support among the general public. In the case of a community intervention, additional planning data may include key informant interviews, focus groups, or coalition member surveys.[134]

Developing an Action Plan and Implementing Interventions

This aspect of the process again deals largely with strategic planning issues. Once an option has been selected, a set of goals and objectives should be developed. A goal is a long-term desired change in the status of a priority health need, and an objective is a short-term, measurable, specific activity that leads toward achievement of a goal. The course of action describes how the goals and objectives will be achieved, what resources are required, and how responsibility for achieving objectives will be assigned.

Evaluating the Program or Policy

In simple terms, evaluation is the determination of the degree to which program or policy goals and objectives are met. If they follow any research design, most public health programs and policies are often evaluated through "quasi-experimental" designs (i.e., those lacking random assignment to intervention and comparison groups). In general, the strongest evaluation designs acknowledge the roles of both quantitative and qualitative evaluation. Furthermore, evaluation designs need to be flexible and sensitive enough to assess intermediate changes, even those that fall short of changes in behavior. Genuine change takes place incrementally over time, in ways that are often not visible to those too close to the intervention.

The seven-stage framework of EBPH summarized in this chapter is similar to an eight-step approach first described by Jenicek.[33] An additional logical step focuses on teaching others how to practice EBPH.[33]

Table 1-4. Potential Barriers and Solutions for Use of Evidence-Based Decision Making in Public Health

Barrier	Potential Solution
Lack of resources	Commitment to increase funding for prevention and rectifying staff shortages
Lack of leadership and instability in setting a clear and focused agenda for evidence-based approaches	Commitment from all levels of public health leaders to increase the understanding of the value of EBPH approaches
Lack of incentives for using evidence-based approaches	Identification of new ways of shaping organizational culture to support EBPH
Lack of a view of the long-term "horizon" for program implementation and evaluation	Adoption and adherence to causal frameworks and formative evaluation plans
External (including political) pressures drive the process away from an evidence-based approach	Systematic communication and dissemination strategies
Inadequate training in key public health disciplines	Wider dissemination of new and established training programs, including use of distance learning technologies
Lack of time to gather information, analyze data, and review the literature for evidence	Enhanced skills for efficient analysis and review of the literature, computer searching abilities, use of systematic reviews
Lack of evidence on the effectiveness of certain public health interventions for special populations	Increased funding for applied public health research; better dissemination of findings
Lack of information on implementation of interventions	A greater emphasis on building the evidence base for external validity

BARRIERS TO MORE EXTENSIVE USE OF EVIDENCE IN DECISION MAKING

There are several barriers to more effective use of data and analytic processes in decision making[4,8,135] (Table 1-4). Possible approaches for overcoming these barriers have been discussed by others.[13,123,136] Leadership is needed from public health practitioners on the need and importance of evidence-based decision making. Such leadership is evident in training programs, such as the regional leadership network for public health practitioners,[137] and the ongoing efforts under way to develop and disseminate evidence-based guidelines for interventions.[21]

SUMMARY

The successful implementation of EBPH in public health practice is both a science and an art. The science is built on epidemiologic, behavioral, and policy research showing the size and scope of a public health problem and which interventions are likely to be effective in addressing the problem. The art of decision making often involves knowing what information is important to a particular stakeholder at the right time. Unlike solving a math problem, significant decisions in public health must balance science and art, because rational, evidence-based decision making often involves choosing one alternative from among a set of rational choices. By applying the concepts of EBPH outlined in this chapter and book, decision making and, ultimately, public health practice can be improved.

Key Chapter Points

- To achieve state and national objectives for improved population health, more widespread adoption of evidence-based strategies is recommended.
- There are several important distinctions between EBPH and clinical disciplines, including the volume of evidence, study designs used to inform research and practice, the setting or context where the intervention is applied, and the training and certification of professionals.
- Key components of EBPH include making decisions based on the best available, peer-reviewed evidence; using data and information systems systematically; applying program-planning frameworks; engaging the community in decision making; conducting sound evaluation; and disseminating what is learned.
- Numerous analytic tools and approaches that can enhance the greater use of EBPH include public health surveillance, systematic reviews, economic evaluation, health impact assessment, and participatory approaches.
- To increase the dissemination and implementation of EBPH in practice settings (e.g., health departments) several important barriers should be considered: organizational culture, the role of leadership, political challenges, funding challenges, and workforce training needs.

ACKNOWLEDGMENT

Parts of this chapter were adapted with permission from the *Annual Review of Public Health*, Volume 30 ©2009 by Annual Reviews www.annualreviews.org

SUGGESTED READINGS AND SELECTED WEBSITES

Suggested Readings

Brownson, RC, Fielding JE, Maylahn CM. Evidence-based public health: a fundamental concept for public health practice. *Annu Rev Public Health.* 2009;30:175–201.

Fielding JE, Briss PA. Promoting evidence-based public health policy: can we have better evidence and more action? *Health Aff (Millwood)*. 2006;25(4):969–978.

Glasziou P, Longbottom H. Evidence-based public health practice. *Austral NZ J Public Health*. 1999;23(4):436–440.

Green LW, Ottoson JM, Garcia C, Hiatt RA. Diffusion theory and knowledge dissemination, utilization, and integration in public health. *Annu Rev Public Health*. 2009.

Guyatt GH, Rennie D. 2007. *Users' Guides to the Medical Literature: A Manual for Evidence-Based Clinical Practice*. Chicago: American Medical Association.

Muir Gray JA. *Evidence-Based Healthcare: How to Make Health Policy and Management Decisions*. New York and Edinburgh: Churchill Livingstone, 1997.

Sackett DL, Rosenberg WMC, Gray JAM, et al. Evidence based medicine: what it is and what it isn't. *Br Med J*. 1996;312:71–72.

Selected Websites

American Public Health Association <http://www.apha.org>. The American Public Health Association (APHA) is the oldest and most diverse organization of public health professionals in the world, representing more than 50,000 members. The Association and its members have been influencing policies and setting priorities in public health since 1872. The APHA site provides links to many other useful websites.

Evidence-based behavioral practice <http://www.ebbp.org/>. The EBBP.org project creates training resources to bridge the gap between behavioral health research and practice. An interactive website offers modules covering topics such as the EBBP process, systematic reviews, searching for evidence, critical appraisal, and randomized controlled trials. This site is ideal for practitioners, researchers and educators.

Canadian Task Force on Preventive Health Care <http://www.ctfphc.org/>. This website is designed to serve as a practical guide to health care providers, planners and consumers for determining the inclusion or exclusion, content, and frequency of a wide variety of preventive health interventions, using the evidence-based recommendations of the Canadian Task Force on Preventive Health Care.

Cancer Control P.L.A.N.E.T. <http://cancercontrolplanet.cancer.gov/index.html>. Cancer Control P.L.A.N.E.T. acts as a portal to provide access to data and resources for designing, implementing and evaluating evidence-based cancer control programs. The site provides five steps (with links) for developing a comprehensive cancer control plan or program.

CDC Community Health Resources <http://www.cdc.gov/community healthresources>. This searchable site provides access to CDC's best resources for planning, implementing, and evaluating community health interventions and programs to address chronic disease and health disparities issues. The site links to hundreds of useful planning guides, evaluation frameworks, communication materials, behavioral and risk factor data, fact sheets, scientific articles, key reports, and state and local program contacts.

The Guide to Community Preventive Services (the *Community Guide*) <http:// www.thecommunityguide.org/index.html>. The *Guide* provides guidance in choosing evidence-based programs and policies to improve health and prevent disease at the community level. The Task Force on Community Preventive Services, an independent, nonfederal, volunteer body of public health and prevention experts appointed by the director of the Centers for Disease Control and Prevention, has systematically reviewed more than 200 interventions to produce the recommendations and findings available at this site. The topics covered in the *Guide* currently include adolescent health, alcohol, asthma, birth defects, cancer, diabetes, HIV/AIDS, STIs and pregnancy, mental health, motor vehicle, nutrition, obesity, oral health, physical activity, social environment, tobacco, vaccines, violence, and worksite.

Johns Hopkins Center for Global Health <http://www.hopkinsglobalhealth. org/>. The Johns Hopkins Center for Global Health site maintains an extensive list of links to global health organizations and resources. This site includes health-related statistics by country, including background information on the country and basic health statistics.

National Registry of Evidence-based Programs and Practices (NREPP) <http:// www.nrepp.samhsa.gov/>. Developed by the Substance Abuse and Mental Health Services Administration, NREPP is a searchable database of interventions for the prevention and treatment of mental and substance use disorders. The interventions have been reviewed and rated by independent reviewers.

Partnership for Prevention <http://www.prevent.org/>. Working to emphasize disease prevention and health promotion in national policy and practice, Partnership for Prevention is a membership association of businesses, nonprofit organizations, and government agencies. The site includes action guides that translate several of the *Community Guide* recommendations into easy to follow implementation guidelines.

U.S. Preventive Services Task Force <http://www.ahrq.gov/CLINIC/uspstfix. htm>. The U.S. Preventive Services Task Force (USPSTF) conducts standardized reviews of scientific evidence for the effectiveness of a broad range of clinical preventive services, including screening, counseling, and preventive medications. Its recommendations are considered the "gold standard" for clinical preventive services in the United States. Available at this site are USPSTF clinical recommendations by topic and a pocket guide to the *Guide to Clinical Preventive Services, 2009.*

UCLA Health Impact Assessment Clearinghouse Learning and Information Center <http://www.ph.ucla.edu/hs/hiaclic/>. This site contains summaries of health impact assessments (HIAs) conducted in the United States, HIA-related news, and information about HIA methods and tools. An online training manual is provided.

WHO Health Impact Assessments <http://www.who.int/hia/en/>. The World Health Organization provides health impact assessment (HIA) guides and examples from several countries. Many links are provided to assist in understanding and conducting HIAs.

REFERENCES

1. National Center for Health Statistics. *Health, United States, 2000 with Adolescent Health Chartbook*. Hyattsville, MD: Centers for Disease Control and Prevention, National Center for Health Statistics; 2000.
2. Centers for Disease Control and Prevention. *Public Health in the New American Health System. Discussion Paper*. Atlanta, GA: Centers for Disease Control and Prevention; March 1993.
3. Muir Gray JA. *Evidence-Based Healthcare: How to Make Health Policy and Management Decisions*. New York and Edinburgh: Churchill Livingstone; 1997.
4. Brownson RC, Baker EA, Leet TL, et al. *Evidence-Based Public Health*. New York: Oxford University Press; 2003.
5. Glasziou P, Longbottom H. Evidence-based public health practice. *Austral NZ J Public Health.* 1999;23(4):436–440.
6. McMichael C, Waters E, Volmink J. Evidence-based public health: what does it offer developing countries? *J Public Health (Oxf).* 2005;27(2):215–221.
7. Fielding JE, Briss PA. Promoting evidence-based public health policy: can we have better evidence and more action? *Health Aff (Millwood).* 2006;25(4):969–978.
8. Kahn EB, Ramsey LT, Brownson RC, et al. The effectiveness of interventions to increase physical activity. A systematic review (1,2). *Am J Prev Med.* 2002;22 (4 Suppl 1):73–107.
9. Kohatsu ND, Melton RJ. A health department perspective on the Guide to Community Preventive Services. *Am J Prev Med.* 2000;18(1 Suppl):3–4.
10. Brownson RC, Gurney JG, Land G. Evidence-based decision making in public health. *J Public Health Manag Pract.* 1999;5:86–97.
11. Carlson SA, Fulton JE, Lee SM, et al. Physical education and academic achievement in elementary school: data from the early childhood longitudinal study. *Am J Public Health.* 2008;98(4):721–727.
12. Fielding JE. Where is the evidence? *Annu Rev Public Health.* 2001;22:v–vi.
13. Institute of Medicine Committee for the Study of the Future of Public Health. *The Future of Public Health*. Washington, DC: National Academies Press; 1988.
14. Anderson J. "Don't confuse me with facts…": evidence-based practice confronts reality. *Med J Aust.* 1999;170(10):465–466.
15. Baker EL, Potter MA, Jones DL, et al. The public health infrastructure and our nation's health. *Annu Rev Public Health.* 2005;26:303–318.
16. Haynes B, Haines A. Barriers and bridges to evidence based clinical practice. *BMJ.* 1998;317(7153):273–276.
17. Catford J. Creating political will: moving from the science to the art of health promotion. *Health Promot Int.* 2006;21(1):1–4.

18. Black BL, Cowens-Alvarado R, Gershman S, et al. Using data to motivate action: the need for high quality, an effective presentation, and an action context for decision-making. *Cancer Causes Control.* 2005;(16 Suppl 1):15–25.

19. Curry S, Byers T, Hewitt M, eds. *Fulfilling the Potential of Cancer Prevention and Early Detection.* Washington, DC: National Academies Press; 2003.

20. Briss PA, Brownson RC, Fielding JE, Zaza S. Developing and using the Guide to Community Preventive Services: lessons learned about evidence-based public health. *Annu Rev Public Health.* 2004;25:281–302.

21. Zaza S, Briss PA, Harris KW, eds. *The Guide to Community Preventive Services: What Works to Promote Health?* New York: Oxford University Press; 2005.

22. Agency for Healthcare Research and Quality. *Guide to Clinical Preventive Services,* 3rd ed. Retrieved October 22, 2005, from http://www.ahrq.gov/clinic/gcpspu.htm

23. Cancer Control PLANET. Cancer Control PLANET. Links resources to comprehensive cancer control. Retrieved May 26, 2008, from http://cancercontrolplanet.cancer.gov/index.html

24. SAMHSA. SAMHSA's National Registry of Evidence-based Programs and Practices. Retrieved August 16, 2008, http://www.nrepp.samhsa.gov/

25. Kohatsu ND, Robinson JG, Torner JC. Evidence-based public health: an evolving concept. *Am J Prev Med.* 2004;27(5):417–421.

26. Green LW. Public health asks of systems science: to advance our evidence-based practice, can you help us get more practice-based evidence? *Am J Public Health.* 2006;96(3):406–409.

27. Kerner J, Rimer B, Emmons K. Introduction to the special section on dissemination: dissemination research and research dissemination: how can we close the gap? *Health Psychol.* 2005;24(5):443–446.

28. Dreisinger M, Leet TL, Baker EA, et al. Improving the public health workforce: evaluation of a training course to enhance evidence-based decision making. *J Public Health Manag Pract.* 2008;14(2):138–143.

29. McGlynn EA, Asch SM, Adams J, et al. The quality of health care delivered to adults in the United States. *N Engl J Med.* 2003;348(26):2635–2645.

30. Thacker SB, Ikeda RM, Gieseker KE, et al. The evidence base for public health informing policy at the Centers for Disease Control and Prevention. *Am J Prev Med.* 2005;29(3):227–233.

31. Jenicek M. Epidemiology, evidence-based medicine, and evidence-based public health. *J Epidemiol Commun Health.* 1997;7:187–197.

32. Rychetnik L, Hawe P, Waters E, et al. A glossary for evidence based public health. *J Epidemiol Commun Health.* 2004;58(7):538–545.

33. Satterfield JM, Spring B, Brownson RC, et al. Toward a transdisciplinary model of evidence-based practice. *Milbank Q.* 2009;87(2):368–390.

34. McKean E, ed. *The New Oxford American Dictionary.* 2nd ed. New York, NY: Oxford University Press; 2005.

35. McQueen DV. Strengthening the evidence base for health promotion. *Health Promot Int.* 2001;16(3):261–268.

36. Chambers D, Kerner J. Closing the gap between discovery and delivery. Dissemination and Implementation Research Workshop: Harnessing Science to Maximize Health, Rockville, MD, 2007.

37. McQueen DV, Anderson LM. What counts as evidence? Issues and debates. In: Rootman, ed. Evaluation in Health Promotion: Principles and Perspectives. Copenhagen, Denmark: World Health Organization; 2001:63–81.

38. Rimer BK, Glanz DK, Rasband G. Searching for evidence about health education and health behavior interventions. *Health Educ Behav.* 2001;28(2):231–248.
39. Kerner JF. Integrating research, practice, and policy: what we see depends on where we stand. *J Public Health Manag Pract.* 2008;14(2):193–198.
40. Mulrow CD, Lohr KN. Proof and policy from medical research evidence. *J Health Polit Policy Law.* 2001;26(2):249–266.
41. Sturm R. Evidence-based health policy versus evidence-based medicine. *Psychiatr Serv.* 2002;53(12):1499.
42. Brownson RC, Royer C, Ewing R, et al. Researchers and policymakers: travelers in parallel universes. *Am J Prev Med.* 2006;30(2):164–172.
43. Nutbeam D. How does evidence influence public health policy? Tackling health inequalities in England. *Health Promot J Aust.* 2003;14:154–158.
44. Ogilvie D, Egan M, Hamilton V, Petticrew M. Systematic reviews of health effects of social interventions: 2. Best available evidence: how low should you go? *J Epidemiol Community Health.* 2005;59(10):886–892.
45. Sanson-Fisher RW, Campbell EM, Htun AT, Bailey LJ, Millar CJ. We are what we do: research outputs of public health. *Am J Prev Med.* 2008;35(4):380–5.
46. Glasgow RE, Green LW, Klesges LM, et al. External validity: we need to do more. *Ann Behav Med.* 2006;31(2):105–108.
47. Green LW, Glasgow RE. Evaluating the relevance, generalization, and applicability of research: issues in external validation and translation methodology. *Eval Health Prof.* 2006;29(1):126–153.
48. Castro FG, Barrera M, Jr., Martinez CR, Jr. The cultural adaptation of prevention interventions: resolving tensions between fidelity and fit. *Prev Sci.* 2004;5(1):41–45.
49. Kerner JF, Guirguis-Blake J, Hennessy KD, et al. Translating research into improved outcomes in comprehensive cancer control. *Cancer Causes Control.* 2005;16 (Suppl 1):27–40.
50. Rychetnik L, Frommer M, Hawe P, et al. Criteria for evaluating evidence on public health interventions. *J Epidemiol Commun Health.* 2002;56(2):119–127.
51. Glasgow RE. What types of evidence are most needed to advance behavioral medicine? *Ann Behav Med.* 2008;35(1):19–25.
52. Kemm J. The limitations of "evidence-based" public health. *J Eval Clin Pract.* 2006;12(3):319–324.
53. Dobrow MJ, Goel V, Upshur RE. Evidence-based health policy: context and utilisation. *Soc Sci Med.* 2004;58(1):207–217.
54. Maslov A. A theory of human motivation. *Psychol Rev.* 1943;50:370–396.
55. Pawson R, Greenhalgh T, Harvey G, et al. Realist review—a new method of systematic review designed for complex policy interventions. *J Health Serv Res Policy.* 2005;10(Suppl 1):21–34.
56. Millward L, Kelly M, Nutbeam D. *Public Health Interventions Research: The Evidence.* London: Health Development Agency; 2003.
57. Petticrew M, Roberts H. Systematic reviews—do they "work" in informing decision-making around health inequalities? *Health Econ Policy Law.* 2008;3(Pt 2): 197–211.
58. Petticrew M, Cummins S, Ferrell C, et al. Natural experiments: an underused tool for public health? *Public Health.* 2005;119(9):751–757.
59. Tones K. Beyond the randomized controlled trial: a case for "judicial review." *Health Educ Res.* 1997;12(2):i–iv.

60. Steckler A, McLeroy KR, Goodman RM, et al. Toward integrating qualitative and quantitative methods: an introduction. *Health Educ Q.* 1992;19(1):1–8.
61. Dorfman LE, Derish PA, Cohen JB. Hey girlfriend: An evaluation of AIDS prevention among women in the sex industry. *Health Educ Q.* 1992;19(1):25–40.
62. Hugentobler M, Israel BA, Schurman SJ. An action research approach to workplace health: Integrating methods. *Health Educ Q.* 1992;19(1):55–76.
63. Goodman RM, Wheeler FC, Lee PR. Evaluation of the Heart to Heart Project: lessons from a community-based chronic disease prevention project. *Am J Health Promot.* 1995;9:443–455.
64. McQueen DV. The evidence debate. *J Epidemiol Commun Health.* 2002;56(2):83–84.
65. Suppe F. *The Structure of Scientific Theories.* 2nd ed. Urbana, IL: University of Illinois Press; 1977.
66. Cavill N, Foster C, Oja P, et al. An evidence-based approach to physical activity promotion and policy development in Europe: contrasting case studies. *Promot Educ.* 2006;13(2):104–111.
67. Fielding JE. Foreword. In: Brownson RC, Baker EA, Leet TL, Gillespie KN, eds. *Evidence-Based Public Health.* New York: Oxford University Press; 2003:v–vii.
68. Presidential Task Force on Evidence-Based Practice. Evidence-based practice in psychology. *Am Psychol.* 2006;61(4):271–285.
69. Gambrill E. Evidence-based practice: Sea change or the emperor's new clothes? *J Soc Work Educ.* 2003;39(1):3–23.
70. Mullen E, Bellamy J, Bledsoe S, et al. Teaching evidence-based practice. *Res Soc Work Pract.* 2007;17(5):574–582.
71. Melnyk BM, Fineout-Overholt E, Stone P, et al. Evidence-based practice: the past, the present, and recommendations for the millennium. *Pediatr Nurs.* 2000;26(1):77–80.
72. Evidence-Based Medicine Working Group. Evidence-based medicine. A new approach to teaching the practice of medicine. *JAMA.* 1992;17:2420–2425.
73. Cochrane A. *Effectiveness and Efficiency: Random Reflections on Health Services.* London: Nuffield Provincial Hospital Trust; 1972.
74. Guyatt G, Cook D, Haynes B. Evidence based medicine has come a long way. *BMJ.* 2004;329(7473):990–991.
75. Canadian Task Force on the Periodic Health Examination. The periodic health examination. Canadian Task Force on the Periodic Health Examination. *Can Med Assoc J.* 1979;121(9):1193–1254.
76. US Preventive Services Task Force. *Guide to Clinical Preventive Services: An Assessment of the Effectiveness of 169 Interventions.* Baltimore: Williams & Wilkins; 1989.
77. Taubes G. Looking for the evidence in medicine. *Science.* 1996;272:22–24.
78. Oldenburg BF, Sallis JF, French ML, et al. Health promotion research and the diffusion and institutionalization of interventions. *Health Educ Res.* 1999;14(1):121–130.
79. Tilson H, Gebbie KM. The public health workforce. *Annu Rev Public Health.* 2004;25:341–356.
80. Turnock BJ. *Public Health: What It Is and How It Works.* 3rd ed. Gaithersburg, MD: Aspen Publishers; 2004.
81. Hausman AJ. Implications of evidence-based practice for community health. *Am J Commun Psychol.* 2002;30(3):453–467.
82. McGinnis JM. Does proof matter? why strong evidence sometimes yields weak action. *Am J Health Promot.* 2001;15(5):391–396.

83. Thacker SB. Public health surveillance and the prevention of injuries in sports: what gets measured gets done. *J Athl Train.* 2007;42(2):171–172.

84. Chriqui JF, Frosh MM, Brownson RC, et al. Measuring policy and legislative change. *Evaluating ASSIST: A Blueprint for Understanding State-Level Tobacco Control.* Bethesda, MD: National Cancer Institute; 2006.

85. Masse LC, Chriqui JF, Igoe JF, et al. Development of a Physical Education-Related State Policy Classification System (PERSPCS). *Am J Prev Med.* 2007;33(4, Suppl 1): S264–S276.

86. Masse LC, Frosh MM, Chriqui JF, et al. Development of a School Nutrition-Environment State Policy Classification System (SNESPCS). *Am J Prev Med.* 2007;33(4, Suppl 1):S277–S291.

87. National Institute on Alcohol and Alcoholism. Alcohol Policy Information System. http://alcoholpolicy.niaaa.nih.gov/.

88. McLeroy KR, Bibeau D, Steckler A, et al. An ecological perspective on health promotion programs. *Health Educ Q.* 1988;15:351–377.

89. Stokols D. Translating social ecological theory into guidelines for community health promotion. *Am J Health Promot.* 1996;10(4):282–298.

90. Glanz K, Bishop DB. The role of behavioral science theory in the development and implementation of public health interventions. *Annu Rev Public Health.* 2010;31:391–418.

91. Cargo M, Mercer SL. The value and challenges of participatory research: Strengthening its practice. *Annu Rev Public Health.* 2008;29:325–350.

92. Israel BA, Schulz AJ, Parker EA, et al. Review of community-based research: assessing partnership approaches to improve public health. *Annu Rev Public Health.* 1998;19:173–202.

93. Green LW, Mercer SL. Can public health researchers and agencies reconcile the push from funding bodies and the pull from communities? *Am J Public Health.* 2001;91(12):1926–1929.

94. Leung MW, Yen IH, Minkler M. Community based participatory research: a promising approach for increasing epidemiology's relevance in the 21st century. *Int J Epidemiol.* 2004;33(3):499–506.

95. Land G, Romeis JC, Gillespie KN, et al. Missouri's Take a Seat, Please! and program evaluation. *J Public Health Manage Pract.* 1997;3(6):51–58.

96. Thacker SB, Berkelman RL. Public health surveillance in the United States. *Epidemiol Rev.* 1988;10:164–190.

97. Thacker SB, Stroup DF. Public health surveillance. In: Brownson RC, Petitti DB, eds. *Applied Epidemiology: Theory to Practice.* 2nd ed. New York, NY: Oxford University Press; 2006:30–67.

98. Annest JL, Pirkle JL, Makuc D, et al. Chronological trend in blood lead levels between 1976 and 1980. *N Engl J Med.* 1983;308:1373–1377.

99. Tobacco Education and Research Oversight Committee for California. Confronting a Relentless Adversary: A Plan for Success: Toward a Tobacco-Free California, 2006–2008. In: Health CDoP, ed. Sacramento, CA; 2006.

100. Biener L, Harris JE, Hamilton W. Impact of the Massachusetts tobacco control programme: population based trend analysis. *BMJ.* 2000;321(7257):351–354.

101. Hutchison BG. Critical appraisal of review articles. *Can Fam Physician.* 1993;39:1097–1102.

102. Milne R, Chambers L. Assessing the scientific quality of review articles. *J Epidemiol Commun Health.* 1993;47(3):169–170.
103. Mulrow CD. The medical review article: state of the science. *Ann Intern Med.* 1987;106(3):485–488.
104. Oxman AD, Guyatt GH. The science of reviewing research. *Ann N Y Acad Sci.* 1993;703:125–133; discussion 133–124.
105. Mullen PD, Ramirez G. The promise and pitfalls of systematic reviews. *Annu Rev Public Health.* 2006;27:81–102.
106. Waters E, Doyle J. Evidence-based public health practice: improving the quality and quantity of the evidence. *J Public Health Med.* 2002;24(3):227–229.
107. Gold MR, Siegel JE, Russell LB, et al. *Cost-Effectiveness in Health and Medicine.* New York: Oxford University Press; 1996.
108. Carande-Kulis VG, Maciosek MV, Briss PA, et al. Methods for systematic reviews of economic evaluations for the Guide to Community Preventive Services. Task Force on Community Preventive Services. *Am J Prev Med.* 2000;18(1 Suppl):75–91.
109. Harris P, Harris-Roxas B, Harris E, et al. *Health Impact Assessment: A Practical Guide.* Sydney: Australia: Centre for Health Equity Training, Research and Evaluation (CHETRE). Part of the UNSW Research Centre for Primary Health Care and Equity, UNSW; August 2007.
110. Cole BL, Wilhelm M, Long PV, et al. Prospects for health impact assessment in the United States: new and improved environmental impact assessment or something different? *J Health Polit Pol Law.* 2004;29(6):1153–1186.
111. Kemm J. Health impact assessment: a tool for healthy public policy. *Health Promot Int.* 2001;16(1):79–85.
112. Mindell J, Sheridan L, Joffe M, et al. Health impact assessment as an agent of policy change: improving the health impacts of the mayor of London's draft transport strategy. *J Epidemiol Commun Health.* 2004;58(3):169–174.
113. Green LW, George MA, Daniel M, et al. *Review and Recommendations for the Development of Participatory Research in Health Promotion in Canada.* Vancouver, British Columbia: The Royal Society of Canada; 1995.
114. Soriano FI. *Conducting Needs Assessments. A Multdisciplinary Approach.* Thousand Oaks, CA: Sage Publications; 1995.
115. Sederburg WA. Perspectives of the legislator: allocating resources. *MMWR Morb Mortal Wkly Rep.* 1992,41(Suppl).37–48.
116. Hallfors D, Cho H, Livert D, et al. Fighting back against substance abuse: are community coalitions winning? *Am J Prev Med.* 2002;23(4):237–245.
117. Brownson RC, Diem G, Grabauskas V, et al. Training practitioners in evidence-based chronic disease prevention for global health. *Promot Educ.* 2007;14(3):159–163.
118. Tugwell P, Bennett KJ, Sackett DL, et al. The measurement iterative loop: a framework for the critical appraisal of need, benefits and costs of health interventions. *J Chronic Dis.* 1985;38(4):339–351.
119. Birkhead GS, Davies J, Miner K, et al. Developing competencies for applied epidemiology: from process to product. *Public Health Rep.* 2008;123(Suppl 1):67–118.
120. Birkhead GS, Koo D. Professional competencies for applied epidemiologists: a roadmap to a more effective epidemiologic workforce. *J Public Health Manag Pract.* 2006;12(6):501–504.

121. Gebbie K, Merrill J, Hwang I, et al. Identifying individual competency in emerging areas of practice: an applied approach. *Qual Health Res.* 2002;12(7):990–999.

122. Brownson R, Ballew P, Kittur N, et al. Developing competencies for training practitioners in evidence-based cancer control. *J Cancer Educ.* 2009;24(3):186–193.

123. Baker EA, Brownson RC, Dreisinger M, et al. Examining the role of training in evidence-based public health: a qualitative study. *Health Promot Pract.* 2009;10(3):342–348.

124. Maxwell ML, Adily A, Ward JE. Promoting evidence-based practice in population health at the local level: a case study in workforce capacity development. *Aust Health Rev.* 2007;31(3):422–429.

125. Maylahn C, Bohn C, Hammer M, et al. Strengthening epidemiologic competencies among local health professionals in New York: teaching evidence-based public health. *Public Health Rep.* 2008;123(Suppl 1):35–43.

126. Oliver KB, Dalrymple P, Lehmann HP, et al. Bringing evidence to practice: a team approach to teaching skills required for an informationist role in evidence-based clinical and public health practice. *J Med Libr Assoc.* 2008;96(1):50–57.

127. Pappaioanou M, Malison M, Wilkins K, et al. Strengthening capacity in developing countries for evidence-based public health: the data for decision-making project. *Soc Sci Med.* 2003;57(10):1925–1937.

128. Linkov F, LaPorte R, Lovalekar M, et al. Web quality control for lectures: Supercourse and Amazon.com. *Croat Med J.* 2005;46(6):875–878.

129. Brownson RC, Ballew P, Brown KL, et al. The effect of disseminating evidence-based interventions that promote physical activity to health departments. *Am J Public Health.* 2007;97(10):1900–1907.

130. Proctor EK. Leverage points for the implementation of evidence-based practice. *Brief Treatment Crisis Intervent.* 2004;4(3):227–242.

131. Chambers LW. The new public health: do local public health agencies need a booster (or organizational "fix") to combat the diseases of disarray? *Can J Public Health.* 1992;83(5):326–328.

132. Bryan RL, Kreuter MW, Brownson RC. Integrating Adult Learning Principles into Training for Public Health Practice. *Health Promot Pract.* Apr 2 2008.

133. Ginter PM, Duncan WJ, Capper SA. Keeping strategic thinking in strategic planning: macro-environmental analysis in a state health department of public health. *Public Health.* 1992;106:253–269.

134. Florin P, Stevenson J. Identifying training and technical assistance needs in community coalitions: a developmental approach. *Health Educ Res.* 1993;8:417–432.

135. Jacobs J, Dodson E, Baker E, et al. Barriers to evidence-based decision making in public health: a national survey of chronic disease practitioners. *Public Health Rep.* 2010;In press.

136. Institute of Medicine Committee on Public Health. *Healthy Communities: New Partnerships for the Future of Public Health.* Washington, DC: National Academies Press; 1996.

137. Wright K, Rowitz L, Merkle A, et al. Competency development in public health leadership. *Am J Public Health.* 2000;90(8):1202–1207.

2

Assessing Scientific Evidence
for Public Health Action

> It is often necessary to make a decision on the basis of information sufficient
> for action but insufficient to satisfy the intellect.
>
> —Immanuel Kant

In most areas of public health and clinical practice, decisions on when to intervene and which program or policy to implement are not simple and straightforward. These decisions are often based on three fundamental questions: (1) Should public health action be taken to address a particular public health issue (Type 1, etiologic evidence)? (2) What action should be taken (Type 2, intervention evidence)? (3) How can a particular program or policy most effectively be implemented in a local setting (Type 3, contextual evidence)? This chapter primarily explores the first and second questions. That is, it focuses on several key considerations in evaluating scientific evidence and determining when a scientific basis exists for some type of public health action. It deals largely with the interpretation of epidemiologic studies that seek to identify health risks and intervention programs and policies that seek to improve population health. The third question is explored in more detail in later chapters (especially Chapters 8 and 9).

Public health information for decision making is founded on science, and science is based on the collection, analysis, and interpretation of data.[1,2] Data in public health are generally derived from two overlapping sources: research studies and public health surveillance systems. Here, we focus on information from research studies; an emphasis on public health surveillance is provided in Chapter 6. Research studies are primarily conducted in five broad areas[3]: (1) to understand the (etiologic) links between behaviors and health (For example, does fruit and vegetable intake influence the risk of coronary heart disease?); (2) to develop methods for measuring the behavior (What are the most valid and reliable methods by which to measure fruit and vegetable consumption?); (3) to identify the factors that influence the behavior (Which populations are at highest risk of low consumptions of fruits and vegetables?); (4) to determine whether public health interventions are successful in meeting their stated objectives for risk reduction (Is a media campaign to increase fruit and vegetable intake effective?); and (5) to translate (or disseminate) research to practice (How does one "scale-up" an effective intervention promoting fruit and vegetable consumption so it will widely improve population health?). In general, too much emphasis has been placed on the discovery of etiologic knowledge compared with the development, adaptation, and dissemination of effective interventions.[4,5]

BACKGROUND

In this era when public and media interest in health issues is intense, the reasons for not taking action based on an individual research study, even if it was carefully designed, successfully conducted, and properly analyzed and interpreted, need to be emphasized. Public health research is incremental, with a body of scientific evidence building up over years or decades. Therefore, while individual studies may contribute substantially to public health decision making, a single study rarely constitutes a strong basis for action. The example in Box 2-1 regarding toxic shock syndrome is unusual because rapid action was taken based on a small but convincing body of scientific evidence.[6–8]

When considering the science, strong evidence from epidemiologic (and other) studies may suggest that prevention and control measures be taken.

Box 2-1. Toxic Shock Syndrome in the United States

In the case of an infectious agent transmitted by a fomite (i.e., an inanimate object that may harbor a pathogen), the illness known as toxic shock syndrome was reported to the Centers for Disease Control by individual physicians and five state health departments beginning in October 1979.[6] Toxic shock syndrome began with high fever, vomiting, and profuse watery diarrhea and progressed to hypotensive shock. Among the first 55 cases, the case-fatality ratio was 13%. The bacterium *Staphylococcus aureus* was found to be responsible for the syndrome. Through a nationwide case-control study of 52 cases and 52 matched controls, the mode of transmission was determined to be the use of high absorbency (fluid capacity) tampons in women.[7] The findings of epidemiologic studies led to public health recommendations to women regarding safe use of tampons, a voluntary removal of the Rely brand, and subsequent lowering of absorbency of all brands of tampons.[8] These actions in turn led to substantial reductions in the incidence of toxic shock syndrome since the early observations of the association between tampon use and toxic shock syndrome.

Conversely, evidence may be equivocal, so that taking action would be premature. Often the strength of evidence is suggestive but not conclusive, yet one has to make a decision about the desirability of taking action. Here, other questions come to mind:

- Is the public health problem large and growing?
- Are there effective interventions for addressing the problem?
- Is a particular program or policy worth instituting (i.e., is it better than alternatives?), and will it provide a satisfactory return on investment, measured in monetary terms or in health impacts?
- What information about the local context related to this particular intervention is helpful in deciding its potential use in the situation at hand?

If the answer to the first three questions is "yes," then the decision to take action is relatively straightforward. In practice, unfortunately, decisions are seldom so simple.

EXAMINING A BODY OF SCIENTIFIC EVIDENCE

As practitioners, researchers, and policy makers committed to improving population health, we have a natural tendency to scrutinize the scientific literature for new findings that would serve as the basis for prevention or intervention programs. In fact, the main motivation for conducting research should be to stimulate appropriate public health action. Adding to this inclination to intervene may be claims from investigators regarding the critical importance of their findings, media interpretation of the findings as the basis for immediate action, political pressure for action, and community support for responding to the striking new research findings with new or modified programs. The importance of community action in motivating public health efforts was shown in the Long Island Breast Cancer Study Project (LIBCSP). Community advocates in Long Island raised concerns about the high incidence of breast cancer and possible linkages with environmental chemicals and radiation. More than 10 research projects are being conducted by the New York State Health Department, along with scientists from universities and the National Institutes of Health. In each Long Island–area county, breast cancer incidence increased over a 10-year period, while mortality from breast cancer decreased.[9] To date, the LIBCSP has not identified a set of specific environmental agents that could be responsible for the high rates of breast cancer incidence. The exceptions may be breast cancer risk associated with exposure to polyaromatic hydrocarbon exposure and living in proximity to organochlorine-containing hazardous waste sites.[10] The LIBCSP is an important example of participatory research in which patient advocates play important roles in shaping the research (participatory approaches are discussed in more detail in Chapters 4 and 9).

Finding Scientific Evidence

Chapter 7 describes systematic methods for seeking out credible, peer-reviewed scientific evidence. Modern information technologies have made searching the scientific literature quick and accessible. There are also numerous websites that summarize research and provide ready access to surveillance data. The ready access to information may also present a paradox, in that more access is better to the extent one can synthesize contrary findings and recognize good science and advice versus bad findings. Often, various tools are helpful in examining and synthesizing an entire body of evidence, rather than reviewing the literature on a study-by-study basis. These summary approaches, described in Chapter 3, include systematic reviews of the literature, evidence-based guidelines, summaries of best practices, health impact assessments, and economic evaluations.

The Roles of Peer Review and Publication Bias

In assessing evidence, it is important to understand the role of peer review. Peer review is the process of reviewing research proposals, manuscripts submitted for publication by journals, and abstracts submitted for presentation at scientific meetings. These materials are judged for scientific and technical merit by other scientists in the same field.[11] Reviewers are commonly asked to comment on such issues as the scientific soundness of the methods used, innovation, generalizability, and appropriateness of a scientific article to the audience. Although peer review has numerous limitations, including a large time commitment, complexity, and expense, it remains the closest approximation to a gold standard when determining the merits of scientific endeavor.

Through the process of peer review and dissemination of science, it is important to guard against publication bias—that is, the higher likelihood for journal editors to publish positive or "new" findings in contrast to negative studies or those that do not yield statistically significant results. Studies have shown that positive findings tend to get published more often and more quickly.[12] Recent work provides direct empirical evidence for the existence of publication bias.[13] There are numerous possible reasons for publication bias, including researchers' tendency to submit positive rather than negative studies, peer reviewers who are more likely to recommend publication of positive studies, and journal editors who favor publication of positive studies.[14] The net effect of publication bias may be an overrepresentation of false-positive findings in the literature.

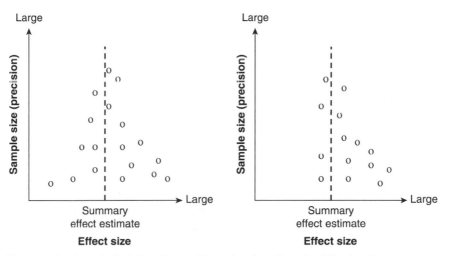

FIGURE 2-1. Hypothetical funnel plots illustrating the effect of publication bias.

It is also important to be aware of potential publication bias when reading or conducting meta-analyses that rely solely on the published literature and do not seek out unpublished studies. When a sufficient number of studies is available, funnel plots may be an effective method by which to determine whether publication bias is present in a particular body of evidence.[14,15] Figure 2-1 presents hypothetical data showing the effects of publication bias. In the plot on the right side, smaller studies are represented in the literature only when they tend to show a positive effect. Thus, the left side of the inverted funnel is missing, and publication bias may be present. Steps to address publication bias include making strenuous efforts to find all published and unpublished work when conducting systematic reviews[16] and the establishment of reporting guidelines that specifically address publication bias.[17]

ASSESSING CAUSALITY IN ETIOLOGIC RESEARCH

A cause of a disease is an event, condition, characteristic, or combination of factors that plays an important role in the development of the disease or health condition.[18] An epidemiologic study assesses the extent to which there is an association between these factors and the disease or health condition. An intervention (program, policy, or other public health action) is based on the presumption that the associations found in these epidemiologic studies are causal rather than arising through bias or for some other spurious reason.[19] Unfortunately, in most instances in observational research, there is no opportunity to prove absolutely that an association is causal. Nonetheless, numerous frameworks have been developed that are useful in determining whether a cause-and-effect relationship exists between a particular risk factor and a given health outcome. This is one of the reasons for assembling experts to reach scientific consensus on various issues.

Criteria for Assessing Causality

The earliest guidelines for assessing causality for infectious diseases were developed in the 1800s by Jacob Henle and Robert Koch. The Henle-Koch Postulates state that (1) the agent must be shown to be present in every case of the disease by isolation in pure culture; (2) the agent must not be found in cases of other disease; (3) once isolated, the agent must be capable of reproducing the disease in experimental animals; and (4) the agent must be recovered from the experimental disease produced.[11,20] These postulates have proved less useful in evaluating causality for more contemporary health conditions because most noninfectious diseases have long periods of induction and multifactorial causation.

Subsequently, the U.S. Department of Health, Education, and Welfare,[21] Hill,[22] Susser,[23] and Rothman[24] have all provided insights into causal criteria, particularly in regard to causation of chronic diseases such as heart disease, cancer, and arthritis. Although criteria have sometimes been cited as checklists for assessing causality, they were intended as factors to consider when examining an association: they have value but only as general guidelines. Several criteria relate to particular cases of refuting biases or drawing on nonepidemiologic evidence. These criteria have been discussed in detail elsewhere.[19,25,26] In the end, belief in causality is based on an individual's judgment, and different individuals may in good faith reach different conclusions based on the same available information. The six key issues that follow have been adapted from Hill[22] and Weed.[27] Each is described by a definition and a rule of evidence. These are also illustrated in Table 2-1 by examining two risk factor/disease relationships.

1. Consistency
   Definition: The association is observed in studies in different settings and populations, using various methods.
   Rule of evidence: The likelihood of a causal association increases as the proportion of studies with similar (positive) results increases.
2. Strength
   Definition: This is defined by the size of the relative risk estimate. In some situations, meta-analytic techniques are used to provide an overall, summary risk estimate.

Table 2-1. Degree to Which Causal Criteria Are Met for Two Contemporary Public
Health Issues

Issue	Physical Activity and Coronary Heart Disease (CHD)	Extremely Low Frequency Electromagnetic Fields (EMFs) and Childhood Cancer[a]
Consistency	Over 50 studies since 1953; vast majority of studies show positive association.	Based on a relatively small number of studies, the preponderance of the evidence favors a judgment of no association.
Strength	Median relative risk of 1.9 for a sedentary lifestyle across studies, after controlling for other risk factors.	Early studies showed relative risks in the range of 1.5 to 2.5. Most subsequent studies with larger sample sizes and more comprehensive exposure methods have not shown positive associations.
Temporality	Satisfied, based on prospective cohort study design.	Not satisfied; very difficult to assess because of ubiquitous exposure and the rarity of the disease.
Dose-response relationship	Most studies show an inverse relationship between physical activity and risk of CHD.	Since there is little biological guidance into what component(s) of EMF exposure may be problematic, exposure assessment is subject to a high degree of misclassification. True dose gradients are therefore very hard to classify reliably.
Biological plausibility	Biological mechanisms are demonstrated, including atherosclerosis, plasma/lipid changes, blood pressure, ischemia, and thrombosis.	No direct cancer mechanism is yet known, as EMFs produce energy levels far too low to cause DNA damage or chemical reactions.
Experimental evidence	Trials have not been conducted related to CHD but have been carried out for CHD intermediate factors such as blood pressure, lipoprotein profile, insulin sensitivity, and body fat.	Numerous experimental studies of EMF exposure have been conducted to assess indirect mechanisms for carcinogenesis in animals and via in vitro cell models. The few positive findings to date have not been successfully reproduced in other laboratories.

[a]Predominantly childhood leukemia and brain cancer.

Rule of evidence: The likelihood of a causal association increases as the summary relative risk estimate increases. Larger effect estimates are generally less likely to be explained by unmeasured bias or confounding.

3. *Temporality*

Definition: This is perhaps the most important criterion for causality—some consider it an absolute condition. Temporality refers to the temporal relationship between the occurrence of the risk factor and the occurrence of the disease or health condition.

Rule of evidence: The exposure (risk factor) must precede the disease.

4. *Dose-response relationship*

Definition: The observed relationship between the dose of the exposure and the magnitude of the relative risk estimate.

Rule of evidence: An increasing level of exposure (in intensity and/or time) increases the risk when hypothesized to do so.

5. *Biological plausibility*

Definition: The available knowledge on the biological mechanism of action for the studied risk factor and disease outcome.

Rule of evidence: There is not a standard rule of thumb except that the more likely the agent is biologically capable of influencing the disease, then the more probable is it that a causal relationship exists.

6. *Experimental evidence*

Definition: The presence of findings from a prevention trial in which the factor of interest is removed from randomly assigned individuals.

Rule of evidence: A positive result (i.e., reduction in a health condition) after removal of the risk factor provides evidence of a causal association.

In practice, evidence for causality is often established through the elimination of noncausal explanations for an observed association. For example, some studies have suggested that alcohol use might increase the risk of breast cancer. Other studies have not found such an association. Further studies would need to be conducted to determine if there might be confounding or other biases that account for the findings. By whittling away alternative explanations, the hypothesis that asserts alcohol use causes breast cancer becomes increasingly credible. It is the job of researchers to propose and test noncausal explanations, so that when the association has withstood a series of such challenges, the case for causality is strengthened.

Because most associations involve unknown confounders, a key issue becomes the extent to which causal conclusions or public health recommendations should be delayed until all or nearly all potential confounders are discovered and/or better measured.[28] As noted earlier, those who argue that causality must be established with absolute certainty before interventions are attempted may fail to appreciate that their two alternatives—action and inaction—each have risks and benefits. When searching for causal relationships, researchers generally seek those that are modifiable and potentially amenable to some type of public health intervention. For example, if researchers studied youth and discovered that age of initiation of smoking was strongly related to the ethnicity of the teen and exposure to advertising, the latter variable would be a likely target of intervention efforts.

INTERVENTION STUDY DESIGN AND EXECUTION: ASSESSING INTERNAL VALIDITY

As described in Chapter 1, public health practitioners are often interested in finding Type 2 and Type 3 evidence (e.g., Which interventions are effective? How do I implement the intervention?). A body of intervention research is often judged on the basis of internal validity, which is the degree to which the treatment or intervention effects changed the dependent variable. For a study or program evaluation to be internally valid, the study and comparison groups should be selected and compared in a way that the observed differences in dependent variables are attributed to the hypothesized effects under study (apart from sampling error).[11] In other words, can the observed results be attributed to the risk factor being studied or intervention being implemented? These concepts are illustrated in Figure 2-2.

While it is beyond the scope of this chapter to discuss these issues in detail, an overview of key issues (so-called threats to validity) is provided, along with entry points into a larger body of literature. The internal validity of a given study can be assessed based on the study design and study execution.

In public health research, a variety of study designs is used to assess health risks and to measure intervention effectiveness. Commonly, these are not "true" experiments in which study participants are randomized to an intervention or control condition. These generally quasi-experimental or observational designs are described in Chapter 6. A hierarchy of designs shows that a randomized trial tends to be the strongest type of study, yet such a study is often not feasible in community settings[29,30] (Table 2-2). Interestingly, when summary results from the same topic were based on observational studies and on randomized controlled trials, the findings across study designs were remarkably similar.[31]

The quality of a study's execution can be determined by many different standards. In general, internal validity is threatened by all types of systematic error,

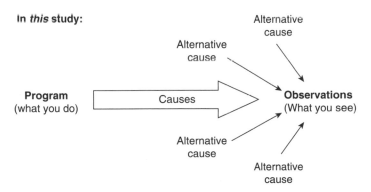

FIGURE 2-2. Illustration of internal validity in establishing a cause-and-effect relationship. (*Source*: < http://www.socialresearchmethods.net/kb/>.)

Table 2-2. Hierarchy of Study Designs

Suitability	Examples	Attributes
Greatest	Randomized group or individual trial; prospective cohort study; time-series study with comparison group	Concurrent comparison groups and prospective measurement of exposure and outcome
Moderate	Case-control study; time series study without comparison group	All retrospective designs or multiple premeasurements or postmeasurements but no concurrent comparison group
Least	Cross-sectional study; case series; ecologic study	Before-after studies with no comparison group or exposure and outcome measured in a single group at the same point in time

Source: Adapted from Briss et al.[29,30]

and error rates are influenced by both study design and study execution. Systematic error occurs when there is a tendency within a particular study to produce results that vary in a systematic way from the true values.[18] Dozens of specific types of bias have been identified. Among the most important are the following[11]:

1. Selection bias—error due to systematic differences in characteristics between those who take part in the study and those who do not
2. Information bias—a flaw in measuring exposure or outcomes that results in different quality (accuracy) of information between study groups
3. Confounding bias—distortion of the estimated effect of an exposure on an outcome, caused by the presence of an extraneous factor associated with both the exposure and the outcome

In ongoing work of the U.S. Public Health Service,[32] study execution is assessed according to six categories, each of which may threaten internal validity: (1) study population and intervention descriptions; (2) sampling; (3) exposure and outcome measurement; (4) data analysis; (5) interpretation of results (including follow-up, bias, and confounding); and (6) other related factors.

THE NEED FOR A STRONGER FOCUS ON EXTERNAL VALIDITY

Most research in public health to date has tended to emphasize internal validity (e.g., well-controlled efficacy trials) while giving limited attention to external validity (i.e., the degree to which findings from a study or set of studies can be generalizable to and relevant for populations, settings, and times other than those in which the original studies were conducted).[33] Green succinctly summarized a key challenge related to external validity in 2001:

"Where did the field get the idea that evidence of an intervention's efficacy from carefully controlled trials could be generalized as THE best practice for widely varied populations and settings?" (p. 167)[34]

Much of the information needed to assess external validity relates to so-called Type 3 (or contextual) evidence,[35] as described in Chapter 1. Too often, this evidence is incomplete or missing completely in the peer-reviewed literature. For example, Klesges and colleagues[36] reviewed 19 childhood obesity studies to assess the extent to which dimensions of external validity were reported. Importantly, the work of Klesges and colleagues shows that some key contextual variables (e.g., cost, program sustainability) are missing entirely in the peer-reviewed literature on obesity prevention. This finding is likely to apply across most other areas of public health.

To develop a stronger literature base for external validity, there is a need for guidelines and better reporting of key variables.[37,38] The essential questions are outlined in Table 2-3 and follow the SPOT guidelines (Settings and populations; Program/policy implementation and adaptation; Outcomes for decision making; *Time*: Maintenance and institutionalization).[39] By answering these questions, public health practitioners can better determine whether a program or study is relevant to their particular setting. This often includes consideration of the target audience, available resources, staff capacity, and availability of appropriate measures.

For public health practitioners, these data on external validity are likely to be as important as information on the internal validity of a particular program or policy, yet detailed information on external validity is often missing in journal articles. Similarly, systematic reviews have difficulty in examining whether factors that may affect external validity (e.g., training and involvement of staff, organizational characteristics) function as important effect modifiers.[40] For certain public health issues, documentation is available on how to implement programs that have been shown to be internally valid. Such guidance is sometimes called an implementation guide, which might assist a practitioner in adapting a scientifically proven intervention to local contextual conditions. Implementation guides have been developed for many areas of public health.

In other cases, it is worth the effort to seek additional data on external validity. This gathering of information relates to the concept of "pooling"—that is, a step in the intervention process where one reviews and pools the best experience from prior attempts at behavioral, environmental, and/or policy change.[41] Key informant interviews are one useful tool to collect these data.[42] Persons to interview may

Table 2-3. Quality Rating Criteria for External Validity

1. Settings and populations
   A. Participation: Are there analyses of the participation rate among potential (a) settings, (b) delivery staff, and (c) patients (consumers)?
   B. Target audience: Is the intended target audience stated for adoption (at the intended settings such as worksites, medical offices, etc.) and application (at the individual level)?
   C. Representativeness—Settings: Are comparisons made of the similarity of settings in study to the intended target audience of program settings—or to those settings that decline to participate?
   D. Representativeness—Individuals: Are analyses conducted of the similarity and differences between patients, consumers, or other subjects who participate versus either those who decline, or the intended target audience?

2. Program or policy implementation and adaptation
   A. Consistent implementation: Are data presented on level and quality of implementation of different program components?
   B. Staff expertise: Are data presented on the level of training or experience required to deliver the program or quality of implementation by different types of staff?
   C. Program adaptation: Is information reported on the extent to which different settings modified or adapted the program to fit their setting?
   D. Mechanisms: Are data reported on the process(es) or mediating variables through which the program or policy achieved its effects?

3. Outcomes for decision making
   A. Significance: Are outcomes reported in a way that can be compared to either clinical guidelines or public health goals?
   B. Adverse consequences: Do the outcomes reported include quality of life or potential negative outcomes?
   C. Moderators: Are there any analyses of moderator effects—including of different subgroups of participants and types of intervention staff—to assess robustness versus specificity of effects?
   D. Sensitivity: Are there any sensitivity analyses to assess dose-response effects, threshold level, or point of diminishing returns on the resources expended?
   E. Costs: Are data on the costs presented? If so, are standard economic or accounting methods used to fully account for costs?

4. Time: Maintenance and institutionalization
   A. Long-term effects: Are data reported on longer-term effects, at least 12 months following treatment?
   B. Institutionalization: Are data reported on the sustainability (or reinvention or evolution) of program implementation at least 12 months after the formal evaluation?
   C. Attrition: Are data on attrition by condition reported, and are analyses conducted of the representativeness of those who drop out?

Source: From Green and Glasgow.[39]

include stakeholders at the local level (e.g., program delivery agents, target populations) who have indigenous wisdom about the context for a particular intervention[39] or the lead investigator or project manager in a research study. Less intensive (yet more superficial) ways to gather this information may involve emailing colleagues or posting specific questions on Listservs.

OTHER IMPORTANT ISSUES WHEN CONSIDERING PUBLIC HEALTH ACTION

In addition to understanding scientific causality and validity (both internal and external), several related issues are important to consider when weighing public health action.

Overarching Factors Influencing Decision Making in Public Health

There are many factors that influence decision making in public health[19,43,44] (Table 2-4). Some of these factors are under the control of the public health practitioner, whereas others are nearly impossible to modify. A group of experts may systematically assemble and present a persuasive body of scientific evidence such as recommendations for clinical or community-based interventions, but even when they convene in a rational and evidence-based manner, the process is imperfect, participants may disagree, and events may become politically charged, as noted in Table 2-5 and Box 2-2.[45-51] In addition, one may have little control over

Table 2-4. Factors Influencing Decision Making among Public Health Administrators, Policy Makers, and the General Public

Category	Influential Factor
Information	• Sound scientific basis, including knowledge of causality • Source (e.g., professional organization, government, mass media, friends)
Clarity of contents	• Formatting and framing • Perceived validity • Perceived relevance • Cost of intervention • Strength of the message (i.e., vividness)
Perceived values, preferences, beliefs	• Role of the decision maker • Economic background • Previous education • Personal experience or involvement • Political affiliation • Willingness to adopt innovations • Willingness to accept uncertainty • Willingness to accept risk • Ethical aspect of the decision
Context	• Culture • Politics • Timing • Media attention • Financial or political constraints

Source: Adapted from Bero et al.[43] and Anderson et al.[44]

Table 2-5. Chronology and Selected Statements from the Development of Consensus Breast Cancer Screening Guidelines for Women Aged 40 to 49 Years, 1997

Date	Source	Statement or Quote
January 23, 1997	NIH Consensus Development Panel (called for and cosponsored by the National Cancer Institute)	Every woman should decide for herself "based not only on objective analysis of scientific evidence and consideration of her individual medical history, bus also on how she perceives and weighs each potential risk and benefits, the values she places on each and how she deals with uncertainty."
January 24, 1997	American Cancer Society	"The confusion surrounding the important question of whether women in their 40s should have regular mammograms had not been cleared up and perhaps was made even murkier by the recent announcement."
February 4, 1997	U.S. Senator Mikulski	"I could not believe when an NIH advisory panel decided that women in this age group might not need mammograms. This flies in the face of what we know."
February 4, 1997	U.S. Senator Snowe	"Women and their doctors look to the Nation's preeminent cancer research institute—the National Cancer Institute—for clear guidance and advice on this issue. By rescinding its guideline, NCI produced wide-spread confusion and concern among women and physicians regarding the appropriate age at which to seek mammograms."
February 4, 1997	US Senate Resolution 47	"... we say enough is enough. We should take time out, go back to our science, go back to our research, go back to the National Institutes of Health and ask them to come up with the recommendation that we need."
March 27, 1997	National Cancer Institute	"The NCI advises women age 40-49 who are of average risk of breast cancer to have screening mammograms every year or two."

the timing of some major public health event (e.g., prostate cancer diagnosis in an elected leader) that may have a large impact on the awareness and behaviors of the general public and policy makers.[52] Therefore, for success in the policy process, one often needs to proactively analyze and assemble data so that evidence is ready when a policy window or opportunity emerges.[53] Generally, evidence for public policy decisions should be viewed across a continuum of certainty (i.e., a range of rational policy options) rather than as a dichotomy.[19]

Estimating Population Burden and the Prevented Fraction

As noted earlier, many factors enter into decisions about public health interventions, including certainty of causality, validity, relevance, economics, and political climate (Table 2-4). Measures of burden may also contribute substantially to

Box 2-2. The Evolution of Breast Cancer Screening Guidelines

Breast cancer screening guidance for women aged 40 to 49 years has been the subject of considerable debate and controversy. Breast cancer is the most common cancer type among U.S. women, accounting for 184,450 new cases and 40,930 annual deaths.[46] It is suggested that appropriate use of screening mammography may lower death rates due to breast cancer up to 30%. Official expert guidance from the U.S. government was first issued in 1977 when the National Cancer Institute (NCI) recommended annual mammography screening for women aged 50 and older but discouraged screening for younger women.[47] In 1980, the American Cancer Society dissented from this guidance and recommended a baseline mammogram for women at age 35 years and annual or biannual mammograms for women in their 40s.[48] The NCI and other professional organizations differed on recommendations for women in their 40s throughout the late 1980s and 1990s. To resolve disagreement, the director of the National Institutes of Health called for a Consensus Development Conference in January 1997. Based on evidence from randomized, controlled trials, the consensus group concluded that the available data did not support a blanket mammography recommendation for women in their 40s. The panel issued a draft statement that largely left the decision regarding screening up to the woman[49] (Table 2-5). This guidance led to widespread media attention and controversy. Within 1 week, the U.S. Senate passed a 98-to-0 vote resolution calling on the NCI to express unequivocal support for screening women in their 40s, and within 60 days, the NCI had issued a new recommendation.

The controversy regarding breast cancer screening resurfaced in 2009. The U.S. Preventive Services Task Force was first convened by the Public Health Service in 1984. Since its inception, it has been recognized as an authoritative source for determining the effectiveness of clinical preventive services, and its methods have been adapted by guidelines groups worldwide. In December 2009, the Task Force revised its guideline on mammography screening, which in part recommended against routine screening mammography in women aged 40 to 49 years.[50] The change from the earlier guideline was based on benefit-risk calculations including the likelihood of false-positive tests that result in additional radiographs, unnecessary biopsies, and significant anxiety. This recommendation was met with unprecedented media attention and charges by some groups (like the American College of Radiology) that the guidelines were changed in response to the Obama Administration's wish to save health care dollars.[51] The US Department of Health and Human Services, which appoints and vets the Task Force, also distanced itself from the updated recommendation. This example points to the interplay of science, politics, timing, and health communication when assessing the evidence for public health interventions.

science-based decision making. The burden of infectious diseases, such as measles, has been primarily assessed through incidence, measured in case numbers or rates. For chronic or noninfectious diseases like cancer, burden can be measured in terms of morbidity, mortality, and disability. The choice of measure should depend on the characteristics of the condition being examined. For example, mortality rates are useful in reporting data on a fatal condition such as lung cancer. For a common, yet generally nonfatal condition such as arthritis, a measure of disability would be more useful (e.g., limitations in "activities of daily living"). When available, measures of the population burden of health conditions are extremely useful (e.g., quality-adjusted life years [QALYs]).

When assessing the scientific basis for a public health program or policy, quantitative considerations of preventable disease can help us make a rational choice. This can be thought of as "preventable burden." When presented with an array of potential causal factors for disease, we need to evaluate how much might be gained by reducing or eliminating each of the hazards. For example, can we predict in numerical terms the benefits that one or more interventions might yield in the community?

Epidemiologic measures, such as relative risk estimates, indicate how strongly exposure and disease are associated, but they do not indicate directly the benefits that could be gained through modifying the exposure. Of still greater potential value is the incorporation of information into how common the exposure is. Although some exposures exert a powerful influence on individuals (i.e., a large relative risk), they are so rare that their public health impact is minimal. Conversely, some exposures have a modest impact but are so widespread that their elimination could have great benefit. To answer the question, "What proportion of disease in the total population is a result of the exposure?" the *population attributable risk* (PAR) is used. The PAR is calculated as follows:

$$\frac{P_e \,(\text{relative risk} - 1)}{1 + P_e \,(\text{relative risk} - 1)}$$

where P_e represents the proportion of the population that is exposed. Assuming that the relative risk of lung cancer due to cigarette smoking is 15 (i.e., smokers have 15 times the risk of lung cancer compared with nonsmokers) and that 30% of the population are smokers, the population attributable risk is 0.81 or 81%. This would suggest that 81% of the lung cancer burden in the population is caused by cigarette smoking and could be eliminated if the exposure were eliminated. Table 2-6 describes a variety of risk factors for coronary heart disease.[54] This list demonstrates that the greatest population burden (PAR) would be affected by eliminating elevated cholesterol and physical inactivity, even though the relative risk values for these risk factors are in the moderate or weak range.[54]

A related metric is the prevented fraction (PF). In an intervention in which "exposure" to a program or policy may protect against disease, the PF is the proportion of disease occurrence in a population averted due to a protective risk factor or public health intervention.[55] The PF is calculated as follows:

$$P_e \,(1 - \text{relative risk})$$

where P_e represents the prevalence of exposure to the protective factor and relative risk is a protective effect estimate (i.e., exposure to the preventive measure protects

Table 2-6. Modifiable Risk Factors for Coronary Heart Disease, United States ©
American Public Health Association

Magnitude	Risk Factor	Best Estimate, % of population (Attributable Risk, range)
Strong (relative risk >4)	None	
Moderate (relative risk 2–4)	High blood pressure (>140/90 mm Hg)	25 (20–29)
	Cigarette smoking	22 (17–25)
	Elevated cholesterol (>200 mg/dL)	43 (39–47)
	Diabetes (fasting glucose S140 mg/dL)	8 (1–15)
Weak (relative risk <2)	Obesity[a]	17 (7–32)
	Physical inactivity	35 (23–46)
	Environmental tobacco smoke exposure	18 (8–23)
	Elevated plasma C-reactive protein (>3.0 mg/L)	19 (11–25)
	Elevated fibrinogen (>3.74 g/L)	21 (17–25)
	Elevated plasma homocysteine (>15 μmol/L)	5 (2–9)
Possible	Psychological factors	
	Alcohol use[b]	
	Infectious agents	

Source: From Newschaffer et al.[54]

[a]Based on body mass index >30 kg/m².

[b]Moderate to heavy alcohol use may increase risk, whereas light use may reduce risk.

against acquiring a specific health problem). This formula for the PF is the same
one used to calculate vaccine efficacy and also has been used to estimate the benefits of disease screening programs.[56] Thacker and colleagues[57] examined 702
population-based interventions and found PF data on only 31 (4.4%), suggesting
the need to expand the evidence base on prevention.

Assessing Time Trends

There are numerous other factors that may be considered when weighing the need
for public health action. One important factor to consider involves temporal trends.
Public health surveillance systems can provide information on changes over time
in a risk factor or disease of interest. Through the use of these data, one may determine whether the condition of interest is increasing, decreasing, or remaining
constant. One may also examine the incidence or prevalence of a condition in relation to other conditions of interest. For example, if a public health practitioner
were working with a statewide coalition to control cancer, it would be useful to
plot both the incidence and mortality rates for various cancer sites[58] (Figure 2-3).
The researcher might reach different conclusions on the impact and changing

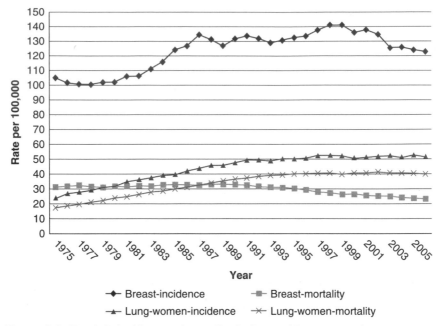

FIGURE 2-3. Trends in incidence and mortality for lung and breast cancer in women, United States, 1975–2006. (Source: Horner et al.[58])

magnitude of various cancers when examining incidence versus mortality rates across the state. When working at a local level, however, it would be important to note that sample sizes might be too small for many health conditions, making rates unstable and subject to considerable fluctuations over time. In addition, a formal time-series analysis requires numerous data points (approximately 50 for the most sophisticated statistical methods). A simple and often useful time-series analysis can often be conducted with ordinary least-squares regression techniques, which are amenable to fewer data points than formal time-series analyses.

Priority Setting via National Health Goals

Determining public health and health care priorities in a climate of limited resources is a demanding task. In some cases, priority setting from experts and government bodies can help to focus areas for public health action. These efforts are particularly useful in evaluating Type 1 evidence (i.e., something must be done on a particular health topic). They are often less helpful for Type 2 evidence (i.e., this specific intervention should be conducted within a local area).

Public health leaders began to formulate concrete public health objectives as a basis for action during the post–World War II era. This was a clear shift from earlier efforts as emphasis was placed on quantifiable objectives and explicit time limits.[59] A few key examples illustrate the use of public data in setting and measuring progress toward health objectives. A paper by the Institute of Medicine[60] sparked a U.S. movement to set objectives for public health.[59] These initial actions by the Institute of Medicine led to the 1979 "Healthy People. The Surgeon General's Report on Health Promotion and Disease Prevention," which set five national goals—one each for the principal life stages of infancy, childhood, adolescence and young adulthood, adulthood, and older adulthood.[61] Over approximately the same time period, the World Health Organization published "Health Targets for Europe" in 1984 and adopted a Health for All policy with 38 targets.[62]

More recently, the U.S. Public Health Service established four overarching health goals for 2020: (1) eliminate preventable disease, disability, injury, and premature death; (2) achieve health equity, eliminate disparities, and improve the health of all groups; (3) create social and physical environments that promote good health for all; and (4) promote healthy development and healthy behaviors across every stage of life.[63] As discussed in the final chapter in this book, addressing social and physical determinants of health raises important questions about the types of evidence that are appropriate and how we track progress.

SUMMARY

The issues covered in this chapter highlight one of the continuing challenges for public health practitioners and policy makers—determining when scientific evidence is sufficient for public health action. In nearly all instances, scientific studies cannot demonstrate causality with absolute certainty.[22,64] The demarcation between action and inaction is seldom distinct and requires careful consideration of scientific evidence as well as assessment of values, preferences, costs, and benefits of various options. The difficulty in determining scientific certainty was eloquently summarized by A. B. Hill[22]:

All scientific work is incomplete—whether it be observational or experimental. All scientific work is liable to be upset or modified by advancing knowledge. That does not confer upon us a freedom to ignore the knowledge we already have, or to postpone the action that it appears to demand at a given time.

Because policy cannot wait for perfect information, one must consider actions wherein the benefit outweighs the risk. This was summarized by Szklo[65] as: "How much do we stand to gain if we are right?" and "How much do we stand to lose if we are wrong?"

In many instances, waiting for absolute scientific certainty would mean delaying crucial public health action. For example, the first cases of acquired immunodeficiency syndrome (AIDS) were described in 1981 yet the causative agent (a retrovirus) was not identified until 1983.[66] Studies in epidemiology and prevention research therefore began well before gaining a full understanding of the molecular biology of AIDS transmission.

For success in evidence-based public health, strong skills are crucial in understanding causality and interpreting the ever-expanding evidence basis for action.

Key Chapter Points

- When considering public health measures, it is helpful to consider the consequences of taking action or no action.
- Advances in public health research are generally incremental, suggesting the need for intervention as a body of literature accumulates.
- When evaluating literature and determining a course of action, both internal and external validity should be considered.
- A set of standardized criteria can be useful in assessing the causality of an association.
- Many factors beyond science, such as resource constraints, sources of information, timing, and politics, influence decision making in public health.

SUGGESTED READINGS AND SELECTED WEBSITES

Suggested Readings

Green LW, Glasgow RE. Evaluating the relevance, generalization, and applicability of research: issues in external validation and translation methodology. *Eval Health Prof.* 2006;29(1):126–153.

Rothman KJ. Causes. *Am J Epidemiol.* 1976;104:587–592.

Remington PL, Brownson RC, Savitz DA. Methods in chronic disease epidemiology. In: Remington PL, Brownson RC, Wegner M, eds. *Chronic Disease Epidemiology and Control.* 3rd ed. Washington, DC: American Public Health Association; 2010.

Weed DL. On the use of causal criteria. *Int J Epidemiol.* 1997;26(6):1137–1141.

Zaza S, Briss PA, Harris KW, eds. *The Guide to Community Preventive Services: What Works to Promote Health?* New York: Oxford University Press; 2005.

Selected Websites

Disease Control Priorities Project <http://www.dcp2.org>. The Disease Control Priorities Project (DCPP) is an ongoing effort to assess disease control priorities and produce evidence-based analysis and resource materials to inform health policy making in developing countries. DCPP has produced three volumes providing technical resources that can assist developing countries in improving their health systems and, ultimately, the health of their people.

Health Evidence Network (WHO Regional Office for Europe) <http://www.euro.who.int/HEN>. The Health Evidence Network (HEN) is an information service primarily for public health and health care policy makers in the European Region. HEN synthesizes the huge quantity of information and evidence available in the fields of public health and health care that are dispersed among numerous databases and other sources. HEN provides summarized information from a wide range of existing sources: websites, databases, documents, and national and international organizations and institutions. It also produces its own reports on topical issues.

Healthy People <http://www.healthypeople.gov/>. Healthy People provides science-based, 10-year national objectives for promoting health and preventing disease in the United States. Since 1979, Healthy People has set and monitored national health objectives to meet a broad range of health needs, encourage collaborations across sectors, guide individuals toward making informed health decisions, and measure the impact of prevention activity.

Office of the Surgeon General <http://www.surgeongeneral.gov/>. The U.S. Surgeon General serves as America's chief health educator by providing Americans the best scientific information available on how to improve their health and reduce the risk of illness and injury. The U.S. Surgeon General's public health priorities, reports, and publications are available on this site.

Partners in Information Access for the Public Health Workforce <http://phpartners.org/>. Partners in Information Access for the Public Health Workforce represent a collaboration of U.S. government agencies, public health organizations, and health sciences libraries that provides timely, convenient access to selected public health resources on the Internet.

The Research Methods Knowledge Base <http://www.socialresearchmethods.net/kb/>. The Research Methods Knowledge Base is a comprehensive web-based textbook that covers the entire research process, including formulating research questions; sampling; measurement (surveys, scaling, qualitative, unobtrusive); research design (experimental and quasi-experimental); data analysis; and writing the research paper. It uses an informal, conversational style to engage both the newcomer and the more experienced student of research.

UCSF School of Medicine: Virtual Library in Epidemiology <http://www.epibiostat.ucsf.edu/epidem/epidem.html>. The University of California, San Francisco maintains an extensive listing of websites in epidemiology and related fields. Among the categories are government agencies and international organizations, data sources, and university sites.

World Health Organization <http://www.who.int/en/>. The World Health Organization (WHO) is the directing and coordinating authority for health within the United Nations system. It is responsible for providing leadership on global health matters, shaping the health research agenda, setting norms and standards, articulating evidence-based policy options, providing technical support to countries, and monitoring and assessing health trends. From this site, one can access *The World Health Report*, WHO's leading publication that provides an expert assessment on global health with a focus on a specific subject each year.

REFERENCES

1. Brownson RC, Fielding JE, Maylahn CM. Evidence-based public health: a fundamental concept for public health practice. *Annu Rev Public Health*. 2009;30:175–201.
2. Fielding JE, Briss PA. Promoting evidence-based public health policy: can we have better evidence and more action? *Health Aff (Millwood)*. 2006;25(4):969–978.
3. Sallis JF, Owen N, Fotheringham MJ. Behavioral epidemiology: a systematic framework to classify phases of research on health promotion and disease prevention. *Ann Behav Med*. 2000;22(4):294–298.
4. Brownson RC, Kreuter MW, Arrington BA, True WR. Translating scientific discoveries into public health action: how can schools of public health move us forward? *Public Health Rep*. 2006;121(1):97–103.
5. Oldenburg BF, Sallis JF, French ML, Owen N. Health promotion research and the diffusion and institutionalization of interventions. *Health Educ Res*.1999;14(1): 121–130.
6. Centers for Disease Control. Toxic-shock syndrome—United States. *MMWR*. 1980;29:229–230.
7. Shands KN, Schmid GP, Dan BB, et al. Toxic-shock syndrome in menstruating women: association with tampon use and Staphylococcus aureus and clinical features in 52 cases. *N Engl J Med*. 1980;303:1436–1442.
8. Schuchat A, Broome CV. Toxic shock syndrome and tampons. *Epidemiol Rev*. 1991;13:99–112.
9. US Department of Health and Human Services. *Interim Report of the Long Island Breast Cancer Study Project*. Bethesda, MD: National Institutes of Health; 2000.
10. Winn DM. Science and society: the Long Island Breast Cancer Study Project. *Nat Rev Cancer*. 2005;5(12):986–994.
11. Porta M, ed. *A Dictionary of Epidemiology*. 5th ed. New York: Oxford University Press; 2008.
12. Olson CM, Rennie D, Cook D, et al. Publication bias in editorial decision making. *JAMA*. 2002;287(21):2825–2828.
13. Dwan K, Altman DG, Arnaiz JA, et al. Systematic review of the empirical evidence of study publication bias and outcome reporting bias. *PLoS One*. 2008;3(8):e3081.
14. Guyatt G, Rennie D, eds. *Users' Guides to the Medical Literature. A Manual for Evidence-Based Clinical Practice*. Chicago, IL: American Medical Association Press; 2002.
15. Petitti DB. *Meta-analysis, Decision Analysis, and Cost-Effectiveness Analysis: Methods for Quantitative Synthesis in Medicine*. 2nd ed. New York: Oxford University Press; 2000.

16. Sterne JA, Egger M, Smith GD. Systematic reviews in health care: investigating and dealing with publication and other biases in meta-analysis. *BMJ*. 2001;323(7304):101–105.
17. Moher D, Simera I, Schulz KF, et al. Helping editors, peer reviewers and authors improve the clarity, completeness and transparency of reporting health research. *BMC Med*. 2008;6:13.
18. Bonita R, Beaglehole R, Kjellstrom T. *Basic Epidemiology*. 2nd ed. Geneva, Switzerland: World Health Organization; 2006.
19. Savitz DA. *Interpreting Epidemiologic Evidence. Strategies for Study Design and Analysis*. New York, NY: Oxford University Press; 2003.
20. Rivers TM. Viruses and Koch's postulates. *J Bacteriol*. 1937;33:1–12.
21. US Dept of Health, Education, and Welfare. *Smoking and Health. Report of the Advisory Committee to the Surgeon General of the Public Health Service*. Publication (PHS) 1103. Washington, DC: Centers for Disease Control; 1964.
22. Hill AB. The environment and disease: association or causation? *Proc R Soc Med*. 1965;58:295–300.
23. Susser M. *Causal Thinking in the Health Sciences: Concepts and Strategies in Epidemiology*. New York: Oxford University Press; 1973.
24. Rothman KJ. Causes. *Am J Epidemiol*. 1976;104:587–592.
25. Kelsey JL, Whittemore A, Evans A, Thompson W. *Methods in Observational Epidemiology*. 2nd ed. New York: Oxford University Press; 1996.
26. Rothman K, Greenland S, Lash T. *Modern Epidemiology*. Philadelphia, PA: Lippincott Williams & Wilkins; 2008.
27. Weed DL. Epidemiologic evidence and causal inference. *Hematol/Oncol Clin N Am*. 2000;14(4):797–807.
28. Weed DL. On the use of causal criteria. *Int J Epidemiol*. 1997;26(6):1137–1141.
29. Briss PA, Zaza S, Pappaioanou M, et al. Developing an evidence-based Guide to Community Preventive Services—methods. The Task Force on Community Preventive Services. *Am J Prev Med*. 2000;18(1 Suppl):35–43.
30. Briss PA, Brownson RC, Fielding JE, Zaza S. Developing and using the Guide to Community Preventive Services: lessons learned about evidence-based public health. *Annu Rev Public Health*. 2004;25:281–302.
31. Concato J, Shah N, Horwitz RI. Randomized, controlled trials, observational studies, and the hierachy of research designs. *N Engl J Med*. 2000;342:1887–1892.
32. Zaza S, Briss PA, Harris KW, eds. *The Guide to Community Preventive Services: What Works to Promote Health?* New York: Oxford University Press; 2005.
33. Green LW, Ottoson JM, Garcia C, Hiatt RA. Diffusion theory, and knowledge dissemination, utilization, and integration in public health. *Annu Rev Public Health*. 2009;30:151–174.
34. Green LW. From research to "best practices" in other settings and populations. *Am J Health Behav*. 2001;25(3):165–178.
35. Rychetnik L, Hawe P, Waters E, et al. A glossary for evidence based public health. *J Epidemiol Commun Health*. 2004;58(7):538–545.
36. Klesges LM, Dzewaltowski DA, Glasgow RE. Review of external validity reporting in childhood obesity prevention research. *Am J Prev Med*. 2008;34(3):216–223.
37. Glasgow RE. What types of evidence are most needed to advance behavioral medicine? *Ann Behav Med*. 2008;35(1):19–25.

38. Glasgow RE, Green LW, Klesges LM, et al. External validity: we need to do more. *Ann Behav Med.* 2006;31(2):105–108.
39. Green LW, Glasgow RE. Evaluating the relevance, generalization, and applicability of research: issues in external validation and translation methodology. *Eval Health Prof.* 2006;29(1):126–153.
40. Green LW, Glasgow RE, Atkins D, Stange K. Making evidence from research more relevant, useful, and actionable in policy, program planning, and practice slips "twixt cup and lip." *Am J Prev Med.* 2009;37(6 Suppl 1):S187–191.
41. Green LW, Kreuter MW. *Health Promotion Planning: An Educational and Ecological Approach.* 4th ed. New York, NY: McGraw-Hill; 2005.
42. Yin RK. Case Study Research: Design and Methods. 3rd ed. Thousand Oaks, CA: Sage Publications; 2003.
43. Bero LA, Jadad AR. How consumers and policy makers can use systematic reviews for decision making. In: Mulrow C, Cook D, eds. *Systematic Reviews. Synthesis of Best Evidence for Health Care Decisions.* Philadelphia, PA: American College of Physicians; 1998:45–54.
44. Anderson LM, Brownson RC, Fullilove MT, et al. Evidence-based public health policy and practice: promises and limits. *Am J Prev Med.* 2005;28(5 Suppl): 226–230.
45. Ernster VL. Mammography screening for women aged 40 through 49—a guidelines saga and a clarion call for informed decision making. *Am J Public Health.* 1997;87(7):1103–1106.
46. American Cancer Society. *Cancer Facts and Figures 2008.* Atlanta, GA: American Cancer Society; 2008.
47. Breslow L, et al. Final Report of NCI Ad Hoc Working Groups on Mammography in Screening for Breast Cancer. *J Natl Cancer Inst.* 1977;59(2):469–541.
48. American Cancer Society. Report on the Cancer-Related Health Checkup. *CA: A Cancer J Clin.* 1980;30:193–196.
49. National Institutes of Health Consensus Development Panel. National Institutes of Health Consensus Development Conference Statement: Breast Cancer Screening for Women Ages 40–49, January 21–23, 1997. *J Natl Cancer Inst.* 1997;89: 1015–1026.
50. Screening for breast cancer: U.S. Preventive Services Task Force recommendation statement. *Ann Intern Med.* 2009;151(10):716–726, W-236.
51. Kolata G. Mammogram Debate Took Group by Surprise. *The New York Times.* November 20, 2009.
52. Oliver TR. The politics of public health policy. *Annu Rev Public Health.* 2006;27:195–233.
53. Brownson RC, Chriqui JF, Stamatakis KA. Understanding evidence-based public health policy. *Am J Public Health.* 2009;99(9):1576–1583.
54. Newschaffer CJ, Liu L, Sim A. Cardiovascular disease. In: Remington PL, Brownson RC, Wegner M, eds. *Chronic Disease Epidemiology and Control.* 3rd ed. Washington, DC: American Public Health Association; 2010: 383–428.
55. Gargiullo PM, Rothenberg RB, Wilson HG. Confidence intervals, hypothesis tests, and sample sizes for the prevented fraction in cross-sectional studies. *Stat Med.* 1995;14(1):51–72.
56. Straatman H, Verbeek AL, Peeters PH. Etiologic and prevented fraction in case-control studies of screening. *J Clin Epidemiol.* 1988;41(8):807–811.

57. Thacker SB, Ikeda RM, Gieseker KE, et al. The evidence base for public health informing policy at the Centers for Disease Control and Prevention. *Am J Prev Med.* 2005;29(3):227–233.
58. Horner M, Ries L, Krapcho M, et al. *SEER Cancer Statistics Review*, 1975–2006. Bethesda, MD: National Cancer Institute; 2009.
59. Breslow L. The future of public health: prospects in the United States for the 1990s. *Annu Rev Public Health.* 1990;11:1–28.
60. Nightingale EO, Cureton M, Kamar V, Trudeau MB. *Perspectives on Health Promotion and Disease Prevention in the United States* [staff paper]. Washington, DC: Institute of Medicine, National Academy of Sciences; 1978.
61. US Dept of Health, Education, and Welfare,. *Healthy People. The Surgeon General's Report on Health Promotion and Disease Prevention.* Washington, DC: US Dept of Health, Education, and Welfare; 1979. Publication 79–55071.
62. Irvine L, Elliott L, Wallace H, Crombie IK. A review of major influences on current public health policy in developed countries in the second half of the 20th century. *J R Soc Promot Health.* 2006;126(2):73–78.
63. Fielding J, Kumanyika S. Recommendations for the concepts and form of Healthy People 2020. *Am J Prev Med.* 2009;37(3):255–257.
64. Susser M. Judgement and causal inference: criteria in epidemiologic studies. *Am J Epidemiol.* 1977;105:1–15.
65. Szklo M. Translating epi data into public policy is subject of Hopkins symposium. Focus is on lessons learned from experience. Epidemiol Monitor. 1998(August/September).
66. Wainberg MA, Jeang KT. 25 Years of HIV-1 research: progress and perspectives. *BMC Med.* 2008;6:31

3

Understanding and Applying Analytic Tools

> There are in fact two things: science and opinion. One begets knowledge, the latter ignorance.
>
> —Hippocrates

The preceding chapters have underlined the desirability of using evidence to inform decision making in public health. Chapter 1 gave an overview and definitions of evidence-based practice. Chapter 2 described the scientific factors to consider when determining whether some type of public health action is warranted. This chapter describes several useful tools for evidence-based public health practice, such as systematic reviews and economic evaluation, which help practitioners answer the question, "Is this program or policy worth doing?"

Chapter 3 has five main parts. First, we describe some context and processes for developing systematic reviews and economic evaluations. Then we discuss several analytic tools for measuring intervention impact and effectiveness (e.g., systematic reviews, meta-analysis). The third part describes economic evaluation, a set of methods for comparing benefits and costs. One particular type of economic evaluation, cost-utility analysis, is described in greater detail. In the fourth section, several challenges and opportunities in using these analytic tools are discussed. The chapter concludes with a short discussion of processes for translating evidence into public health action (e.g., expert panels, practice guidelines). A major goal of this chapter is to help readers develop an understanding of these evidence-based methods and an appreciation of their usefulness. We seek to assist practitioners in becoming informed users of various analytic tools for decision making. The chapter does not provide detailed descriptions of the mechanics of conducting various types of analytic reviews—readers are referred to several excellent sources for these elements.[1-9]

BACKGROUND

A review can be thought of as a more comprehensive, modern-day equivalent of the encyclopedia article. Traditionally, an encyclopedia article was written by a person knowledgeable in a subject area, who was charged with reviewing the literature and writing a summary assessment of the current state of the art on that particular topic.

A systematic review uses a formal approach to identify and synthesize the existing knowledge base and prespecifies key questions of interest in an attempt to find all of the relevant literature addressing those questions. It also systematically assesses the quality of identified papers. Systematic reviews can address any number of problems and have recently been used in advertising, astronomy, criminology, ecology, entomology, and parapsychology.[10] In this chapter, the focus is on reviews of the effectiveness of interventions to improve health. The goal of a systematic review is an unbiased assessment of a particular topic, such as interventions to improve vaccination rates or to reduce smoking rates, that summarizes a large amount of information, identifies beneficial or harmful interventions, and points out gaps in the scientific literature.[8,11] Systematic reviews can be conducted in many ways—by an individual, a small team of researchers, or a larger expert panel. It is sometimes stipulated that such a review include a quantitative synthesis (i.e., meta-analysis) of the data. In this chapter, however, the outcome of the systematic review process is defined as a narrative (qualitative) assessment of the literature, a practice guideline, or a quantitative statistical combination of results like a meta-analysis.[12]

Economic evaluation aims at improving the allocation of scarce resources. Given that we cannot afford to do everything, how do we choose among projects? Economic evaluation identifies and weighs the relative costs and benefits of competing alternatives so that the project with the least costs for a given benefit, or the greatest benefits for a given cost, can be identified and chosen. Like systematic reviews, economic evaluations can use the existing literature to forecast the impact of a proposed program or policy. However, economic evaluations can also use prospective data to determine the cost-effectiveness of a new project.

As a result, economic evaluations are increasingly being conducted alongside interventions.[13,14] The essential difference between the two methods is their aim. Systematic reviews can cover any of a broad array of topics, such as the epidemiology of a particular disease or condition, the effectiveness of an intervention, or the economic costs of a particular treatment. Economic evaluations have a narrower focus and deal primarily with costs and benefits: What benefits will be gained at what cost?

TOOLS FOR ASSESSING INTERVENTION IMPACT AND EFFECTIVENESS

A number of analytic tools are available to assess risk of exposure to a particular factor (e.g., cigarette smoking, lack of mammography screening). Other tools are focused less on etiologic research and more on measuring the effectiveness of a particular public health intervention. To provide an overview of several useful tools, we will describe systematic reviews, meta-analysis, pooled analysis, risk assessment, and health impact assessment.

Systematic Reviews

As noted earlier, systematic reviews are syntheses of comprehensive collections of information on a particular topic. Reading a good review can be one of the most efficient ways to become familiar with state-of-the-art research and practice for many specific topics in public health, as well as a way to inform health policy.[15–17]

The use of explicit, systematic methods in reviews limits bias and reduces chance effects, thus providing more reliable results on which to make decisions.[8] Numerous approaches are used in developing systematic reviews. All systematic reviews have important common threads as well as important differences but this chapter focuses primarily on the similarities. General methods used in a systematic review as well as several types of reviews and their practical applications are described later; more detailed descriptions of these methods are available elsewhere.[15,18–20] Several authors have provided checklists that can be useful in assessing the methodological quality of a systematic review article[19,21–23] (Table 3-1).

Methods for Conducting a Systematic Review.   The goal of this section is not to teach readers how to conduct a systematic review but rather to provide a basic understanding of the six common steps in conducting a systematic review. Each is briefly summarized and some selected differences in approaches are discussed.

Identify the Problem.   The first step in a systematic review is the identification of the problem. Reviewing the literature, considering the practical aspects of the problem, and talking to experts in the area are all ways to begin to develop a concise statement of the problem (see Chapter 5). Systematic reviews focusing on effectiveness typically begin with a formal statement of the issue to be addressed. This usually includes statements of the intervention under study, the population in which it might be used, the outcomes being considered, and the relevant comparison. For example, the problem might be to determine the effectiveness of screening for Type 2 diabetes in adult African American men to reduce the occurrence of macrovascular and microvascular complications of diabetes compared to

Table 3-1. "Checklist" for Evaluating the Methodological Quality of a Systematic Review[a]

What are the methods?
- Are decision rules for the systematic review explicit, transparent, and clearly described?
- Do the methods take into account study design?
- Is study execution considered?

Are the results valid?
- Were the results similar from study to study?
- How precise were the results?
- Do the pooled results allow me to examine subgroups differences?
- Did the review explicitly address a focused and answerable question?
- Based on the search process, is it likely that important, relevant studies were missed?
- Were the primary studies of high methodological quality?
- Were assessments of studies reproducible?
- Can a causal association be inferred from the available data?

How can I apply the results to population health and/or patient care?
- How can I best interpret the results to apply them to the populations that I serve in my public health agency or to care of patients in my practice?
- Were all outcomes of clinical and public health importance considered?
- Are the benefits worth the costs and potential risks?
- Did the authors provide explicit consideration of external validity?

---

[a]Adapted from: Kelsey et al.,[22] Guyatt and Rennie,[19] Briss et al.,[21] and Liberati et al.[23]

usual care. Problem identification should also include a description of where the information for the systematic review will be obtained (e.g., information will come from a search of the literature over the last 10 years).

Search the Literature.   There are numerous electronic databases available, and one or more of these should be systematically searched. Several of these are excellent sources of published literature as well. These databases and the method for literature searching are described in detail in Chapter 7. For a variety of reasons, however, limiting searching to electronic databases can have drawbacks:

- Most systematic reviews use the published literature as the source of their data. Databases, however, may not include technical or final reports. If these are thought to be important relative to the intervention being considered, then a source for these documents should be identified and searched.
- Published studies may be subject to publication bias—the tendency of research with statistically significant results to be submitted and published over results that are not statistically significant and/or null.[7] To reduce the likelihood of publication bias, some reviews go to considerable lengths to find additional unpublished studies (see Chapter 2, section on publication bias).

- Even the best database searches typically find only one-half to two-thirds of the available literature. Reviews of reference lists and consultations with experts are very helpful in finding additional sources. Often, advice from experts in the field, national organizations, and governmental public health agencies can be very helpful.

Apply Inclusion and Exclusion Criteria.   The third step is to develop inclusion and exclusion criteria for those studies to be reviewed. This step often leads to revision and further specification of the problem statement. Common issues include the study design, the level of analysis, the type of analysis, and the source(s) and time frame for study retrieval. The inclusion and exclusion criteria should be selected so as to yield those studies most relevant to the purpose of the systematic review. If the purpose of the systematic review is to assess the effectiveness of interventions to increase physical activity rates among school-aged children, for example, then interventions aimed at representative populations (e.g., those including adults) would be excluded. Ideally, as the inclusion and exclusion criteria are applied, at least a portion of the data retrieval should be repeated by a second person, and results should be compared. If discrepancies are found, the inclusion and exclusion criteria are probably not sufficiently specific or clear. They should be reviewed and revised as needed.

Study Design.   The first issue to consider is the type of study. Should only randomized controlled trials be included? Some would answer "yes" because randomized controlled trials are said to provide the most reliable data and to be specially suited for supporting causal inference. Others would argue that randomized controlled trials also have their limitations, such as contamination or questionable external validity, and that including a broader range of designs could increase the aggregate internal and external validity of the entire body of evidence. An additional problem with limiting public health systematic reviews to randomized trials is that there are many public health areas in which this would result in no studies being possible (because trials would be unethical or infeasible). Observational and quasi-experimental studies are appropriate designs for many intervention topics. There may also be characteristics of a study that are necessary for inclusion, such as that baseline and follow-up assessment be made in conjunction with the intervention and/or that a comparison group be used.

Level of Analysis.   The inclusion and exclusion criteria for level of analysis should match the purpose of the systematic review. The most salient feature for public health is whether studies are at the individual or the community level. A potentially confusing problem, especially if one is interested in assessing community-based interventions, is what to do with "mixed" studies—those that include interventions aimed at both the community and the individual. A good strategy in that case is to include all related studies in the data searching and then use the data abstraction form (described later) to determine whether the study should remain in the data set.

Type of Analysis.   Evaluations of interventions can use several methods. Some, like the use of focus groups, are more qualitative; others, such as regression modeling, are more quantitative. Often, the specification of the question will make some types of studies relevant and others off-topic. Some questions can be addressed in varied ways, and when this is true, broad inclusiveness might give more complete answers. However, the more disparate the methodologies included, the more difficult it is to combine and consolidate the results. A qualitative approach to the review tends to be more inclusive, collecting information from all types of analysis. Meta-analysis, because it consolidates results using a statistical methodology, requires quantitative analysis.

Data Sources and Time Frame.   The final items to be specified are where a search for studies will be conducted and the time period to be covered. The natural history of the intervention should help determine the time frame. A major change in the delivery of an intervention, for example, makes it difficult to compare results from studies before and after the new delivery method. In this case, one might limit the time to the "after" period. An additional factor influencing time frame is the likely applicability of the results. Sometimes, substantial changes in context have occurred over time. For example, results from the 1980s may be of questionable relevance to the current situation. In that case, one might limit the review to more recent data. A pragmatic factor influencing the selection of a time frame is the availability of electronic databases.

Conduct Data Abstraction.   Once the inclusion and exclusion criteria have been specified, the next step is to find the studies that fit the framework, and then to extract a common set of information from them. In general, a data abstraction form should be used. This form should direct the systematic extraction of key information about the elements of the study so that they can be consolidated and assessed. Typical elements include the number of participants, the type of study, a precise description of the intervention, and the results for the study. If the data abstraction form is well designed, the data consolidation and assessment can proceed using only the forms. The exact format and content of the abstraction form depend on the intervention and the type of analysis being used in the systematic review. An excellent and comprehensive example of an abstraction form is provided by the Task Force on Community Preventive Services.[9]

Consolidate the Evidence.   The next step in a systematic review is an assessment of whether data from the various studies can be combined. (Often they should not if, for example, all of the available studies have serious flaws or if the interventions or outcomes are too disparate.) If data can be combined to reach an overall conclusion, it may be done either qualitatively or quantitatively.

Assessment and Conclusion.   Once the evidence has been consolidated, the final step is to assess it and reach a conclusion. For example, suppose that the intervention being reviewed is the launching of mass media campaigns to increase physical activity rates among adults. Further, assume that a meta-analysis of this topic reveals that a majority of studies find that community-based interventions improve physical activity rates. However, the effect size is small. What should the review conclude?

The review should consider both the strength and weight of the evidence and the substantive importance of the effect. This assessment can be done by the reviewer using his or her own internal criteria or by using explicit criteria that were set before the review was conducted. An example of the latter approach is the method used by the U.S. Preventive Services Task Force (USPSTF).[24] The USPSTF looks at the quality and weight of the evidence (rated Good, Fair, or Poor), and the net benefit, or effect size, of the preventive service (rated Substantial, Moderate, Small, and Zero/negative). Their overall rating and recommendation reflect a combination of these two factors. For example, if a systematic review of a preventive service finds "Fair" evidence of a "Substantial" effect, the Task Force gives it a recommendation of "B," or a recommendation that clinicians routinely provide the service to eligible patients.

If no formal process for combining the weight of the evidence and the substantive importance of the findings has been specified beforehand, and the systematic review yields mixed findings, then it is useful to seek help with assessing the evidence and drawing a conclusion. The analyst might ask experts in the field to review the evidence and reach a conclusion or make a recommendation.

After completing the systematic review, the final step is to write up a report and disseminate the findings. The report should include a description of all of the just-discussed steps. Ideally, the systematic review should be disseminated to the potential users of the recommendations. The method of dissemination should be targeted to the desired audience. Increasingly, this means putting reports on the Internet so that they are freely accessible or presenting the findings to a community planning board. However, it is also important to submit reviews for publication in peer-reviewed journals. This provides one final quality check. Various methods for disseminating the results of systematic reviews are described later in this chapter.

Meta-analysis

Over the past three decades, meta-analysis has been increasingly used to synthesize the findings of multiple research studies. Meta-analysis was originally developed in the social sciences in the 1970s when hundreds of studies existed on the same topics.[7] The key contribution of meta-analysis has been to provide a systematic, replicable, and objective method of integrating the findings of individual studies.[25] Meta-analysis uses a quantitative approach to summarize evidence, in which results from separate studies are pooled to obtain a weighted average summary result.[7] Its use has appeal because of its potential to pool a group of smaller studies, enhancing statistical power. It also may allow researchers to test subgroup effects (e.g., by gender or age group) that are sometimes difficult to assess in a single, smaller study. Suppose there were several studies examining the effects of exercise on cholesterol levels, with each reporting the average change in cholesterol levels, the standard deviation of that change, and the number of study participants. These average changes could be weighted by sample size and pooled to obtain an average of the averages change in cholesterol levels. If this grand mean showed a significant decline in cholesterol levels among exercisers, then the meta-analyst would conclude that the evidence supported exercise as a way to lower cholesterol levels. Box 3-1 describes a recent meta-analysis of the relationship between alcohol consumption and breast cancer.[26]

Similar to the method described above for conducting a systematic review, Petitti[7] notes four essential steps in conducting a meta-analysis: (1) identifying relevant studies; (2) deciding upon inclusion and exclusion criteria for studies under consideration; (3) abstracting the data; and (4) conducting the statistical analysis, including exploration of heterogeneity.

Meta-analysis includes several different statistical methods for aggregating the results from multiple studies. The method chosen depends on the type of analysis used in the original studies, which, in turn, is related to the type of data analyzed. For example, continuous data, such as cholesterol levels, can be analyzed by comparing the means of different groups. Continuous data could also be analyzed with multiple linear regression. Discrete (dichotomous) data are often analyzed with relative risks or odds ratios, although a range of other options also exists.

An important issue for meta-analysis is the similarity of studies to be combined. This similarity, or homogeneity, is assessed using various statistical tests. If studies are too dissimilar (high heterogeneity), then combining their results is problematic. One approach is to combine only homogeneous subsets of studies. While statistically appealing, this to some extent defeats the purpose of the systematic review because a single summary assessment of the evidence is not reported. An alternative approach is to use meta-analytic methods that allow the addition of control variables that measure the differences among studies. For example, studies

Box 3-1. Meta-Analysis of the Effect of Alcohol Consumption on the Risk of Breast Cancer

The relationship between alcohol consumption and the risk of breast cancer has been examined in numerous studies over the years. After all of these studies, what can we conclude? Does alcohol consumption increase the risk of breast cancer? A meta-analysis found that the answer to this question is a mild "yes": alcohol use increases the risk of breast cancer, but by a small amount.[26]

To arrive at this answer, the authors searched MEDLINE, an electronic database, from 1966 to 1999 for studies of the relationship between alcohol consumption and breast cancer. They then looked at the references cited in these articles to find additional articles. This approach identified seventy-four publications. Next, they reviewed the publications to see if they met the inclusion and exclusion criteria they had specified. Inclusion criteria included such requirements as reporting alcohol intake in a manner that could be converted to grams of alcohol per day and reporting data from an original cohort or case-control study. Exclusion criteria included items such as reports that were published only as letters to the editor or abstracts and studies that had implausible results. After applying the inclusion and exclusion criteria, 42 reports remained.

These 42 reports were then carefully reviewed and abstracted. The number of participants, alcohol consumption, incidence of breast cancer, and presence of several confounders for the group were extracted from each study. The authors used regression analysis to combine the aggregate data from the various studies and estimate a dose-response relationship between alcohol consumption and breast cancer risk. Using regression analysis also allowed them to control for and examine the effects of various confounders, such as study site (hospital-based or other) and type of alcoholic beverage. In comparison with nondrinkers, women consuming an average of 6 grams of alcohol per day (approximately one-half of a typical alcoholic drink) had a 4.9% increased risk of breast cancer (95% confidence interval [CI], 1.03% to 1.07%). Women consuming one (12 grams of alcohol) or two (24 grams of alcohol) drinks per day had increased risks of 10% (95% CI, 1.06% to 1.14%) and 21% (95% CI, 1.13% to 1.30%), respectively.

may differ by type of study design. If so, then a new variable could be created to code different study design types, such as observational and randomized controlled trials.

The statistical issue of the similarity of studies is related to the inclusion and exclusion criteria. These criteria are selected to identify a group of studies for review that are similar in a substantive way. If the meta-analysis finds that the studies are not statistically homogeneous, then the source of heterogeneity should be investigated. This part of the meta-analysis thus forces a reconsideration of the inclusion and exclusion criteria.[27] A careful search for the sources of heterogeneity and a consideration of their substantive importance can improve the overall systematic review.

Meta-analysis has generated a fair amount of controversy, particularly when it is used to combine results of observational studies.[7,28] However, the quality of meta-analyses has improved, perhaps due to the dissemination and adoption of guidelines for their conduct.[29,30] Journal articles based on meta-analysis need to be read in the same critical manner as articles based on original research. Despite its limitations, a properly conducted meta-analysis provides a rigorous way of integrating the findings of several studies. Because it follows a set of specified guidelines, it can be less subjective than the usual qualitative review that weights and combines studies based on the expert opinion of the authors.

Pooled Analysis

Unlike meta-analysis, which uses data aggregated at the study level, pooled analysis refers to the analysis of data from multiple studies at the level of the individual participant. The goals of a pooled analysis are the same as a meta-analysis (i.e., obtaining a quantitative estimate of effect). This type of systematic review is much less common than others described in this chapter and has received less formal treatment in the literature. Nonetheless, it has proved informative in characterizing dose-response relationships for certain environmental risks that may be etiologically related to a variety of chronic diseases. For example, pooled analyses have been published on radiation risks for nuclear workers,[31] the relationship between alcohol, smoking, and head and neck cancer,[32] and whether vitamin D can prevent fractures.[33]

Risk Assessment

Quantitative risk assessment is a widely used term for a systematic approach to characterizing the risks posed to individuals and populations by environmental pollutants and other potentially adverse exposures.[34] In the United States, its use is either explicitly or implicitly required by a number of federal statutes, and its application worldwide is increasing. Risk assessment has become an established process through which expert scientific input is provided to agencies that regulate environmental or occupational exposures.[35] Four key steps in risk assessment are hazard identification, risk characterization, exposure assessment, and risk estimation. An important aspect of risk assessment is that it frequently results in classification schemes that take into account uncertainties about exposure-disease relationships. For example, the U.S. Environmental Protection Agency (EPA) developed a five-tier scheme for classifying potential and proved cancer-causing agents that includes the following: (1) Carcinogenic to Humans, (2) Likely to Be Carcinogenic to Humans; (3) Suggestive Evidence of Carcinogenic Potential; (4) Inadequate Information to Assess Carcinogenic Potential; and (5) Not Likely to Be Carcinogenic to Humans.[36]

Health Impact Assessment

A relatively new assessment tool is the health impact assessment (HIA), which measures the impact of a nonhealth intervention on the health of a community.[37–39] For example, zoning changes to require sidewalks can increase physical activity, thus improving the health of the community. The number of existing HIAs is small but growing rapidly, and there have been calls for more use of this methodology.[40] In the United States, this method can be viewed as an extension of the environmental impact statement, an assessment of the intended and unintended consequences of new development on the environment required for some projects.

Dannenberg and colleagues[40] reviewed 27 HIAs completed in the United States from 1999 to 2007. Topics studied ranged from policies about living wages and after-school programs to projects about power plants and public transit. Within this group of 27 HIAs, an excellent illustration is the assessment of a Los Angeles living wage ordinance.[41] Researchers used estimates of the effects of health insurance and income on mortality to project and compare potential mortality reductions attributable to wage increases and changes in health insurance status among workers covered by the Los Angeles City living wage ordinance.[41] Estimates demonstrated that the health insurance provisions of the ordinance would have a much larger health benefit than the wage increases, thus providing valuable information for policy makers who may consider adopting living wage ordinances in other jurisdictions or modifying existing ordinances.

There are five steps to an HIA: screening, scoping, appraisal, reporting, and monitoring.[39] The screening step is used to determine whether the proposed program or intervention will have significant impacts on health, necessitating an HIA. In the scoping step, the relevant community and the health impacts associated with the proposed program are identified. Next, the health impacts on the community are projected and measured. This appraisal step can be done in a relatively quick manner or can be accomplished with a more detailed comprehensive approach such as computer modeling or systematic review. In the fourth step, reporting, the positive and negative health impacts of the proposed program are reported, along with suggestions on how best to mitigate negative outcomes and enhance positive ones. Finally, if the proposed program is implemented, its actual impact on health should be monitored and reported to add to the existing evidence base.

TOOLS FOR COMPARING OPTIONS AND WEIGHING BENEFITS VERSUS COSTS

When comparing a variety of options for intervention, decision analysis and economic evaluation may be particularly useful.

Decision Analysis

Decision analysis is a derivative of operations research and game theory that involves the identification of all available choices and potential outcomes of each in a visual series of decisions.[42] Along with each choice in the "decision tree," probabilities of outcomes are estimated that arise at decision nodes. An example of a decision tree is shown in Figure 3-1. This tree is based upon a study of oseltamivir (Tamiflu) treatment for influenza among patients at high risk for complications.[43] The study estimated what would happen in the Netherlands if persons with a high risk of complications from influenza were treated with oseltamivir or were not treated. To estimate the effects of oseltamivir treatment, the authors had to identify all of the outcomes relevant to influenza (the branches of the tree) and use the literature to find the prevalence of these events within 1 year (the probabilities below the branches of the tree). This study could help inform pandemic preparedness.

Decision analysis has historically been used to help inform complex decisions under conditions of uncertainty. It has been widely used by clinicians to make decisions about individual patients. Increasingly, decision analysis has been used to develop policies about the management of groups of patients by looking for the "best" outcome for the most value and is often a fundamental component of an economic evaluation.[2] In the latter case, the tree is modified to include the costs and benefits of each branch as well as the probabilities.

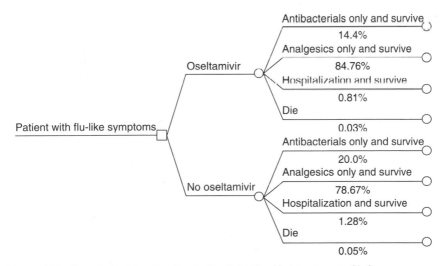

FIGURE 3-1. Sample decision tree for oseltamivir (Tamiflu) treatment of influenza among persons at high risk of complications. (Based on data from Postma et al.[43])

There are five steps in a decision analysis[44]:

1. Identifying and bounding the problem
2. Structuring the problem
3. Gathering information to fill the decision tree
4. Analyzing the decision tree
5. Harnessing uncertainty by conducting a sensitivity analysis

The first two steps help one to draw the decision tree. Step 3, "gathering information," can be done by using new data or by surveying the literature. For a standard decision tree, the probability of reaching each branch and the number of persons who will enter the tree are the two essential pieces of information. For an economic evaluation, the tree must also include the costs and benefits of each branch.

The decision tree is analyzed by starting a number of persons at the base of the tree. The number of persons could be derived from population data or a hypothetical cohort. Based on the probabilities found at each branching point, a certain number of persons go to different branches. The process stops when all of the persons have reached one of the far right-hand branches, which represent the final outcomes. For example, suppose that 10,000 persons in the Netherlands are at high risk of complications from influenza. If oseltamivir is prescribed to all of these persons, 3 will die from influenza (10,000 * 0.0003). If, alternatively, these persons do not receive oseltamivir, 5 of them will die from influenza (10,000 * 0.0005). The numbers of people at the final outcomes of interest are then compared and a conclusion reached. Using Figure 3-1 and comparing the number of influenza-related deaths by treatment with oseltamivir, one could conclude that oseltamivir reduces the number of deaths by 40%.[43]

The fifth step is to conduct a sensitivity analysis. Decision analysis in medicine arose in part to reflect and analyze the uncertainty of treatment outcomes. The probability assigned to each branch is the average likelihood of that particular outcome. In practice, the actual probability may turn out to be higher or lower. Sensitivity analysis varies the probability estimates and reanalyzes the tree. The less the outcomes vary as the probabilities are altered, the more robust is the result. There are several ways to conduct a sensitivity analysis, and this technique is discussed further in the context of economic evaluation later in this chapter.

Decision analysis is especially useful for a clinical or policy decision under the following conditions:

• The decision is complex and information is uncertain.
• Viable choices exist that are legal, ethical, and not cost prohibitive.
• The decision is a close call and consequences are important.

Decision analysis can be informative because it forces the analyst to explicitly list all the potential outcomes and pathways and the likelihood of each. Often, the process itself is illuminating, especially if there are complex pathways involved.

Economic Evaluation

Economic evaluation is the comparison of costs and benefits to determine the most efficient allocation of scarce resources. We undertake economic evaluations all the time in everyday life, although we seldom think of the process explicitly. For example, ordering dinner at a restaurant requires weighing the costs (monetary and caloric) versus the benefits (nutrition and flavor) of all of the options. Then, we choose an entree that is the "best" use of our resources—the best value for the money. This implicit weighing of costs and benefits is almost automatic, although we have probably all faced a menu that offered too many options at one time or another. In most public health applications, however, weighing the costs and benefits does not occur so automatically.

What are the distinguishing features of public health that require a formal economic evaluation? Consider three features of the restaurant example. First, the costs and benefits are all borne by one person, the diner, who has an incentive to compare costs and benefits and make a wise choice. Second, the information needed for the choice is fairly easy to obtain. The entrees are described on the menu, the prices are listed, and the diner knows his or her own palate and preferences. Finally, the stakes are fairly low. A bad decision can be remedied by sending the meal back to the kitchen or by avoiding the entree or restaurant the next time the diner eats out.

All three of these characteristics are absent from most public health decisions. First, by their nature, public health programs are aimed at improving the health of a community, so benefits will be spread over a large number of people. Costs are also typically spread over a large group, often through taxation. Second, the information about costs and benefits may not be easy to obtain. Benefits and costs must be measured over many people. Often, the benefits include hard-to-measure items like improved health status. Third, the stakes are often relatively high. Programs may be expensive and resources scarce, so only a few of a large range of interventions may be funded. A bad choice cannot easily be remedied.

Types of Economic Evaluation.   There are four interrelated types of economic evaluation: cost-benefit analysis (CBA), cost-effectiveness analysis (CEA), cost-utility analysis (CUA), and cost-minimization analysis (CMA). This chapter explains CUA in greater detail; the other methods are then compared briefly to it. CUA is singled out because it is the recommended method of the U.S. Public

Health Service Panel on Cost-Effectiveness Analysis[3] and the most commonly used method today.

The four methods differ primarily in the way that they measure benefits. CBA measures benefits in monetary units (e.g., dollars, Euros), whereas CEA measures benefits in an appropriate health unit (e.g., lives saved). CUA is a type of CEA in which benefits (e.g., life years saved) are adjusted for quality of life and quantified with a health utility measure (usually quality-adjusted life years [QALYs]). CMA is only used when the benefits of the two interventions are identical, so the unit of measurement of benefits is not an issue. Because CBA uses the most "generic" outcome measure (many things can be measured in currency, including the value of transportation projects and educational interventions), it allows for the comparison of the most programs. As we move to CEA, then to CUA, and finally to CMA, the range of programs that can be compared narrows.

Outcomes of an Economic Evaluation.   Figure 3-2 shows the potential outcomes of an economic evaluation.[2] Consider the four quadrants of the graph. Programs that improve health and save money (Quadrant IV) are obviously worthwhile and should be undertaken. Similarly, programs that worsen health and add to costs (Quadrant II) are undesirable and should not be initiated or continued. The remaining two quadrants (I and III) are where the dilemmas lie and where economic evaluation can be informative.

Historically, as public health systems and nations develop, interventions and programs begin in Quadrant IV, with those programs that are both cost saving and improve health. Many early public health interventions, such as sanitation systems, fall in Quadrant IV. Once these interventions are exploited and implemented,

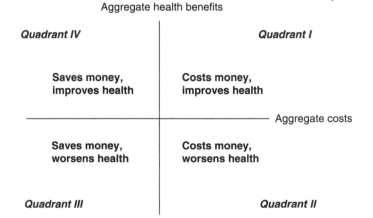

FIGURE 3-2. Possible outcomes of an economic evaluation. (Adapted from Drummond et al.[2])

attention turns to Quadrant I, programs that improve health at some cost. Eventually, as budgetary pressures increase, Quadrant III programs are considered: programs that reduce costs, but at some loss of health status. For both of these quadrants, the question is, What is the return on the investment (or disinvestment) of the public's funds? Economic evaluation provides a way to answer this question so that programs with the greatest return on investment can be selected.

Conceptual Framework for Economic Evaluation.   In the influenza example above, several key conceptual elements of economic evaluation can be identified. Before considering the mechanics of conducting an economic evaluation, it may be useful to determine the general elements and approach of all economic evaluations.

The first element is the selection of the perspective of the economic evaluation. Any intervention can be considered from several points of view, often characterized as moving from narrow to broad. The narrowest perspective is that of the agency or organization directly involved in delivering the proposed intervention. A next level might be the perspective of insurers, or payers, especially in health, where consumers and payers are often two separate groups. The broadest perspective is that of society as a whole. The Public Health Service Panel on Cost-Effectiveness Analysis[3] recommends this broad perspective for all economic evaluations, and it is required in several countries with national health systems. The societal perspective is the most appropriate in public health because interventions are designed to benefit the public and taxpayers who fund the costs.

The next stage is the identification and measurement of all costs, including incremental costs of a program, option, or intervention. Incremental costs are the additional costs related to the program. If such costs are concentrated among a small group of people, this step will be relatively easy. As costs are more dispersed, it may become more difficult to identify all potential costs. Measurement of the identified costs may similarly be complicated by issues of units of measurement (e.g., monetary wages versus donated labor time) and timing (e.g., costs incurred over a 5-year interval).

The third conceptual element is the identification and measurement of all benefits. Again, the incremental benefits are of interest: What additional benefits will this program provide, compared with some specified alternative? This step is often more complicated than the identification and measurement of costs. In public health, benefits can include improved health status (cases prevented) and improved mortality outcomes (deaths averted). Clearly, these benefits will be difficult to measure and will be partially subjective.

A fourth element is the comparison of costs and benefits. One can think of placing costs on one side of a balance, or scale, and benefits on the other. To which side does the scale tip? If the costs and benefits are measured in the same units (e.g., Euros), then this question is easy to answer. If, as is usually the case, the costs are in monetary units and the benefits are in some health outcome measure, then it is difficult to see whether the balance is tipping toward the costs or the benefits side. Instead of placing costs and benefits on the two sides of a scale, the best assessment that can be made is that it costs X monetary units per unit of health benefit. This is found by forming a ratio, with costs in the numerator and benefits in the denominator:

$$\text{Economic evaluation ratio} = \frac{\text{Incremental costs}}{\text{Incremental benefits}}$$

The final conceptual element is the interpretation of the results. If one finds, for example, that a program costs $27,000 per life saved, is the program worthwhile? There are numerous ways to approach this question, involving ethics, practical considerations, political realities, and economics. One could argue that, clearly, a life is worth $27,000 and the program is worthwhile. If, however, there is another program that costs $15,000 per life saved and the budget allows only one to be funded, an argument can be made that the latter program is more worthwhile than the former.

Determining Costs.   The first step in an economic evaluation is to identify and determine all the costs of the intervention. These will be summed to form the numerator of the cost-utility (or cost-benefit or cost-effectiveness) ratio. Table 3-2 shows the types of costs and their usual measures. The labels and definitions for the types of costs vary across disciplines and across textbooks. The important objective of the cost portion of the analysis is the identification and determination of *all* costs, regardless of their labels.

The first category of costs is direct, or program, costs. One caution in stating these costs is that the true economic cost of providing the program should be identified. This is the resource cost of the program, also referred to as the opportunity cost. If this program is undertaken, what other program will we forego? What opportunity must be passed up in order to fund this program? In health, there is often a distinction between *charges* and *costs*. For example, a screening test for diabetes may be billed at $200; however, the cost of providing the test is $150. The $150 figure should be used.

Direct costs include labor costs, often measured by the number of full-time equivalent employees (FTEs) and their wages and fringe benefits. If volunteers will be used, the value of their time should be imputed using either their own wage rates or the average wage rate for similarly skilled work within the community. Other direct costs are supplies and overhead. (Figure 9-3 provides a detailed worksheet for determining direct costs.)

Indirect costs are the other main component of costs. These can be subdivided into five categories. Three of these (time and travel costs, the cost of treating side

Table 3-2. Types of Costs Included in Economic Evaluations

Category of Cost	Usual Measures and Examples
Direct or program costs	
Labor	Wages and fringe benefits
Supplies	Supplies for the intervention, including office supplies, screening tests, and materials
Overhead	Allocation for office space, rent, and utilities
Indirect costs	
Positive indirect costs; to be added to costs	
Time and travel costs	Time costs to participants, including lost wages
	Travel costs to participants, including transportation and child care
	Caregiver costs, including both time and travel
	Any costs of the program incurred by other budgetary groups
Cost of treating side effects	Cost of treatment; using actual cost or charge data or imputed, using local, regional, or national averages
Cost of treatment during gained life expectancy	National data on average cost of treatment per year, multiplied by extended life expectancy
Negative indirect costs (benefits); to be subtracted from costs	
Averted treatment costs	Weighted sum of the cost of treatment, including alternative options and complications. Weights reflect the proportion of people projected to have each alternative treatment or complication. Data can be from administrative databases, such as claims data, or imputed, using local, regional, or national average costs or charges.
Averted productivity losses	Wages and fringe benefits of participants; for persons not in the labor force, average wages of similarly aged persons or local, regional, or national average wages

effects, and the cost of treatment during gained life expectancy) are positive costs and are added to the numerator. The other two (averted treatment costs and averted productivity losses) are negative costs (i.e., benefits) that are subtracted from the numerator because they directly affect the public health budget.

The first category of costs is the time and travel costs to the participants. From a societal standpoint, these costs should be attributed to the program. Often, to obtain these costs, a survey of program participants must be conducted. In addition, if other family members or friends are involved as caregivers to the program participants, their time and travel costs should be included. The second category of indirect costs is the cost of treating side effects. If the intervention causes any side effects, the cost of treating them should be charged to the intervention.

The third component of indirect costs is the cost of treatment during gained life expectancy. If a person's life is extended due to an intervention, he or she will consume additional health care resources in those additional years. Should these costs be added to the numerator of the cost-utility ratio? Proponents of their inclusion argue that these costs are part of the health budget and will affect its future size. Those opposed point out that these persons will also be paying taxes, thus helping to support their additional consumption of health care. Why single out one aspect of their future spending? The U.S. Public Health Service Panel on Cost-Effectiveness Analysis[3] did not make a recommendation with respect to this issue.

The fourth group of indirect costs is averted treatment costs. These are future treatment costs that will be saved as a result of the intervention. For example, screening for diabetes might identify cases earlier and thus limit or prevent some complications and early mortality. These are complications that will not need to be treated (if prevented) or that will not need to be treated as expensively (if delayed). The onset of diabetes and the incidence of complications with and without the program must be estimated and then multiplied by the costs of treatment to obtain the averted treatment costs.

The fifth category is averted productivity losses. These represent the savings to society from avoiding lost work time. Ideally, these are measured directly using the wages and fringe benefits of participants. Often, this information is not available–either it was not collected or it does not exist because the participants are not in the labor force. In this case, the average wages and fringe benefits of similar persons, or of the average person, can be used to estimate this negative cost. This cost is used in CBA and CEA but not in CUA. Benefits in a CUA are measured in terms of health utility, which in turn depends on a person's ability to work and earn an income. Thus, the negative costs of averted productivity losses are incorporated in the benefit measure in CUA.

Determining benefits.   The next step in the analysis is the identification and measurement of benefits. Here, the selection of the relevant time period is important, especially for public health. The aim of a program or intervention is the improvement of health, so the output to be measured is improved health status. This is a final outcome that may take many years to achieve. Often, a program can only track participants for a brief period of time and any evaluation will, of necessity, measure intermediate outcomes, such as the number of cases identified. In such cases, the literature can often be used to extrapolate the effect of the intermediate outcome on health. For example, suppose that one were evaluating a program designed to increase physical activity levels. Other studies have demonstrated that increased physical activity reduces the risk of cardiac events. These studies can be used to estimate the anticipated final outcomes of the intervention.

The benefits of the program or intervention are the improvement in health and are thus conceptually identical, regardless of the type of economic evaluation.

However, the unit of measurement and the specific elements included differ by type of evaluation. CBA measures the benefits in money. Thus, improvements to health must be converted to currency amounts. If years of life are saved, then these years must be valued in monetary units. There are several suggested methods to make this conversion. All of them are subject to heated debate.[3]

In response to dissatisfaction with the measurement of health benefits in monetary units, particularly the wide range of values found using different methods, some analysts argued for measuring benefits in a naturally occurring health unit, such as years of life saved. This led to the development of CEA, which uses a single health measure (years of life saved, cases averted) as the measure of benefits. This has the advantage of not requiring reductions of different outcomes to a single scale, but a single health measure cannot capture all the benefits of most interventions. Most programs yield morbidity and mortality improvements. By being forced to select one health measure, only morbidity or mortality can be used to determine the cost-effectiveness of the project. This underestimates the cost-effectiveness of projects because the total costs are divided by only a portion of the benefits. In addition, only programs with outcomes measured in the same unit (e.g., lives saved) can be compared.

Partly in response to the shortcomings of CEA, some analysts argued for the development of a health utility measure of benefits. Such a measure combines morbidity and mortality effects into a single metric and is based on the utility, or satisfaction, that health status gives to a person. Individuals' self-reports of their valuation of health form the basis of the health utility measure.

Several measures that meet these criteria have been developed. They include the QALY, the disability-adjusted life year, and the healthy year equivalent. The most widely used of these is the QALY, defined as the amount of time in perfect health that would be valued the same as a year with a disease or disability. For example, consider a year with end-stage renal disease, requiring dialysis. Conceptually, the QALY for this condition is the fraction of a year in perfect health that one would value the same as a full year with the condition. Thus, QALYs range from 0 to 1, with 0 defined as dead and 1 as a year in perfect health. The QALY assigned to this condition will vary across persons, with some considering the condition worse than others. If many individuals are surveyed, however, the average QALY assigned to this condition can be obtained.

There are several ways to elicit QALY weights from individuals. These include the visual rating scale, time tradeoff method, and the standard gamble. There is debate over the theoretically appropriate method and the consistency of results obtained from the different methods.[45] With the visual rating scale, survey participants are presented with a list of health conditions. Beside each description of a condition, there is a visual scale, or line, that ranges from 0 to 1. Participants are asked to indicate on the lines their QALY valuation of each health condition by making a mark. A participant might mark "0.6," for example, for the year with end-stage renal disease.

To measure the benefits in CUA, the analyst must identify all the morbidity and mortality effects of the intervention. These are then weighted by the appropriate QALY value. In practice, there are three ways to assign QALY weights to different conditions. The first is to directly elicit QALY weights from participants, as described earlier. The second is to use a multi-attribute utility function, such as the EuroQol 5 Dimension (EQ-5D) or the Health Utilities Index (HUI).[46,47] These are brief survey instruments that ask one to rate various attributes of health. For example, the EQ5D rates five aspects of health (mobility, self-care, usual activities, pain/discomfort, and anxiety/depression) from 1 to 3. The responses are then scored to give a QALY value. The weights used for the scoring were obtained from surveys of the general population. The third way to obtain QALY values is by searching the literature or using the internet. QALY values for many diseases and conditions can be found. Some studies report QALY weights for only one or a few diseases or conditions (e.g., end-stage renal disease), while others include tables of QALY values for numerous health states.[48–51]

For example, suppose that an intervention among 1000 persons yields 50 years of life saved. However, these years saved will be lived with some disability. Review of the literature indicates that this disability has a QALY weight of 0.7. The benefits of the 50 years of life saved would be valued at 50 • 0.7, or 35 QALYs. Similarly, suppose that the intervention also prevents morbidity among 500 of the participants for 1 year. If the QALY weight of the averted condition is 0.9, then (1 − 0.9), or 0.1 QALY, is saved for each of the 500 persons, yielding a benefit of 50 QALYs. The total benefits for this program would be 35 + 50, or 85 QALYs. This summary measure thus combines both the morbidity and the mortality effects of the intervention. An illustration of the use of QALYs in measuring the impact of screening for diabetes is shown in Box 3-2.[52–55]

Comparing Costs to Benefits.   Once the costs and benefits of the intervention have been determined, the next step is the construction of the economic evaluation ratio. For a CUA, this ratio will be

$$\text{Cost per QALY} = \frac{\text{Direct costs} + \text{Indirect costs}}{\text{QALYs}}$$

Using Table 3-2 and substituting the categories of indirect costs into the equation, the numerator can be restated as follows:

Costs = (Direct costs) + (Time and travel costs) + (Costs of treating side effects)
   − (Averted treatment costs)

Note that the costs of treatment during gained life expectancy have not been included. In addition, averted productivity losses are not subtracted from costs

Box 3-2. Costs of Screening for Type 2 Diabetes

Type 2 diabetes is a chronic disease that usually develops during adulthood and can have multiple complications, including blindness, lower leg amputations, kidney failure, and cardiac problems. These complications can be delayed, minimized, or avoided entirely if the disease is well managed, with good control of blood sugar levels and screening for the onset of complications. Because the disease develops slowly, over a period of years, it is often called the "silent killer": people can live with undetected diabetes for several years, and then the disease is more advanced and the complication rate is higher when they are finally diagnosed. Screening for type 2 diabetes is thus an important prevention issue.

In the 1990s the Centers for Disease Control and Prevention formed the Diabetes Cost-Effectiveness Study Group. As one part of their work, the Study Group considered opportunistic screening for type 2 diabetes and estimated its cost-effectiveness.[52] The costs and benefits of screening all adults, aged 25 and older, at a regular physician visit were estimated.

Costs were estimated using national average charges for physician visits, screening tests, and treatments for the various complications. The occurrence of these costs was estimated, using a computer model that followed a hypothetical cohort of 10,000 adults from the age of screening to death. First, the cohort was assumed to have no routine screening. Second, the cohort was assumed to have screening at the next regular physician visit. The two cohorts were then compared with respect to morbidity and mortality. Because of the earlier detection and treatment of diabetes in the second cohort, those persons had slightly lower diabetes-related mortality, a lower incidence of complications, and delayed onset of complications.

The benefits of screening come at a cost, though. Screening of the entire adult U.S. population would cost $236,449 per additional year of life saved, or $56,649 per quality-adjusted life year (QALY). These ratios were relatively high compared to other screening programs and other reimbursed interventions. The Study Group also considered subgroups of adults as candidates for screening and found that it was much more cost-effective to screen African American and younger cohorts. Screening 25- to 34-year-olds was estimated to cost $35,768 per additional life year saved and $13,376 per QALY. For African Americans aged 25 to 34, the ratios were $2219 per life year and $822 per QALY.

Because the American Diabetes Association recommends triannual screening of those aged 45 and older, based on the presence of risk factors,[53] and because the economic evaluation was somewhat sensitive to some key assumptions, the Study Group did not definitively recommend changing screening guidelines. However, it did note that the subgroup analyses strongly suggest that younger cohorts, who have a longer life span over which to accrue benefits, and minority cohorts, who have a higher incidence of diabetes, could benefit the most from screening.

In 2004, with concern over the increasing prevalence of diabetes rising, a new cost-effectiveness of screening for diabetes was published.[53] This analysis followed the methods of the 1998 study, using computer modeling to estimate the costs and benefits of screening the U.S. adult population. However, the authors incorporated new evidence that hypertension is a strong risk factor for diabetes. Subgroup analyses were run for adults with hypertension in 10-year age cohorts. For all ages, the cost-utility ratios were more favorable for persons with hypertension than for the entire population. For example, the cost per QALY for screening 55-year-olds with hypertension was $34,375, while the cost per QALY for screening all persons aged 55 was $360,966. Screening persons with hypertension ages 55 through 75 was cost-effective, with cost-utility ratios below $50,000 per QALY.

In June 2008, the Task Force released updated guidelines, recommending with a grade of B that asymptomatic adults with sustained elevated blood pressure (over 135/80 mm Hg; treated or untreated) be screened.[54] In its recommendation, the Task Force noted that there is evidence that early detection and treatment of diabetes can delay or prevent the onset of macrovascular and microvascular complications, especially in persons with hypertension.

because they enter into the determination of the QALY weights for the condition of interest. The product of a CUA, then, is that it costs $X for each QALY gained.

In CBA, all the costs and benefits are measured in dollars, so the ratio becomes a single number reflecting the ratio of costs to benefits. For example, a ratio of 1.6 means that it will cost $1.60 for each $1.00 saved. In a CEA, benefits are measured in a naturally occurring health unit, so the ratio will be expressed in terms of that unit. For example, a project might cost $25,000 per life saved.

There are two other issues that should be considered in conducting an economic evaluation: discounting and sensitivity analysis. Discounting refers to the conversion of amounts (usually currency) received over different periods to a common value in the current period. For example, suppose that one were to receive $100 on today's date of each year for 5 years. Although the amount of money is the same, most people prefer, and value, the nearer payments more than the distant payments. The payment received today will be the most valuable because it can be spent today. One might be willing to trade a slightly smaller payment received today for the payment to be received 1 year from today, an even slightly smaller payment today for the payment due in 2 years, etc. Discounting is a formal way to determine the current payments that would be equal in value to distant payments.

In economic evaluation, costs occurring in the future should be discounted to current values. This puts outlays, or expenditures, to be paid in the future on an equal footing with current expenditures. The interest rate should reflect the real rate of growth of the economy, or about 3%. The U.S. Public Health Service Panel on Cost-Effectiveness Analysis recommends an interest rate between 0% and 8%,[3] and many studies use rates from 0% to 10%.

Should benefits also be discounted? The U.S. Public Health Service Panel on Cost-Effectiveness Analysis[3] recommends that they should be, arguing that, like money, nearer health states are preferred to farther ones. In other words, saving the life of a person today is more immediate, and hence more valuable, than saving the life of a person 30 years hence.

A final issue to consider is sensitivity analysis. Numerous assumptions are made in constructing the cost-utility ratio. For example, the average effectiveness of an intervention as reported in a review article or meta-analysis may have been used in a CUA. The costs and benefits of the intervention depend on its effectiveness and will vary if the effectiveness is higher or lower than anticipated. Sensitivity analysis provides a way to estimate the effect of changing key assumptions used in the economic evaluation.

There are several ways to conduct a sensitivity analysis. All start by identifying the key assumptions and parameters that have been used in the economic evaluation. One method is to construct best-case and worst-case scenarios for the intervention, systematically varying all of the assumptions to favor and then to bias against the intervention. The cost-utility ratio is recalculated for the best-case and worst-case scenarios and then reported along with the original ratio. Another method is to vary the key assumptions one at a time, recalculating the cost-utility ratio each time. A table or figure is usually provided to report the cost-utility ratios for the different assumptions. Yet a third method is to use statistical techniques, specifying the distributions of key parameters and then randomly sampling from those distributions in multiple simulations. This yields a cost-utility ratio with an estimated confidence interval. Regardless of the method used, a sensitivity analysis is a vital component of an economic evaluation. The less variation there is in the cost-utility ratio as key assumptions are varied, the more confident one can be in the results.

Interpreting and Using the Results.   Once the cost-utility (or cost-effectiveness or cost-benefit) ratio has been determined, it must be interpreted. For example, is a program that costs $15,000 per QALY worthwhile? There are two principal ways to interpret and use the cost-utility ratio. The first compares the cost-utility ratio internally to other competing programs; the other uses external references, comparing the ratio to an established threshold value. Interventions below the threshold are considered worthwhile.

If several economic evaluations of competing programs have been conducted within an organization, or if information on the cost-utility of several interventions can be obtained, then an internal comparison is warranted. The programs can be ranked from the lowest cost-utility ratio to the highest. Programs with the lowest ratios should generally be funded first, after other considerations are taken into account. For example, a program manager and policy maker also need to consider the amount of resources required to establish and maintain a program, the ethics of various approaches, and the sociopolitical environment.

Comparison with similar programs helps the practitioner decide whether the proposed program is relatively efficient. If existing screening programs for diabetes cost $25,000 per QALY and the proposed screening program is estimated to cost $15,000 per QALY, then the proposed program represents a more efficient screening method.

The alternative way to decide whether a given cost-utility ratio justifies a program is to compare that ratio with an external threshold value for the ratio. How is the threshold value determined? There are two main approaches. One looks at programs that have already been funded, reasoning that society must value such programs. Comparison with programs that are already funded helps the practitioner argue for funding by insurers or public agencies. For example, the Medicare program provides mammography for women aged 65 and older. This coverage is partially based on economic evaluations of breast cancer screening that estimated cost-utility ratios of between $12,000 and $20,000 per QALY.[56] In 2009 dollars, these ratios are $22,662 to $37,770 per QALY. A recent extension of this approach in the United States considered all health care spending, whether federally financed or not, and compared it to improvements in health status to determine a threshold range of $184,000 to $264,000 per QALY.[57]

The alternative approach looks at the average wages of workers and their implied preferences about health and well-being. In the United States, Garber and Phelps used this approach to determine a $50,000 per QALY threshold, based on the average wages of American workers and the context of other publicly funded programs.[58] At the time of the study, $50,000 was roughly twice the average annual wage of an American worker. At current dollar values, the $50,000 per QALY threshold would be approximately $100,000 per QALY. Others have argued for two to three times the average wage as a QALY threshold in developing countries.[59,60] The National Institute for Health and Clinical Excellence (NICE) in Great Britain uses a threshold range of £20,000 to £30,000.[61] Regardless of the method used, there is considerable debate over the appropriate threshold value, particularly in the United States.[62-64]

An important final step in a CUA is the reporting of the results, particularly the cost-utility ratio, in the literature. There are now several catalogs of cost-utility ratios available in the literature and on the Internet, many of which are listed in the website section at the end of this chapter. Often, the public health practitioner can refer to these sources to determine what is already known about the cost-effectiveness of a public health intervention.

CHALLENGES AND OPPORTUNITIES IN USING SYSTEMATIC REVIEWS AND ECONOMIC EVALUATIONS

Analytic tools such as systematic reviews and economic evaluation can be extremely valuable for understanding a large body of literature or assessing the cost-effectiveness of an intervention. However, when undertaking or reading a review of the literature or an economic evaluation, several considerations should be kept in mind, as follow.

Ensuring Consistency in Quality

The quality of systematic reviews has been questioned,[65,66] although current evaluations show increasing compliance with recommended methods.[29,30] Therefore, all systematic reviews require critical appraisal to determine their validity and to establish whether and how they will be useful in practice.[67] Similarly, reviews of the economic evaluation literature have found that studies that are labeled economic evaluations are often only cost studies, are only descriptive, or use the methods inappropriately.[68–70]

Addressing Methodological Issues

In both systematic reviews and economic evaluations, there remain areas of debate about the appropriate ways to conduct these evaluations. Analysts can use established methods inappropriately or use methods still being debated and developed. Three particular areas of concern are as follows: combining studies inappropriately, estimating costs, and measuring benefits.

The first issue, combining studies inappropriately, relates to systematic reviews. Methods of synthesis work well for large effect sizes and randomized designs. When effect sizes are small, with high potential for confounding, it is essential that the component studies are of high quality in both design and execution.

Pertaining to economic evaluation, it is difficult to measure or estimate costs accurately in many public health settings.[69] Sometimes costs are estimated from national or regional data sets, and their local applicability may be questionable. In addition, some programs have high fixed costs, such as equipment or personnel, making it difficult to achieve cost-effectiveness.

The most frequently used outcome measure in CUA, the QALY, has been criticized for a number of reasons. First, there are issues related to the precision and consistency of measurement. Any indicator is imperfect and includes some level of error. When ranking interventions, the QALY score used for a particular condition helps determine the cost-utility ratio. Different QALY values may change an intervention's relative cost-effectiveness. There are several QALY score instruments such as the EQ-5D and a growing set of catalogs of QALY weights available. Unfortunately, these do not always report the same values for the same conditions and interventions. Further, the existing instruments and catalogs are sometimes not sufficiently sensitive to detect small changes in QALYs.[71,72]

A second critique of QALYs relates to ethical issues, including concerns that they may favor the young over the old,[73] men over women,[74] the able-bodied over the disabled,[75,76] and the rich over the poor.[77] By design, QALYs reflect societal preferences and are inherently subjective. However, systematic biases and measurement errors should be minimized as much as possible. The use of QALYs has also been criticized because they rely on utilitarianism as their underlying ethical framework.[78] With utilitarianism, the assumed goal of society is the greatest good for the greatest number, regardless of the distribution of good. Weighting schemes have been proposed to incorporate other allocation frameworks and goals, such as a preference for saving lives over avoiding morbidity.[79,80] Regardless of these critiques, the use of QALYs has become widely accepted and provides a useful starting point for discussions of the appropriate allocation of scarce health resources.

Ensuring Effective Implementation

Systematic reviews and economic evaluations can be useful in informing practice and public policy. However, some difficulties can arise in disseminating the results of these types of studies and using the results.

First, there are unclear effects on decision making. In clinical care, there is consistent evidence showing that introduction of new guidelines can have a positive impact on patient care.[81] In population-based public health, there is a small published body of literature on the impacts of systematic reviews on the decision making of policy makers and consumers.[11,16,17,82] For example, research conducted with public health units in Canada shows that organizational characteristics are important predictors of the use of systematic reviews in decision making.[83] Economic evaluations, while used extensively in other countries, particularly those with national health plans, have a checkered history within the United States.[67,84,85]

A second issue is adapting national or state standards for local needs. Systematic reviews and economic evaluations usually strive to take a national societal perspective. To apply the results of these studies, the practitioner has to consider whether there are specific state or local characteristics that would influence implementation of results from national data. For example, suppose that a policy maker has found a systematic review that supports the use of mass media campaigns to increase physical activity levels. If the city or county in which the policy maker works bans billboard advertising, then the systematic review results would have to be adjusted for this restriction.

Finally, there is the matter of training and accessibility. For many in public health, the key question may be, "How does a practitioner learn about or make appropriate use of these tools?" To make better use of systematic reviews, enhanced training is needed both during graduate education and through continuing education of public health professionals working in community settings.

TRANSLATING EVIDENCE INTO RECOMMENDATIONS AND PUBLIC HEALTH ACTION

Several mechanisms and processes have been used recently to translate the findings of evidence-based reviews in clinical and community settings into recommendations for action. Among these are expert panels, practice guidelines, and best practices.

Expert Panels and Consensus Conferences

Systematic reviews and economic evaluations are often developed, refined, and disseminated via expert panels. These panels examine research studies and their relevance to health conditions, diagnostic and therapeutic procedures, planning and health policy, and community interventions. Expert panels are conducted by many government agencies, in both executive and legislative branches, as well as by voluntary (i.e., specialty) health organizations, such as the American Cancer Society. Ideally, the goal of expert panels is to provide peer review by scientific experts of the quality of the science and scientific interpretations that underlie public health recommendations, regulations, and policy decisions. When conducted well, peer review can provide an important set of checks and balances for the policy-making process.

Consensus conferences are related mechanisms that are commonly used to review scientific evidence. The National Institutes of Health (NIH) have used consensus conferences since 1977 to resolve important and controversial issues in medicine and public health. Recently, a consensus conference was held to evaluate the evidence on the prevention, cessation, and control of tobacco use.[86] The RAND corporation has examined the application of the NIH consensus methods in nine countries, resulting in suggestions for improving the process.[87]

Four procedural stages of the expert review/consensus development process can be described[87]:

Context.   The context for the panel includes the nature of the audience, the topics considered, and how the topics are selected. The issues addressed are limited by the amount of available evidence. In most countries, the topics chosen for consideration by an expert group are selected by a standing committee responsible for assessment of technologies.

Prepanel Process.   The prepanel process includes selecting the chairperson, panel members, and presenters. In this stage, background information is prepared Although oral presentations are important components of a panel meeting, a literature review is common during the prepanel process. The literature review provided to panel members can range from a synthesis of the relevant literature to a comprehensive set of readings on the topic(s) of interest. A common limitation across countries is the lack of a systematic review of the existing literature during the prepanel phase. For some panels, specific questions are circulated in advance of the meeting to frame the scope and direction of the panel. A Delphi process can also be helpful during the prepanel stage (see Chapter 8).

Composition of the Panel.   Panels typically range in size from 9 to 18 members. Experts are sought in a variety of scientific disciplines, such as behavioral science, biostatistics, economics, epidemiology, health policy, or medicine, as appropriate for the topic(s) under consideration. In all countries studied by RAND, panels were made up of both scientists and lay persons. Panel members should not have financial or professional conflicts of interest.

For many public health issues, it is important to obtain community participation in the expert panel process. The community may be defined geographically, demographically (e.g., women aged 40 and older), or by disease status (e.g., people who have survived cancer). Community participation may be achieved directly by having one or more community members on the expert panel or in the consensus group. Alternatively, community input may be incorporated by conducting interviews or focus groups and including this information in the packet of materials the panel will consider.

Panel Meeting. This stage involves the activities actually undertaken at the meeting and immediately following it. These details include public and private forums and the group process used to arrive at recommendations and conclusions. Partly because many consensus conferences across countries have been run fairly informally, McGlynn and colleagues[87] suggest that it is important to formalize and document the group process used to make expert decisions. Draft findings from governmental expert panels are often released for public review and comment prior to final recommendations. Resulting statements or recommendations are widely disseminated in an attempt to make an impact on public health practice and research. Expert panels work best when they publish, along with their recommendations, the rationale for their recommendations and the evidence underlying that rationale.

All expert panels are not created equal. Some, such as the U.S. Preventive Services Task Force (USPSTF) and the Task Force on Community Preventive Services, are explicit about linking recommendations to evidence. In general, we would argue that this explicitness is an advantage over more traditional use of "expert opinion" or "global subjective judgment" because "a clear analytic rationale for recommending certain interventions will enhance the ability of ... users to assess whether recommendations are valid and prudent from their own perspectives ... make sense in their local contexts ... and will achieve goals of importance to them."[21] Evidence-based recommendations should therefore be given greater weight.

Practice Guidelines

A guideline is "a formal statement about a defined task or function."[42] In North America, guideline statements are synonymous with recommendations, whereas in parts of Europe, recommendations are stronger than guidelines. In general, practice guidelines offer advice to clinicians, public health practitioners, managed-care organizations, and the public on how to improve the effectiveness and impact of clinical and public health interventions. Guidelines translate the findings of research and demonstration projects into accessible and useable information for public health practice. To influence community and clinical interventions, guidelines are published by many governmental and nongovernmental agencies. For example, guidelines on screening for hypertension have been published periodically by the National High Blood Pressure Education Program since 1972.[88] Using an evidence-based process and consensus, these guidelines provide recommendations to clinicians. Other examples of evidence-based recommendations follow concerning clinical and community preventive services.

Guidelines for Interventions in Clinical Settings.   Over the past decade, several attempts have been made to take a more evidence-based approach to the development of clinical practice guidelines. There are now organizations contributing to the development of evidence-based clinical practice guidelines in prevention in numerous countries, including the United States, Canada, Great Britain, and Australia and countries in Europe.[89] Two noteworthy efforts are those of the USPSTF and the Canadian Task Force on Preventive Health Care (CTF). The USPSTF and the CTF have collaborated on improving evidence-based clinical prevention for several decades. For each task force, the primary mandate has been to review and synthesize evidence and to form guidelines focused on primary care clinicians.

The USPSTF is now developing its third edition of *The Guide to Clinical Preventive Services,* which represents an excellent example of a process that follows explicit analytic frameworks, takes a systematic approach to data retrieval and extraction, evaluates evidence according to study design and quality, and examines both benefits and harms of intervention.[24] The USPSTF attempts to cast a wide net for each preventive service considered, reviewing multiple types of studies, including randomized controlled trials and observational studies. Recommendations are based in part on a hierarchy of research designs, with the randomized controlled trial receiving the highest score[24] (Table 3-3). When making a recommendation on a particular clinical intervention, the quality of the evidence is placed in a matrix

Table 3-3. Hierarchy of Research Designs Used by the U.S. Preventive Services Task Force

Category	Design
I	Evidence obtained from at least one properly randomized controlled trial
II-1	Evidence obtained from well-designed controlled trials without randomization
II-2	Evidence obtained from well-designed cohort or case-control analytic studies, preferably from more than one center or research group
II-3	Evidence obtained from multiple time series with or without the intervention Dramatic results in uncontrolled experiments (e.g., the results of the introduction of penicillin treatment in the 1940s) could also be regarded as this type of evidence
III	Opinions of respected authorities, based on clinical experience, descriptive studies and case reports, or reports of expert committees

Source: Harris et al.[24]

with the net benefit of the intervention. This results in a rating of "A" (strongly recommended), "B" (recommended), "C" (no recommendation), "D" (recommended against), or "I" (insufficient evidence for a recommendation).

Another important resource is the Cochrane Collaboration, an international initiative begun in 1993 and designed to prepare, maintain, and disseminate systematic reviews of health care interventions.[90] Reviews by the Cochrane Collaboration, updated quarterly, are based exclusively on randomized controlled trials and are available electronically. Cochrane reviews focus primarily on therapeutic interventions, such as the effects of antidepressants for depression in people with physical illness. The Cochrane database catalogs reviews prepared by its members as well as reviews published outside of the collaboration. The database also contains registries on unpublished and ongoing trials that can be used as source data for meta-analyses and other systematic reviews.[90] In addition, the Cochrane Collaboration reviews economic evaluations of effective interventions.

Guidelines for Interventions in Community Settings.   In 2000, an expert panel (the U.S. Public Health Service Task Force on Community Preventive Services), supported by the Centers for Disease Control and Prevention, began publishing *The Guide to Community Preventive Services: Systematic Reviews and Evidence-Based Recommendations* (the *Community Guide*).[9] The underlying reasons for developing the *Community Guide* were as follows: (1) practitioners and policy makers value scientific knowledge as a basis for decision making; (2) the scientific literature on a given topic is often vast, uneven in quality, and inaccessible to busy practitioners; and (3) an experienced and objective panel of experts is seldom locally available to public health officials on a wide range of topics.[91] This effort evaluates evidence related to community, or "population-based," interventions and is intended as a complement to *The Guide to Clinical Preventive Services.* It summarizes what is known about the effectiveness and cost-effectiveness of population-based interventions designed to promote health; prevent disease, injury, disability, and premature death; and reduce exposure to environmental hazards.

Sets of related systematic reviews and recommendations are conducted for interventions in broad health topics, organized by behavior (tobacco product use prevention), environment (the sociocultural environment), or specific diseases, injuries, or impairment (vaccine-preventable diseases). A systematic process is followed that includes forming a review development team, developing a conceptual approach focused around an analytic framework, selecting interventions to evaluate, searching for and retrieving evidence, abstracting information on each relevant study, and assessing the quality of the evidence of effectiveness. Information on each intervention is then translated into a recommendation for or against the intervention or a finding of insufficient evidence. For those interventions where there is insufficient evidence of effectiveness, the *Community Guide* provides guidance for further prevention research. In addition, the *Community Guide* takes a systematic approach to economic evaluation, seeking cost-effectiveness information for those programs and policies deemed effective.[1] (The evidence hierarchy for the *Community Guide* is shown in Chapter 2.)

To date, evidence reviews and recommendations are available for 18 different public health topics, including reducing risk factors (tobacco control), promoting early detection (cancer screening), addressing sociocultural determinants (housing), and promoting health in settings (worksites). Based on dissemination of an early evidence review in the *Community Guide*,[92] health policy has already been positively influenced at the national and state levels[93] (Box 3-3).

Box 3-3. Using Guidelines to Support Health Policy Change for Reducing Alcohol-Related Traffic Fatalities in the United States[a]

A systematic review of the evidence of effectiveness of state laws that lower the allowed blood alcohol concentration (BAC) for motor vehicle drivers from 0.1% to 0.08% found that these laws result in reductions of 7% in fatalities associated with alcohol-impaired driving. The review also identified a study that estimated that approximately 500 lives would be saved annually if all states enacted "0.08% BAC laws." Based on this evidence, the Task Force on Community Preventive Services issued a strong recommendation to state policy makers that they consider enacting this type of law.[93]

In response to requests from members of the U.S. House Appropriations Committee's Transportation Subcommittee for information about the effectiveness of "0.08% BAC laws," this review and recommendation were summarized by the National Safety Council and provided to the subcommittee in late summer 2000. Based in part on this information, the subcommittee voted to include language in the Transportation Appropriations bill requiring states to enact 0.08% BAC laws or risk losing federal highway construction funds. The U.S. House and Senate approved the Transportation Appropriations bill, including the requirement, and the bill was signed into law by President Clinton. Prior to dissemination of the review findings, only 19 states had passed 0.08 BAC laws. By June 30, 2004, all 50 states had enacted these laws.

A case study of this use of evidence from a systematic review was published in 2010.[93] Among the lessons, several stand out: (1) the compelling nature of, and relationships between the policy intervention and health outcomes, (2) the use of a synthesis of the full body of evidence, (3) the use of a recognized and credible process for the synthesis, (4) the participatory engagement of key partners throughout all stages of the process, (5) the use of personalized channels and compelling formats to disseminate the evidence, (6) the ability to involve multiple stakeholders in encouraging uptake and adherence, (7) capitalizing on readiness and teachable moments, and (8) efforts to address sustainability.

---

[a]Contributed by Zaza S. Centers for Disease Control and Prevention, December 2001, and Mercer et al.[93]

"Best Practices" in Public Health

In addition to the analytic approaches discussed thus far, a variety of "best practices" reviews have been conducted and disseminated in recent years. The scope and quality of these reviews vary greatly, making "best practices" an imprecise term. Identification of best practices sometimes occurs when a practitioner informally notes that one intervention activity works better than another.[94] Some researchers have included evidence-based reviews in clinical and community settings under the heading of best practices.[95] Best practices have also involved a grassroots approach toward injury prevention and traffic safety that engaged local citizens in the decision-making process.[96] Other best practices approaches have been a combination of a strictly evidence-based process and expert opinion on what works. An example here is *Best Practices for Comprehensive Tobacco Control Programs,* developed by the Centers for Disease Control and Prevention.[97] In part, this document was developed in response to demand from states that were deciding how to allocate large sums of litigated damages being paid by the tobacco industry[95] and was largely based on the program successes in states that had established comprehensive and effective tobacco control programs—notably California, Massachusetts, Arizona, and Oregon.[98]

Given these variations in how best practices are assembled, readers should carefully scrutinize the process used to develop guidance, particularly when the guidelines do not appear in the peer-reviewed literature.

SUMMARY

This chapter has presented several tools for developing and practicing evidence-based public health, including systematic reviews and economic evaluation. Both are ways to identify, collate, and synthesize what is known about a topic. Systematic reviews give an assessment of state-of-the-art information about a particular intervention and evaluate the efficacy of the intervention ("Does it work?"). Economic evaluation quantifies the costs and benefits of an intervention and provides an assessment of its effectiveness ("Are the costs reasonable to obtain the likely benefits?"). Practice guidelines translate research into information for public health practice ("What recommendations have been issued by expert panels to address the health condition[s] of interest?").

Each of these techniques is relatively sophisticated and is generally carried out by persons with specialized training (e.g., an economist would conduct a CUA). The aim of this chapter has been to explain these techniques to public health practitioners so that they can be educated consumers of these methods.

Key Chapter Points

- Systematic reviews and economic evaluations summarize large amounts of information and can provide reliable tools for decision making among public health professionals and policy makers.
- These techniques are relatively sophisticated, but their underlying logic and structure can be understood.
- The outcome of the systematic review process can be a narrative (qualitative) assessment of the literature or a quantitative meta-analysis, and either can be used to inform guideline development.
- Practice guidelines for clinical and community settings are becoming increasingly common and useful.
- Economic evaluation is the comparison of costs and benefits to determine the most efficient allocation of scarce resources.
- Several challenges (i.e., inconsistent quality, methodological issues, difficulties in implementation) should be kept in mind when considering the use of systematic reviews and economic evaluations.

These methods will be increasingly used, especially in times of limited public health resources, and practitioners must be able to understand them so that they can argue for setting appropriate public health priorities.

SUGGESTED READINGS AND SELECTED WEBSITES

Suggested Readings

Briss PA, Brownson RC, Fielding JE, Zaza S. Developing and using the Guide to Community Preventive Services: lessons learned about evidence-based public health. *Annu Rev Public Health.* 2004,25.281–302.

Drummond MF, Sculpher MJ, Torrance GW, et al. *Methods for the Economic Evaluation of Health Care Programmes.* 3rd ed. New York, NY: Oxford University Press, 2005.

Gold MR, Siegel JE, Russell LB, Weinstein MC. *Cost-Effectiveness in Health and Medicine.* New York, NY: Oxford University Press, 1996.

Haddix AC, Teutsch SM, Corso PS. *Prevention Effectiveness. A Guide to Decision Analysis and Economic Evaluation.* 2nd ed. New York, NY: Oxford University Press; 2002.

Higgins JPT, Green S. *Cochrane Handbook for Systematic Reviews of Interventions.* New York, NY: John Wiley and Sons, 2008.

Kemm J, Parry J, Palmer S, eds. *Health Impact Assessment: Concepts, Theory, Techniques and Applications.* New York, NY: Oxford University Press, 2004.

Muennig P. *Cost-Effectiveness Analysis in Health: A Practical Approach.* San Francisco, CA: Jossey-Bass, 2007.

Petitti DB. *Meta-analysis, Decision Analysis, and Cost-Effectiveness Analysis: Methods for Quantitative Synthesis in Medicine.* 2nd ed. New York, NY: Oxford University Press, 2000.
Petticrew M, Roberts H. *Systematic Reviews in the Social Sciences: A Practical Guide.* Oxford, UK: Blackwell Publishing, 2006.

Selected Websites

Association of Public Health Observatories, The HIA Gateway <http://www.apho. org.uk/default.aspx?QN=P_HIA>. This U.K.-based website provides resources for health impact assessments, including sample causal diagrams and a searchable catalog of HIAs.

Canadian Task Force on Preventive Health Care <http://www.ctfphc.org/>. This website is designed to serve as a practical guide to health care providers, planners, and consumers for determining the inclusion or exclusion, content, and frequency of a wide variety of preventive health interventions, using the evidence-based recommendations of the Canadian Task Force on Preventive Health Care.

The CEA Registry: Center for the Evaluation of Value and Risk in Health, Institute for Clinical Research and Health Policy Studies, Tufts Medical Center <https://research.tufts-nemc.org/cear/default.aspx>. This website includes a detailed database of cost-utility analyses. Originally based on the articles by Tengs et al.,[51,99] the site is continually updated and expanded and now also includes a catalog of QALY weights.

The Cochrane Collaboration <http://www.cochrane.org>. The Cochrane Collaboration is an international organization that aims to help people make well-informed decisions about health care by preparing, maintaining, and promoting the accessibility of systematic reviews of the effects of health care interventions. The Collaboration conducts its own systematic reviews, abstracts the systematic reviews of others, and provides links to complementary databases.

The Guide to Clinical Preventive Services, Third Edition <http://www.ahrq.gov/ clinic/uspstfix.htm>. The U.S. Preventive Services Task Force developed and updates this guide, intended for primary care clinicians, other allied health professionals, and students. It provides recommendations for clinical preventive interventions— screening tests, counseling interventions, immunizations, and chemoprophylactic regimens—for more than 80 target conditions. Systematic reviews form the basis for the recommendations. The Guide is provided through the website of the Agency for Healthcare Research and Quality.

The Guide to Community Preventive Services <http://www.thecommunityguide. org>. Under the auspices of the U.S. Public Health Service, the Task Force on Community Preventive Services developed *The Guide to Community Preventive Services*. The *Community Guide* uses systematic reviews to summarize what is known about the effectiveness of population-based interventions for prevention and control in 18 topical areas. Interventions that are rated effective are then evaluated for cost-effectiveness.

Health Impact Assessment, Centers for Disease Control and Prevention Health Places<http://www.cdc.gov/healthyplaces/hia.htm>. This website provides definitions, examples, and links to other catalogs and archives of HIAs.

National Health Service Centre for Reviews and Dissemination <http://www.york.ac.uk/inst/crd>. Maintained by the University of York, this website distributes information and has searchable databases on intervention effectiveness and intervention cost-effectiveness. The NHS Centre for Reviews and Dissemination is devoted to promoting the use of research-based knowledge in health care. Within the website, one can find the NHS Economic Evaluation Database, which contains 24,000 abstracts of health economics papers including over 7000 quality-assessed economic evaluations. The database aims to assist decision makers by systematically identifying and describing economic evaluations, appraising their quality and highlighting their relative strengths and weaknesses.

The UCLA Health Impact Assessment Clearinghouse Learning Information Center <http://www.ph.ucla.edu/hs/hiaclic>. This site contains a catalogue of HIAs conducted in the United States and information about HIA methods and tools. An online training manual is provided.

World Health Organization Health Impact Assessment <http://www.who.int/hia/en/>. The World Health Organization provides resources, examples, toolkits, and a catalog of worldwide HIAs.

REFERENCES

1. Carande-Kulis VG, Maciosek MV, Briss PA, et al. Methods for systematic reviews of economic evaluations for the Guide to Community Preventive Services. Task Force on Community Preventive Services. *Am J Prev Med.* 2000;18(1 Suppl):75–91.
2. Drummond M, Sculpher M, Torrance G, et al. *Methods for the Economic Evaluation of Health Care Programmes.* 3rd ed. New York, NY: Oxford University Press; 2005.
3. Gold MR, Siegel JE, Russell LB, Weinstein MC. *Cost-Effectiveness in Health and Medicine.* New York, NY: Oxford University Press; 1996.
4. Haddix AC, Teutsch SM, Corso PS. *Prevention Effectiveness. A Guide to Decision Analysis and Economic Evaluation.* 2nd ed. New York, NY: Oxford University Press; 2002.
5. Kemm J, Parry J, Palmer S, eds. *Health Impact Assessment: Concepts, Theory, Techniques and Applications.* New York, NY: Oxford University Press; 2004.
6. Muennig P. *Cost-Effectiveness Analysis in Health: A Practical Approach.* San Francisco, CA: Jossey-Bass; 2007.
7. Petitti DB. *Meta-analysis, Decision Analysis, and Cost-Effectiveness Analysis: Methods for Quantitative Synthesis in Medicine.* 2nd ed. New York, NY: Oxford University Press; 2000.

8. Petticrew M, Roberts H. *Systematic Reviews in the Social Sciences: A Practical Guide*. Oxford, UK: Blackwell Publishing; 2006.
9. Zaza S, Briss PA, Harris KW, eds. *The Guide to Community Preventive Services: What Works to Promote Health?* New York, NY: Oxford University Press; 2005.
10. Petticrew M. Systematic reviews from astronomy to zoology: myths and misconceptions. *BMJ.* 2001;322(7278):98–101.
11. Bero LA, Jadad AR. How consumers and policy makers can use systematic reviews for decision making. In: Mulrow C, Cook D, eds. *Systematic Reviews. Synthesis of Best Evidence for Health Care Decisions*. Philadelphia, PA: American College of Physicians; 1998:45–54.
12. Jackson N, Waters E. Criteria for the systematic review of health promotion and public health interventions. *Health Promot Int.* 2005;20(4):367–374.
13. Marshall DA, Hux M. Design and analysis issues for economic analysis alongside clinical trials. *Med Care.* 2009;47(7 Suppl 1):S14–20.
14. Ramsey S, Willke R, Briggs A, et al. Good research practices for cost-effectiveness analysis alongside clinical trials: the ISPOR RCT-CEA Task Force report. *Value Health.* 2005;8(5):521–533.
15. Bambra C. Real world reviews: A beginner's guide to undertaking systematic reviews of public health policy interventions. *J Epidemiol Commun Health.* Sep 18 2009.
16. Lavis JN. How can we support the use of systematic reviews in policymaking? *PLoS Med.* 2009;6(11):e1000141.
17. Waters E, Doyle J, Jackson N. Evidence-based public health: improving the relevance of Cochrane Collaboration systematic reviews to global public health priorities. *J Public Health Med.* 2003;25(3):263–266.
18. Galsziou P, Irwig L, Bain C, Colditz G. *Systematic Reviews in Health Care: A Practical Guide*. New York, NY: Cambridge University Press; 2001.
19. Guyatt G, Rennie D, eds. *Users' Guides to the Medical Literature. A Manual for Evidence-Based Clinical Practice*. Chicago, IL: American Medical Association Press; 2002.
20. Higgins J, Green S. *Cochrane Handbook for Systematic Reviews of Interventions*. New York, NY: John Wiley and Sons; 2008.
21. Briss PA, Zaza S, Pappaioanou M, et al. Developing an evidence-based Guide to Community Preventive Services—methods. The Task Force on Community Preventive Services. *Am J Prev Med.* 2000;18(1 Suppl):35–43.
22. Kelsey JL, Petitti DB, King AC. Key methodologic concepts and issues. In: Brownson RC, Petitti DB, eds. *Applied Epidemiology: Theory to Practice*. New York, NY: Oxford University Press; 1998:35–69.
23. Liberati A, Altman DG, Tetzlaff J, et al. The PRISMA statement for reporting systematic reviews and meta-analyses of studies that evaluate health care interventions: explanation and elaboration. *J Clin Epidemiol.* 2009;62(10):e1–34.
24. Harris RP, Helfand M, Woolf SH, et al. Current methods of the U.S. Preventive Services Task Force. A review of the process. *Am J Prev Med.* 2001;20(3 Suppl):21–35.
25. Glass GV. Primary, secondary and meta-analysis of research. *Educ Res.* 1976;5:3–8.
26. Ellison RC, Zhang Y, McLennan CE, Rothman KJ. Exploring the relation of alcohol consumption to risk of breast cancer. *Am J Epidemiol.* 2001;154(8):740–747.
27. Weed DL. Interpreting epidemiological evidence: how meta-analysis and causal inference methods are related. *Int J Epidemiol.* 2000;29(3):387–390.

28. Greenland S. Can meta-analysis be salvaged? *Am J Epidemiol.* 1994;140(9):783–787.
29. Gerber S, Tallon D, Trelle S, et al. Bibliographic study showed improving methodology of meta-analyses published in leading journals 1993–2002. *J Clin Epidemiol.* 2007;60(8):773–780.
30. Wen J, Ren Y, Wang L, et al. The reporting quality of meta-analyses improves: a random sampling study. *J Clin Epidemiol.* 2008;61(8):770–775.
31. Cardis E, Vrijheid M, Blettner M, et al. The 15-Country Collaborative Study of Cancer Risk among Radiation Workers in the Nuclear Industry: estimates of radiation-related cancer risks. *Radiat Res.* 2007;167(4):396–416.
32. Lubin JH, Purdue M, Kelsey K, et al. Total exposure and exposure rate effects for alcohol and smoking and risk of head and neck cancer: a pooled analysis of case-control studies. *Am J Epidemiol.* 2009;170(8):937–947.
33. Patient level pooled analysis of 68 500 patients from seven major vitamin D fracture trials in US and Europe. *BMJ.* 340:b5463.
34. Samet JM, White RH, Burke TA. Epidemiology and risk assessment. In: Brownson RC, Petitti DB, eds. *Applied Epidemiology: Theory to Practice.* 2nd ed. New York, NY: Oxford University Press; 2006:125–163.
35. World Health Organization. Environmental Burden of Disease Series, World Health Organization. www.who.int/quantifying_ehimpacts/national. Accessed February 11, 2010.
36. US Environmental Protection Agency. Guidelines for Carcinogen Risk Assessment. EPA/630/P-03/001F:http://cfpub.epa.gov/ncea/cfm/recordisplay.cfm?deid=116283.
37. Cole BL, Fielding JE. Health impact assessment: a tool to help policy makers understand health beyond health care. *Annu Rev Public Health.* 2007;28:393–412.
38. Collins J, Koplan JP. Health impact assessment: a step toward health in all policies. *JAMA.* 2009;302(3):315–317.
39. World Health Organization. Health Impact Assessment http://www.who.int/hia/en/. Accessed February 3, 2010.
40. Dannenberg AL, Bhatia R, Cole BL, et al. Use of health impact assessment in the U.S.: 27 case studies, 1999–2007. *Am J Prev Med.* 2008;34(3):241–256.
41. Cole B, Shimkhada R, Morgenstern H, et al S. Projected health impact of the Los Angeles City living wage ordinance. *J Epidemiol Commun Health.* 2005;59:645–650.
42. Porta M, ed. *A Dictionary of Epidemiology.* 5th ed New York, NY: Oxford University Press; 2008.
43. Postma MJ, Novak A, Scheijbeler HW, et al. Cost effectiveness of oseltamivir treatment for patients with influenza-like illness who are at increased risk for serious complications of influenza: illustration for the Netherlands. *Pharmacoeconomics.* 2007;25(6):497–509.
44. Alemi F, Gustafson D. *Decision Analysis for Healthcare Managers.* Chicago, IL: Health Administration Press; 2006.
45. Martin AJ, Glasziou PP, Simes RJ, Lumley T. A comparison of standard gamble, time trade-off, and adjusted time trade-off scores. *Int J Technol Assess Health Care.* 2000;16(1):137–147.
46. Health Utilities Group. Health Utilities Index: Multiattribute Health Status Classification System: Health Utilities Index Mark 3 (HUI3). http://www-fhs.mcmaster.ca/hug/. Accessed February 3, 2010.
47. The EuroQol Group. EuroQol–What is EQ-5D? . http://www.euroqol.org/contact/contact information.html. Accessed February 2, 2010.

48. Bell CM, Chapman RH, Stone PW, et al. An off-the-shelf help list: a comprehensive catalog of preference scores from published cost-utility analyses. *Med Decis Making.* 2001;21(4):288–294.

49. Sullivan PW, Ghushchyan V. Preference-Based EQ-5D index scores for chronic conditions in the United States. *Med Decis Making.* 2006;26(4):410–420.

50. Sullivan PW, Lawrence WF, Ghushchyan V. A national catalog of preference-based scores for chronic conditions in the United States. *Med Care.* 2005;43(7):736–749.

51. Tengs TO, Wallace A. One thousand health-related quality-of-life estimates. *Med Care.* 2000;38(6):583–637.

52. CDC Diabetes Cost-Effectiveness Study Group. The cost-effectiveness of screening for type 2 diabetes. *JAMA.* 1998;2802(20):1757–1763.

53. American Diabetes Association. Screening for diabetes. *Diabetes Care.* 2002;25(S1): S21–S24.

54. Screening for type 2 diabetes mellitus in adults: U.S. Preventive Services Task Force recommendation statement. *Ann Intern Med.* 2008;148(11):846–854.

55. Hoerger TJ, Harris R, Hicks KA, et al. Screening for type 2 diabetes mellitus: a cost-effectiveness analysis. *Ann Intern Med.* 2004;140(9):689–699.

56. Eddy D. *Breast Cancer Screening for Medicare Beneficiaries.* Washington, DC: Office of Technology Assessment; 1987.

57. Braithwaite RS, Meltzer DO, King JT Jr, et al. What does the value of modern medicine say about the $50,000 per quality-adjusted life-year decision rule? *Med Care.* 2008;46(4):349–356.

58. Garber AM, Phelps CE. Economic foundations of cost-effectiveness analysis. *J Health Econ.* 1997;16(1):1–31.

59. Murray CJ, Evans DB, Acharya A, Baltussen RM. Development of WHO guidelines on generalized cost-effectiveness analysis. *Health Econ.* 2000;9(3):235–251.

60. World Health Organization. *Macroeconomics and Health: Investing in Health for Economic Development.* Geneva, Switzerland: World Health Organization; 2001.

61. McCabe C, Claxton K, Culyer AJ. The NICE cost-effectiveness threshold: what it is and what that means. *Pharmacoeconomics.* 2008;26(9):733–744.

62. Gillick MR. Medicare coverage for technological innovations—time for new criteria? *N Engl J Med.* 2004;350(21):2199–2203.

63. Owens DK. Interpretation of cost-effectiveness analyses. *J Gen Intern Med.* 1998;13(10):716–717.

64. Weinstein MC. How much are Americans willing to pay for a quality-adjusted life year? *Med Care.* 2008;46(4):343–345.

65. Mulrow CD. The medical review article: state of the science. *Ann Intern Med.* 1987;106(3):485–488.

66. Breslow RA, Ross SA, Weed DL. Quality of reviews in epidemiology. *Am J Public Health.* 1998;88(3):475–477.

67. Mullen PD, Ramirez G. The promise and pitfalls of systematic reviews. *Annu Rev Public Health.* 2006;27:81–102.

68. Neumann P. *Using Cost-Effectiveness Analysis to Improve Health Care.* New York, NY: Oxford University Press; 2005.

69. Weatherly H, Drummond M, Claxton K, et al. Methods for assessing the cost-effectiveness of public health interventions: key challenges and recommendations. *Health Policy.* 2009;93(2–3):85–92.

70. Zarnke KB, Levine MA, O'Brien BJ. Cost-benefit analyses in the health-care literature: don't judge a study by its label. *J Clin Epidemiol.* 1997;50(7):813–822.
71. Gerard K, Mooney G. QALY league tables: handle with care. *Health Econ.* 1993;2(1):59–64.
72. Mauskopf J, Rutten F, Schonfeld W. Cost-effectiveness league tables: valuable guidance for decision makers? *Pharmacoeconomics.* 2003;21(14):991–1000.
73. Tsuchiya A. QALYs and ageism: philosophical theories and age weighting. *Health Econ.* 2000;9(1):57–68.
74. Tsuchiya A, Williams A. A "fair innings" between the sexes: are men being treated inequitably? *Soc Sci Med.* 2005;60(2):277–286.
75. Groot W. Adaptation and scale of reference bias in self-assessments of quality of life. *J Health Econ.* 2000;19(3):403–420.
76. Menzel P, Dolan P, Richardson J, Olsen JA. The role of adaptation to disability and disease in health state valuation: a preliminary normative analysis. *Soc Sci Med.* 2002;55(12):2149–2158.
77. Gerdtham UG, Johannesson M. Income-related inequality in life-years and quality-adjusted life-years. *J Health Econ.* 2000;19(6):1007–1026.
78. Dolan P. Utilitarianism and the measurement and aggregation of quality-adjusted life years. *Health Care Anal.* 2001;9(1):65–76.
79. Bleichrodt H, Diecidue E, Quiggin J. Equity weights in the allocation of health care: the rank-dependent QALY model. *J Health Econ.* 2004;23(1):157–171.
80. Cookson R, Drummond M, Weatherly H. Explicit incorporation of equity considerations into economic evaluation of public health interventions. *Health Econ Policy Law.* 2009;4(Pt 2):231–245.
81. Grimshaw J, Eccles M, Thomas R, et al. Toward evidence-based quality improvement. Evidence (and its limitations) of the effectiveness of guideline dissemination and implementation strategies 1966–1998. *J Gen Intern Med.* 2006;21(Suppl) 2:S14–20.
82. Maciosek MV, Coffield AB, Edwards NM, et al. Prioritizing clinical preventive services: a review and framework with implications for community preventive services. *Annu Rev Public Health.* 2009;30:341–355.
83. Dobbins M, Cockerill R, Barnsley J, Ciliska D. Factors of the innovation, organization, environment, and individual that predict the influence five systematic reviews had on public health decisions. *Int J Technol Assess Health Care.* 2001;17(4):467–478.
84. Azimi NA, Welch HG. The effectiveness of cost-effectiveness analysis in containing costs. *J Gen Intern Med.* 1998;13(10):664–669.
85. McDaid D, Needle J. What use has been made of economic evaluation in public health? A systematic review of the literature. In: Dawson S, Morris S, eds. *Future Public Health: Burdens, Challenges and Approaches.* Basingstoke, UK: Palgrave Macmillan; 2009:248–264.
86. National Institutes of Health. NIH State-of-the-Science Conference Statement on Tobacco Use: Prevention, Cessation, and Control. *NIH Consens State Sci Statements.* 2006;23(3):1–26.
87. McGlynn EA, Kosecoff J, Brook RH. Format and conduct of consensus development conferences. Multination comparison. *Int J Technol Assess Health Care.* 1990;6: 450–469.
88. Lenfant C, Chobanian AV, Jones DW, Roccella EJ. Seventh report of the Joint National Committee on the Prevention, Detection, Evaluation, and Treatment of High

Blood Pressure (JNC 7): resetting the hypertension sails. *Hypertension.* 2003;41(6):1178–1179.

89. Feightner JW, Lawrence RS. Evidence-based prevention and international collaboration. *Am J Prev Med.* 2001;20(3 Suppl):5–6.

90. Chalmers I. The Cochrane Collaboration: preparing, maintaining, and disseminating systematic reviews of the effects of health care. *Ann N Y Acad Sci.* 1993;703: 156–163; discussion 163–155.

91. Truman BI, Smith-Akin CK, Hinman AR, et al. Developing the guide to community preventive services: overview and rationale. *Am J Prev Med.* 2000;18(1S):18–26.

92. Shults RA, Elder RW, Sleet DA, et al. Reviews of evidence regarding interventions to reduce alcohol-impaired driving. *Am J Prev Med.* 2001;21(4 Suppl 1):66–88.

93. Mercer S, Sleet DA, Eldew RW, et al. From evidence to policy action: The case for lowering the legal blood alcohol limit for drivers. *Ann Epidemiol.* 2010;20(6): 412–20.

94. Kahan B, Goodstadt M. The Interactive Domain Model of Best Practices in Health Promotion: developing and implementing a best practices approach to health promotion. *Health Promotion Practice.* 2001;2(1):43–67.

95. Green LW. From research to "best practices" in other settings and populations. *Am J Health Behav.* 2001;25(3):165–178.

96. National Highway Traffic Safety Administration. A Safe Communities: A Vision for the Future: A Safe Community in Every Community in America. http://www.nhtsa. dot.gov/portal/site/nhtsa/menuitem.6c6692143d8f3c15fb8e5f8dcba046a0/. Accessed January 28, 2010.

97. Centers for Disease Control and Prevention. *Best Practices for Comprehensive Tobacco Control Programs.* Atlanta, GA: Centers for Disease Control and Prevention, National Center for Chronic Disease Prevention and Health Promotion, Office on Smoking and Health; 2007.

98. Siegel M. The effectiveness of state-level tobacco control interventions: a review of program implementation and behavioral outcomes. *Annu Rev Public Health.* 2002;23:45–71.

99. Tengs TO, Adams ME, Pliskin JS, et al. Five-hundred life-saving interventions and their cost-effectiveness. *Risk Analysis.* 1995;15(3):369–390.

4

Community Assessment

The uncreative mind can spot wrong answers. It takes a creative mind to spot wrong questions.

—A. Jay

Becoming aware of current conditions through a community assessment is one of the first steps in an evidence-based process. The path to the destination depends very much on the starting point. As noted earlier, evidence-based processes include conducting assessments to identify issues within a community, prioritizing these issues, developing interventions to address these issues based on a review of what has worked effectively in other places, and evaluating the process, impact, and outcome of intervention efforts. Because the issues dealt with in public health are complex, each of these steps will require some engagement of community partners and a wide variety of stakeholders. Their level of engagement in each step may vary.

Community assessments may include efforts to identify morbidity and mortality, environmental and organizational conditions, existing policies, and relationships among key stakeholders. In conducting these assessments it is important to attend to not only the needs in the community and problems but also community strengths and assets (similar to the strategic planning considerations outlined in Chapter 5).

While it is ideal to conduct a complete and thorough assessment, this may not be possible in all instances. Choices about what needs to be assessed should be based on the specific questions that are being asked. This may in turn depend on who is asking the questions. Ideally, assessments should be made with a number of stakeholders or partners taking an active role. In reality, some partners may join at a later stage in the evidence-based process. In these cases, partners may bring new perspectives or questions that warrant additional assessments.

This chapter is divided into several sections. The first provides a background on community assessments. The next section describes why a community assessment is critical. The third section discusses a range of partnership models that might be useful in conducting community assessments. The next sections outline who to assess, what to assess, and how to conduct assessments. The final section describes how to disseminate the community assessment findings.

BACKGROUND

Community assessments identify the health concerns in a community, the factors in the community that influence health (i.e., determinants of health), and the assets, resources, and challenges that influence these factors.[1,2] Ideally, assessment is a process in which community stakeholders including community members and a broad array of community-based and government organizations become partners in assessing the community and moving from assessment to action planning[3] (see Chapter 5 for more information on stakeholders). The types of data collected are determined within this partnership and are based on the question(s) this partnership is interested in answering. The data are usually synthesized and provided back to the partnership and the broader community in order to inform future action planning.[1]

WHY CONDUCT COMMUNITY ASSESSMENT

Community assessments are essential to ensure that the right interventions are implemented. This is in part because they can provide insight into the community context so that interventions are designed, planned, and carried out in ways that are acceptable and maximize the benefit to the community. In addition, the assessments can identify (and in some cases build) support for a particular intervention approach. This support is critical for garnering resources and ensuring a successful intervention. Assessments can also provide a baseline measure of a variety of conditions. This baseline, or starting point, is helpful in determining the impact of intervention efforts. In Chapter 10, more information will be provided on how to compare baseline measures to measures collected during and after the intervention to identify differences.

ROLE OF STAKEHOLDERS IN COMMUNITY ASSESSMENT

The role of stakeholders, including community members, community-based organizations, governmental/public agencies, private agencies, and health practitioners, in conducting a community assessment may vary. While some involvement of each of these groups is important, the assessment may be started by one group with others joining in at a later time. Alternately, the assessment may be conducted with a small group of stakeholders, with other partners being asked to join only once a specific intervention has been chosen. Some have argued that engagement of community members and these multiple sectors from the beginning and throughout the process is likely to enhance the relevance and accuracy of the overall assessment and increase the effectiveness of the chosen interventions[4-6] (see Box 4-1).

Coalitions are one way that stakeholders can come together to conduct community assessments. Recognizing that solving complex health issues requires that agencies and community leaders work together effectively, public health professionals have worked with existing or created new coalitions. A *coalition* is defined as a group of community members and/or organizations that join together for a

---

Box 4-1. Community Conversations on Barriers to Quality Health Care in a Rural Community

Engaging multiple stakeholders

The Center for Rural Health in North Dakota held community conversations with 13 rural communities, including five Native American reservations, to determine their barriers to health care and how these could be addressed.[4] The locations of the meetings were determined by the already existing boundaries for service regions in the state. They held meetings on each of the state's Native American reservations and Indian Service areas. The meetings were held in each of the communities with local community members being asked to serve as the host of the meeting in their area. A wide variety of stakeholders were invited from each area, including health care and educational administrators, government representatives and tribal leaders, and community and business leaders.

Multiple methods of data collection

Each meeting lasted 2 hours with time to present the intent of the meeting as well as asking participants to discuss health priorities and how the Center for Rural Health could assist in addressing these. The participants were involved in large- and small-group discussions. In addition, participants were asked to complete a short survey on health care threats, organizational challenges in addressing these, and how the Center for Rural Health might be helpful in addressing these.

Sharing findings and moving to action

Participants noted that the barriers to health care included factors across the ecological framework, including access/transportation, lack of economic growth, uninsured and underinsured, lack of primary prevention activities, and inadequate health care workforce. The Center for Rural Health summarized these findings, compared tribal and nontribal outcomes, and formed workgroups to share results, identify relevant strategies, and recommend interventions.

common purpose.[7,8] Some coalitions are focused on categorical issues, such as diabetes prevention or the reduction of infant mortality rates. Other coalitions form to address broader public health issues (e.g., a partnership for prevention).

Coalitions may differ considerably in the roles and responsibilities of each stakeholder and the types of activities in which they wish to engage.[9] This can be thought of as a continuum of integration.[7,8,10] At one end of the continuum is the desire of agencies and individuals to work together to identify gaps in services, avoid duplication of services, and exchange information to allow for appropriate client referral. This level is characterized by networking and coordination. The next level of integration involves a higher level of cooperation. Agencies maintain their autonomy, agendas, and resources but begin to share these resources to work on an issue that is identified as common to all. The highest level of integration involves collaboration among the agencies as they work together to develop joint agendas, common goals, and shared resources. Before starting a community assessment, it is important for stakeholders to be clear about the level of integration they desire, as each requires progressively higher levels of commitment and resources.

While community coalitions are growing in popularity, their ability to assess their community and create healthful changes depends in part on the coalition's ability to move through various stages of development. There are many recent efforts to define and describe these various stages.[7,11,12] Most often, for these groups to be effective, it is essential that they begin by developing a common vision of what they want to accomplish and a common set of skills to engage in the change process together. In addition, it is important that the individuals involved in the coalition build relationships as individuals and as representatives of their respective community organizations. As with other types of community-based health promotion programs, to be effective, coalitions may need to focus on a variety of issues, such as developing a common set of skills and building trust, at different stages of program implementation. Wolff[13] summarized the unique characteristics that contribute to the development of effective coalitions (Table 4-1). Once coalitions have established these processes they are ready to determine what to assess and how to conduct the assessment.

WHO AND WHAT TO ASSESS

What to assess depends very much on the knowledge to be gained and from whom it will be collected. In terms of the "who" question, it is important to clearly identify the "community" of interest. The community may be defined as individuals who live within a specified geographic region or as individuals who have a common

Table 4-1. Characteristics of Effective Community Coalitions

Characteristic	Description
1. Holistic and comprehensive	Allows the coalition to address issues that it deems as priorities; well illustrated in the Ottawa Charter for Health Promotion.
2. Flexible and responsive	Coalitions address emerging issues and modify their strategies to fit new community needs.
3. Build a sense of community	Members frequently report that they value and receive professional and personal support for their participation in the social network of the coalition.
4. Build and enhance resident engagement in community life	Provides a structure for renewed civic engagement; coalition becomes a forum where multiple sectors can engage with each other.
5. Provide a vehicle for community empowerment	As community coalitions solve local problems, they develop social capital, allowing residents to have an impact on multiple issues.
6. Allow diversity to be valued and celebrated	As communities become increasingly diverse, coalitions provide a vehicle for bringing together diverse group to solve common problems.
7. Incubators for innovative solutions to large problems	Problem solving occurs not only at local levels, but at regional and national levels; local leaders can become national leaders.

Source: Adapted from Wolff.[13]

experience or share a particular social or cultural sense of identity.[14,15] In conducting the assessment, it is also important to identify any subgroups within the community of interest (e.g., youth, lower-income adults) so that the assessments can adequately reflect the range of community members.

The decision regarding what to assess should be guided by the goal of the assessment. For instance, an assessment focusing on youth would include different elements than an assessment focusing on older adults. With that in mind, there are also some general guidelines that are helpful to consider in planning an assessment. In particular, it is important to assess factors along the full range of the ecologic factors that influence population health and well-being, and in doing so, to include the assets in the community—not just the problems.[14,16,17]

Ecologic frameworks (also discussed in Chapter 9) suggest that individual, social, and contextual factors influence individual behavior change and health.[15] Several variations of an ecologic framework have been proposed.[18–21] Based on work conducted by McLeroy and colleagues,[18] it is useful to consider assessment of factors at five levels:

1. Individual factors—characteristics of the individual such as knowledge, attitudes, skills, and a person's developmental history

2. Interpersonal factors—formal and informal social networks and social support systems, including family and friends
3. Organizational factors—social institutions, organizational characteristics, and rules or regulations for operation. Assessments of organizational factors may include not only the existence of these institutions but also organizational capacity and readiness for change (e.g., organizational support, communication within and between organizations, decision making structures, leadership, resources available[14,22–24])
4. Community factors—relationships between organizations, economic forces, the physical environment, and cultural variables that shape behavior
5. Government and policy factors—local, state, and national laws, rules, and regulations

Using an ecologic framework to guide an assessment leads to assessing people in the community (their health and wellness and their behaviors), the organizations and agencies that serve the community, as well as the environment within which the community members reside.[25] In fact, the most effective interventions act at multiple levels because communities are made up of individuals who interact in a variety of social networks and within a particular context; therefore, an assessment needs to provide insight along this wide range of factors. Table 4-2 provides a list of a number of possible indicators for each of these levels of the ecologic framework.

COLLECTING DATA

There are a number of different ways to collect data on each of the indicators listed earlier. Too often community assessment data are collected based on the skills of the individuals collecting the data. If someone knows how to collect survey data, that is the data that are collected. As noted earlier, for any community assessment process to be effective, it is essential to determine the questions that need to be answered and from whom data will be collected. Methods should be used that are best suited to answer the questions—obtaining assistance as needed. Some information may be found using existing data, while other types of information require new data collection. Data are often classified as either quantitative or qualitative. Quantitative data are expressed in numbers or statistics—they answer the "what" question. Qualitative data are expressed in words or pictures and help to understand or explain quantitative data by answering the "why" question. There are different types and different methods of collecting each. More often than not, it is useful to collect multiple types of data as each has certain advantages and disadvantages. Bringing different types of data together is often called triangulation.[26]

Table 4-2. Indicators by Level of an Ecological Framework

Level	Indicators
Individual determinants: characteristics of the individual such as knowledge, attitudes, skills, and a person's developmental history	• Leading causes of death • Leading causes of hospitalization • Behavioral risk and protective factors • Community member skills and talents
Interpersonal determinants: formal and informal social networks and social support systems, including family and friends	• Social connectedness • Group affiliation (clubs, associations) • Faith communities/churches/religious organizations • Cultural/community pride
Organizational determinants: social institutions, organizational characteristics, and rules or regulations for operation	• Number of newspaper/local radio or television/media • Number of public art projects or access to art exhibits/museums • Presence of food pantries • Number and variety of businesses • Number of faith based organizations • Number of civic organizations • Supportive services resource list • Public transportation systems • Number of social services—e.g., food assistance, child care providers, senior centers, housing/shelter assistance • Chamber of Commerce—list of businesses • Number and variety of medical care services: clinics, programs • Number of law enforcement services: e.g., law enforcement agencies; victim services • Number of nonprofit organizations and types of services performed (e.g., The United Way), number of people served (Planned Parenthood), number of people eligible for service • Number of vocational and higher education institutions and fields of study available to students: community college/university • Library
Community and social determinants: relationships between organizations, economic forces, the physical environment, and cultural variables that shape behavior	• Public school system enrollment numbers • Graduation/dropout rates • Test scores • Community history • Community values • Opportunities for structured and unstructured involvement in local decision making • Recreational opportunities: green spaces/parks/waterways/gyms/biking and walking trails • Crosswalks, curb cuts, traffic calming devices • Housing cost, availability • Environmental issues—trash, animals, pollution • Existence of local/citywide strategic planning processes • Employment/unemployment rates • Area economic data • Crime incidence: arrests/convictions, incidence of domestic violence

(continued)

Table 4-2. (Continued)

Level	Indicators
	• Motor vehicle crashes
	• Informal educational opportunities for children and adults
	• Number and types of existing collaborations among organizations
Government and policy factors: local, state, and national laws, rules, and regulations	• Zoning
	• Housing
	• Environmental
	• Economic—minimum wage

Quantitative Data

National, State, and Local Data from Surveillance Systems. These sources of quantitative data are collected through national or statewide initiatives and may include information on morbidity and mortality (cancer registry, death certificates), behavior (Behavioral Risk Factor Surveillance System), or social indicators (European Health for All Database, U.S. Census). The advantage of these data is that they are comparable across geographic regions, allowing comparisons between one community and other communities. The disadvantage of these data is that they may not be a good reflection of a community because of geographic coverage, sampling frames, or method of data collection (e.g., telephone interviews). In addition, these data sets may not include data relevant for answering questions related to a particular assessment or the development of a specific intervention.

Surveys or Quantitative Interviews. These data are collected specifically for a particular community and may include information on demographics, social indicators, knowledge, behavior, attitudes, morbidity, etc. These data may be collected through telephone, mail, face-to-face, or Internet-based interviews. The advantage of these type of data are that one can tailor the survey instrument to specific questions and community of interest. The disadvantage is that one's ability to compare responses to those of other areas depends on many things, including similarity of questions asked and data collection method. In addition, collecting data of this kind can be quite costly. More information on these approaches can be found in Chapter 6.

Community Audits. Community audits are detailed counting of certain factors in a community (e.g., number of recreational centers, supermarkets, fast food restaurants, schools, places of worship, billboards, number of walkers or bikers, cigarette butts, alcohol bottles, and social service and health care facilities).[27–31] Community audits may be conducted using structured check lists or audit tools, or more open-ended processes such as walking or windshield tours of a geographic area.[17] These data are useful in obtaining information about a particular context. However, some data may be influenced by the time of day or time of year (e.g., number of walkers) or observer awareness (e.g., difference between a bottle of soda and a premixed alcohol cocktail container).

Qualitative Data

Interviews.   Interviews may be individual or group conversations. The conversation may be very structured, using a set of questions that are asked of each individual in exactly the same way, or it may be more open, using a general interview protocol that outlines the topics of interest and a variety of probes that may be discussed in the order that seems most appropriate. Group interviews or focus group interviews, as opposed to individual interviews, allow for the influence of social norms to be assessed. The advantages of qualitative data include the potential for enhanced understanding of a particular issue (e.g., not just that someone is inactive but why they are inactive) and participant discussion of the association of various factors on their behavior and health. If a common interview protocol is developed, it is possible for interviews to be compared to each other to determine the range of factors influencing behavior and health. It is also possible to conduct several interviews or focus groups so that some comparisons can be made based different strata (e.g., comparisons across level of physical activity or gender). The disadvantage of qualitative data is that it is often difficult to gather information from as many different individuals and often takes longer to collect the data. The skills of the interviewer to establish rapport with individuals may also have a greater impact in collecting qualitative, as compared to quantitative, data.

Print Media/Written Documents.   Print media also provide a source of qualitative data. For example, newspapers or newsletters may provide insight into the most salient issues within a community. In addition, more recent technological advances allow for review of blogs or listservs as forms of important qualitative data (e.g., the types of support that a breast cancer listserv provides or concerns about medical care within a community). Some have used written diaries as ways to track and log community events or individual actions.

Observation.   Observation is a method of collecting data on a community or an intervention. It entails writing in-depth field notes or descriptions using all of one's sensory perceptions. By collecting these type of data, one can go beyond what a participant says about the program or the community and can gather information on the local context. The data collected may also be beneficial because information may be gathered that individuals are uncomfortable talking about or are not even aware are of interest (like a fish, why talk about the water?). In conducting observations, it is important to consider the benefits and drawbacks of participating and the duration of the observation. It is also useful to recognize that while telling individuals that they are being observed may alter behavior, not telling them will hinder the development of trusting relationships and may be ethically inappropriate. Observational data are a potentially rich source of information but are highly dependent on the skills and the abilities of the observer and may take a great deal of time.

Photovoice.   Photovoice is a type of qualitative data that uses still or video images to document conditions in a community. These images may be taken by community members, community-based organization representatives, or professionals. Once images are taken, they can be used to generate dialogue about the images.[32] These type of data can be very useful in capturing the salient images around certain community topics from the community perspective. As they say, a picture is worth a thousand words. However, it may be difficult to know what the circumstances surrounding the picture are, when it was taken, or why it was taken. What an image means is in the "eye of the beholder."

Community Forums or Listening Sessions.   Community forums are a method of bringing together different segments of the community to have conversations about the most important issues in their community.[4,33,34] These discussions are larger than focus groups. The community may be presented with a short description of the project and then asked one or two key questions focusing on concerns or visions for how improved population health would look. The community may be given the option of responding verbally or through the creation of visual representations.[11,17] The advantage of bringing the community together to discuss community issues in this way is the ability to engage multiple segments of the community and to create rich and complex dialogue of the issues. The difficulty comes in analyzing the data obtained and in ensuring that the sessions allow for multiple voices to be heard.[33]

ANALYSIS OF DATA

Once data have been collected, they need to be analyzed and summarized. Both quantitative and qualitative data analysis requires substantial training far beyond the scope of this book. Chapter 6 will provide an overview of some of the most important analysis considerations when working with quantitative data. Often, in a community assessment, the analysis of most interest involves pattern by person, place, and time. Following is an overview of some of the considerations in analyzing qualitative data.

The analysis of qualitative data, be it analysis of print media, field notes, photovoice, listening sessions, or interviews, is an iterative process of sorting and synthesizing to develop a set of common concepts or themes that occur in the data in order to discern patterns. The process of analysis often begins during data collection. Similarly, as one collects and analyzes the data, there may be interpretations or explanations for patterns seen or linkages among different elements of the data that begin to appear. It is useful to track these as they occur.

There are many different strategies for conducting qualitative data analysis. As with quantitative data, prior to any analysis it is important to ensure that the data are properly prepared. For example, when analyzing interviews it is important that transcripts (verbatim notes often typed from an audio recording) are accurate and complete. The next step in analysis of qualitative data is the development of a set of codes or categories within which to sort different segments of the data. These codes may be predetermined by the questions driving the inquiry, or they may be developed in the process of reviewing the data. Once codes are established, the data are reviewed and sorted into the codes or categories, with new codes or categories developed for data that do not fit into established coding schemes. The data within each code are reviewed to ensure that the assignment is accurate and that any subcategories are illuminated. These codes or categories are then reviewed to determine general themes or findings. There are some methods that allow the comparison across various groups (e.g., development of matrices that compare findings among men and women or health practitioners and community members). For large data sets, there are software packages that allow for these types of comparisons (e.g., NUDIST, ATLAS.TI). (Those interested in further information on qualitative analysis should see additional sources.[35,36]) Whenever possible, before finalizing data analysis it is helpful to conduct "member checking." Member checking is a process of going back to the individuals from whom the data were collected and verifying that the themes and concepts that were derived resonate with the participants.[11]

DISSEMINATING COMMUNITY ASSESSMENT FINDINGS

Community assessments within an evidence-based public health decision-making process should be used to both understand the community of interest and identify the most important issues for this community. The assessment itself should be seen as the first step in a collaborative process of developing and implementing interventions. Therefore, once data are collected, it is important to summarize and present the data back to all partners in a way that is understandable and that integrates the lessons learned from each data source. In doing so, it is important to note the advantages and disadvantages of the data collected as well as the parts of the community the data represent.

There are several ways of presenting data. One can provide information to the community in the form of graphs. These graphs can compare rates of morbidity and mortality in one community to those in other communities or can compare subgroups within a particular community. Maps can also be useful in displaying the data collected. For example, maps can be used to highlight areas in a community that have more or less opportunity to access healthy foods or resources for physical activity. One can similarly use maps to identify the density of food outlets, libraries, schools, or even community organizations.[37-39]

In addition to creating materials to document findings from a community assessment, it is important that all stakeholders have an opportunity to reflect on and discuss the findings. This discussion should include dialogue regarding what is surprising and what is expected, what the data represent and what seems to still be missing. To move toward action, the partnership needs to have confidence that the data they have, while never being all the data that could be gathered, is sufficient to move toward action. From there, a full understanding of the data is important in prioritizing the most important issues to work on and in developing action plans.

SUMMARY

Community assessments are essential to provide information on existing individual, organizational, and community conditions. Because of the complexity of public health concerns, it is important to obtain information at multiple levels of the ecologic framework. Involving stakeholders early on in defining what questions need to be asked, and what existing and new data can be used to answer these questions, can save having to wait to act until additional information is gathered and synthesized. Even when stakeholders are involved in the earliest phases, as data are shared the findings inevitably lead to additional questions. It is critical to remember that an assessment is conducted to point the way to action, not as an end in itself. The best way to move effectively to action is to share data in ways that communicate to a wide audience, recognize the strengths and limitations of the data, and provide the opportunity for dialogue regarding findings in ways that lead to prioritization of issues (see Chapter 8), intervention planning (see Chapter 9), and evaluation (see Chapter 10).

Key Chapter Points

- Assessments should be conducted at all levels of the ecological framework, using methods that are appropriate for the questions asked.
- Key stakeholders should be involved at the earliest phases possible.
- Assessments should be conducted in ways that lead to action.

SUGGESTED READINGS AND SELECTED WEBSITES

Suggested Readings

Kaye G, Wolff T. *From the Ground Up! A Workbook on Coalition Building & Community Development*. Amherst, MA: AHEC/Community Partners; 2002.

Kretzmann JP, McKnight JL. *Building Communities from the Inside Out: A Path toward Finding and Mobilizing a Community's Assets*. Chicago, IL: ACTA Publications; 1993.

Miles MB, Huberman AM. *Qualitative Data Analysis: An Expanded Sourcebook*. Thousand Oaks, CA: Sage Publications, 1994.

North Carolina Department of Health and Human Services. *Community Assessment Guide Book: North Carolina Community Health Assessment Process*. Raleigh, NC; 2002.

Patton, MQ. *Qualitative Research and Evaluation Methods*. Thousand Oaks, CA: Sage Publications; 2002.

Plested BA, Edwards RW, Jumper Thurman P. *Community Readiness: A Handbook for Successful Change*. Fort Collins, CO: Triethnic Center for Prevention Research; 2005.

Selected Websites

AssessNow <http://www.assessnow.info/orientation/toolkit>. AssessNow provides public health staff with information, tools, and resources to improve the practice of community health assessment. The learning resource toolkit is a compilation of web resources, training information, and learning activities, organized by competency.

CDC Social Determinants of Health Maps <http://www.cdc.gov/dhdsp/library/maps/social_determinants.htm>. The social determinants of health maps available at the Centers for Disease Control and Prevention website can be used in conjunction with other data to identify interventions that might positively impact the health of your community of interest.

Community Health Improvement Resources <http://www.dhss.mo.gov/CHIR/>. Maintained by the Missouri Department of Health and Senior Services, Community Health Improvement Resources (CHIR) is an interactive planning system designed for use by public health practitioners and community stakeholders to improve the health of a community. CHIR uses a data-driven, evidence-based public health process to guide decision-making, priority setting, and intervention planning. The process acknowledges that communities have different needs. Sections include community assessment and prioritization, partnerships, readiness, and capacity. While some data sources are specific to Missouri, the site offers tips and resources useful to all.

The Community Toolbox <http://ctb.ku.edu/en/>. The Community Tool Box is a global resource for free information on essential skills for building healthy communities. It offers more than 7000 pages of practical guidance on topics such as leadership, strategic planning, community assessment, advocacy, grant writing, and evaluation. Sections include descriptions of the task, step-by-step guidelines, examples, and training materials.

Conducting a Community Assessment <http://www.ncrel.org/sdrs/areas/issues/envrnmnt/css/ppt/chap2.htm>. This online chapter covers fundamental aspects of community assessments including guiding principles, useful indicators for a community scan, and sources of information on communities.

UCLA Center for Health Policy Research, Health DATA Program <http://www.healthpolicy.ucla.edu/ProgramDetails.aspx?id=3>. The Health DATA (Data. Advocacy. Training. Assistance) Program exists to make data understandable to a wide range of health advocates through trainings, workshops, and technical assistance. The site includes instructional videos, Health DATA publications, and links to free online resources in areas such as community-based participatory research, community assessment, data collection (e.g., asset mapping, focus groups, surveys, key informant interviews), and data analysis and presentation.

Wisconsin Clearinghouse for Prevention Resources <http://wch.uhs.wisc.edu/01-Prevention/01-Prev-Coalition.html>. This site on coalition building from the Wisconsin Clearinghouse for Prevention Resources provides tools and resources for developing and sustaining a coalition of individuals and organizations.

REFERENCES

1. North Carolina Department of Health and Human Services. *Community Assessment Guide Book: North Carolina Community Health Assessment Process.* Raleigh, NC; 2002.
2. Wright J, Williams R, Wilkinson JR. Development and importance of health needs assessment. *BMJ.* 1998;316(7140):1310–1313.
3. Eng E, Strazza-Moore K, Rhodes SD, et al. Insiders and outsiders assess who is "the community." In: Israel BA, Eng E, Schulz AJ, Parker EA, eds. *Methods in Community-Based Participatory Research for Health.* San Francisco, CA: Jossey Bass; 2005.
4. Moulton PL, Miller ME, Offutt SM, Gibbens BP. Identifying rural health care needs using community conversations. *J Rural Health.* 2007;23(1):92–96.

5. Green LW, Mercer SL. Can public health researchers and agencies reconcile the push from funding bodies and the pull from communities? *Am J Public Health.* 2001;91(12):1926–1929.

6. Clark MJ, Cary S, Diemert G, et al. Involving communities in community assessment. *Public Health Nursing.* 2003;20(6):456–463.

7. Butterfoss FD, Goodman RM, Wandersman A. Community coalitions for prevention and health promotion. *Health Educ Res.* 1993;8(3):315–330.

8. Parker EA, Eng E, Laraia B, et al. Coalition building for prevention: lessons learned from the North Carolina Community-Based Public Health Initiative. *J Public Health Manag Pract.* 1998;4(2):25–36.

9. World Health Organization. Ottawa Charter for Health Promotion. International Conference on Health Promotion, Ontario, Canada, 1986.

10. Alter C, Hage J. *Organizations Working Together: Coordination in Interorganizational Networks.* Newbury Park, CA: Sage Publications; 1992.

11. Baker EA, Motton F. Creating understanding and action through group dialogue. In: Israel BA, Eng E, Schultz AJ, Parker EA, eds. *Methods in Community-Based Participatory Research for Health.* San Francisco, CA: Jossey-Bass; 2005.

12. Florin P, Mitchell R, Stevenson J. Identifying training and technical assistance needs in community coalitions: a developmental approach. *Health Educ Res.* 1993;8(3):417–432.

13. Wolff T. Community coalition building—contemporary practice and research: introduction. *Am J Commun Psychol.* 2001;29(2):165–172; discussion 205–111.

14. Paronen O, Oja P. How to understand a community: community assessment for the promotion of health-related physical activity. *Patient Educ Counsel.* 1998;33:S25–S28.

15. Baker EA, Brownson CA. Defining characteristics of community-based health promotion programs. *J Public Health Manag Pract.* 1998;4(2):1–9.

16. Kretzmann JP, McKnight JL. *Building Communities from the Inside Out: A Path toward Finding and Mobilizing a Community's Assets.* Chicago, IL: ACTA Publications; 1993.

17. Sharpe PA, Greaney ML, Lee PR, Royce SW. Assets-oriented community assessment. *Public Health Rep.* 2000;115(2–3):205–211.

18. McLeroy KR, Bibeau D, Steckler A, Glanz K. An ecological perspective on health promotion programs. *Health Educ Q.* 1988;15(4):351–377.

19. Simons-Morton DG, Simons-Morton BG, Parcel GS, Bunker JF. Influencing personal and environmental conditions for community health: a multilevel intervention model. *Fam Commun Health.* 1988;11(2):25–35.

20. Breslow L. Social ecological strategies for promoting healthy lifestyles. *Am J Health Promotion.* 1996;10(4):253–257.

21. Goodman RM, Wandersman A, Chinman M, et al. An ecological assessment of community-based interventions for prevention and health promotion: approaches to measuring community coalitions. *Am J Commun Psychol.* 1996;24(1):33–61.

22. Schulz AJ, Israel BA, Lantz P. Instrument for evaluating dimensions of group dynamics within community-based participatory research partnerships. *Eval Progr Planning.* 2003;26(3):249–262.

23. Plested BA, Edwards RW, Jumper Thurman P. *Community Readiness: A Handbook for Successful Change.* Fort Collins, CO: Triethnic Center for Prevention Research; 2005.

24. Baker EA, Brennan Ramirez LK, Claus JM, Land G. Translating and disseminating research- and practice-based criteria to support evidence-based intervention planning. *J Public Health Manag Pract.* 2008;14(2):124–130.

25. Glanz K. Perspectives on using theory. In: Glanz K, Lewis FM, Rimer BK, eds. *Health Behavior and Health Education*. 2nd ed. San Francisco, CA: Jossey-Bass Publishers; 1997:441–449.
26. Patton MQ. *Qualitative Evaluation and Research Methods*. 2nd ed. Thousand Oaks, CA: Sage Publications, Inc.; 1990.
27. Brownson RC, Hoehner CM, Day K, et al. Measuring the built environment for physical activity: state of the science. *Am J Prev Med*. 2009;36(4 Suppl):S99–S123.
28. Cheadle A, Sterling TD, Schmid TL, Fawcett SB. Promising community-level indicators for evaluating cardiovascular health-promotion programs. *Health Educ Res*. 2000;15(1):109–116.
29. Cheadle A, Wagner E, Koepsell T, et al. Environmental indicators: a tool of evaluating community-based health-promotion programs. *Am J Prev Med*. 1992;8:345–350.
30. Hausman AJ, Becker J, Brawer R. Identifying value indicators and social capital in community health partnerships. *J Commun Psychol*. 2005;33(6):691–703.
31. McKinnon RA, Reedy J, Morrissette MA, et al. Measures of the food environment: a compilation of the literature, 1990–2007. *Am J Prev Med*. 2009;36(4 Suppl): S124–S133.
32. Wang C, Burris MA. Photovoice: concept, methodology, and use for participatory needs assessment. *Health Educ Behav*. 1997;24(3):369–387.
33. North Carolina Department of Health and Human Services. *Healthy Carolinas: North Carolina Community Health Assessment Process*. NC Division of Public Office of Healthy Carolinas/Health Education & State Center for Health Statistics; 2008; Raleigh, NC.
34. Minkler M, Hancock. Community driven asset identification and issue selection. In: Minkler M, Wallerstein N, eds. *Community-Based Participatory Research for Health: From Process to Outcomes*. San Francisco, CA: Jossey-Bass; 2008; 135–154.
35. Huberman M, Miles M. *The Qualitative Researcher's Companion*. London, UK: Sage Publications; 2002.
36. Patton MQ. *Qualitative Evaluation and Research Methods*. 3rd ed. Thousand Oaks, CA: Sage; 2002.
37. Plescia M, Koontz S, Laurent S. Community assessment in a vertically integrated health care system. *Am J Public Health*. 2001;91(5):811–814.
38. Zenk SN, Lachance LL, Schulz AJ, et al. Neighborhood retail food environment and fruit and vegetable intake in a multiethnic urban population. *Am J Health Promot*. 2009;23(4):255–264.
39. Baker EA, Schootman M, Barnidge E, et al. The role of race and poverty in access to foods that enable individuals to adhere to dietary guidelines. *Prevent Chron Dis*. 2006;3(3):A76.

5

Developing an Initial Statement
of the Issue

If you don't know where you are going, you will wind up somewhere else.
—Yogi Berra

An early step in an evidence-based process is to develop a concise statement of the issue being considered. A clear articulation of the problem at hand will enhance the likelihood that a systematic and focused planning process can be followed, leading to successful outcomes and achievement of objectives. A clear statement of the issue provides a concrete basis for a priority setting process that is objective, which then leads to better program planning, intervention, and evaluation. A fully articulated issue statement includes a complete description of the problem, potential solutions, data sources, and health-related outcomes. While this may seem straightforward, developing a sound issue statement can be challenging. In fact, the development of well-stated and answerable clinical questions has been described as the most difficult step in the practice of evidence-based medicine.[1]

Issue statements can be initiated in at least three different ways. They might be part of a section on background and objectives of a grant application for external support of a particular intervention or program. Since this is generally the first portion of a grant application to be viewed by funders, a clear delineation of the issue under consideration is crucial. An issue statement might also be in response to a request from an administrator or elected official about a particular issue. For example, a governor or minister of health might seek input from agency personnel on a specific problem. Your task might be to develop a politically and scientifically acceptable issue statement within a short time period in response. Or, a program or agency might define issues as a result of a community assessment or as part of a strategic planning process that could take several months to implement and evaluate. Each scenario demonstrates a different set of reasons and circumstances for defining a particular public health issue. In all cases, it is essential that the initial statement of the issue be clear, articulate, and well understood by all members of the public health team, as well as other relevant parties.

This chapter is divided into two major sections. The first examines some lessons and approaches that can be learned from the processes of community assessment and strategic planning. The second describes a systematic approach to developing an issue statement by breaking it into four component parts: background/epidemiologic data; questions about the program or policy; solutions being considered; and potential outcomes. It should be remembered that an initial issue statement is likely to evolve as more information is gathered in the course of program implementation and policy development.

BACKGROUND

Developing a concise and useful issue statement can be informed by the processes of community assessment and strategic planning. In a community assessment, issues emerge and are defined in the process of determining the health needs or desires of a population. In strategic planning, the identification of key strategic issues helps define the priorities and direction for a group or organization. In addition, issue definition is closely linked with the objective setting steps involved in developing an action plan for a program (see Chapter 9) and forms part of the foundation of an effective evaluation strategy (see Chapter 10).

Important Aspects of Community Assessment

Community (or needs) assessment was discussed in more detail in Chapter 4. In brief, a needs assessment is "a systematic set of procedures undertaken for the purpose of setting priorities and making decisions about program or organizational improvement and allocation of resources. The priorities are based on identified needs."[2] A community assessment may involve a variety of different data types, including epidemiologic (quantitative) data, qualitative information, data on health inequalities, and patterns of health resource utilization.[3]

The initial aspects of a community assessment are especially pertinent when defining an issue or problem. A typical community assessment would begin by considering sources of baseline or background data on a health problem or a community. These sources might include primary and/or secondary data. Primary data involve collection of new information for a particular program or study through such methods as a community survey, interviews, focus groups, etc. Collection of primary data often occurs over a relatively long period of time, sometimes years, although a local community assessment survey can be done in 3 to 6 months. Community assessments often rely on secondary data sources—that is, data routinely collected at a local, state, or national level. The greatest advantages of using secondary data rather than collecting primary data are time and cost. Many government, university, and nonprofit agencies spend years and many dollars collecting and maintaining data. These agencies also have the technical expertise that ensures that data are high quality. Several important sources of secondary data are readily available and are listed with their websites at the end of this chapter. One disadvantage of secondary data is that detailed local information may not be available for smaller or less populous areas. Community health assessments often use a mix of primary and secondary data. In addition to quantitative secondary data on morbidity, mortality, and health behaviors, they may make use of qualitative primary data collected via interviews or focus group methods.

Key Aspects of Strategic Planning

Strategic planning is a disciplined effort to produce decisions and actions that shape and guide what an organization is, what it does, and why it does it.[4] It is a continuous process for identifying intended future outcomes and how success will be measured, often with a 3- to 5-year time horizon. A complete discussion of strategic planning benefits and methods is available elsewhere.[4-7] Rational strategic planning is based on three deceptively simple questions: "Where are we?" "Where do we want to be?" "How do we get there?"[6] In this section, specific aspects that help shape issue definition within an evidence-based public health framework are reviewed.

   In many senses, problem definition is similar to the early steps in a strategic planning process, which often involve reaching consensus on the mission and values of the organization, analyzing the internal and external environments, involving people affected by the plan in the process, and creating a common vision for the future. As noted in Chapter 1, the public health environment is ever-changing and shaped by new science and information, policies, and social forces. In particular, the early phases of a strategic planning process often involve an environmental assessment. This assessment may include an analysis of political, economic, social, and technological (PEST) trends in the larger environment. Such an analysis is important to understand the context in which specific problems are embedded and within which they must be addressed. A TOWS analysis (identification of an organization's external Threats, Opportunities, internal Weaknesses and Strengths) is often prepared as well (Figure 5-1). The TOWS analysis brings the organization into focus and assesses the impact of external forces (threats and opportunities) in relation to the gaps and resources (weaknesses and strengths). As an issue becomes more clearly defined using the methods detailed in the next section, it is important to remember the context in which the issue is being addressed. Some of the questions and areas that may be considered early in an environmental assessment are

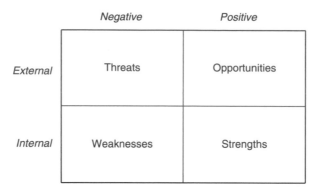

FIGURE 5-1. Components of a TOWS analysis.

shown in Table 5-1.[8] Later, when strategies are known, a comprehensive assessment of resources—financial and nonfinancial—is needed. A well-done community assessment and/or environmental analysis can increase the likelihood of asking the right questions that will later guide an evidence-based process.

DIVIDING AN ISSUE INTO ITS COMPONENT PARTS

When beginning to define an issue, several fundamental questions should be asked and answered:

• What was the basis for the initial statement of the issue? This may include the social/political/health circumstances at the time the issue was originated and how it was framed. This provides the context for the issue.

Table 5-1. Important Questions to Consider in an Environmental Analysis

Area of Interest	Questions to Consider
External assessment	Will the community accept and support addressing this issue? Are there government regulations and other legal factors affecting the issue? Have the views of each important stakeholder been taken into account? Are there other external groups addressing this issue with success or lack of success (both current and in the past)?
Internal assessment	Is this issue relevant to the mission and values of the organization? What, if anything, are we already doing to address the issue? Does the organization have the desire and ability to address this issue? Who in the agency has an interest in seeing the issue addressed? If so, how high is the priority of this issue for the organization?

Source: Adapted from Timmreck.[8]

- Who was the originator of the concern? The issue may have developed internally within a community or organization or may be set as an issue by a policy
  maker or funder.
- Should/could the issue be stated in the epidemiologic context of person (How
  many people are affected and who are they?), place (What is the geographic
  distribution of the issue?), and time (How long has this issue been a problem?
  What are anticipated changes over time?)?[9]
- Is there a consensus among stakeholders that the problem is properly stated?

This section will begin to address these and other questions that one may
encounter when developing an initial issue statement. A sound issue statement
may draw on multiple disciplines, including biostatistics, epidemiology, health
communication, health economics, health education, management, medicine,
planning, and policy analysis. An issue statement should be stated as a quantifiable question (or series of questions) leading to an analysis of root causes or likely
intervention approaches. It should also be unbiased in its anticipated course of
action. Figure 5-2 describes the progression of an issue statement along with some
of the questions that are crucial to answer. One question along the way is "Do we
need more information?" The answer to that question is nearly always yes, so the
challenge becomes where to find the most essential information efficiently. It is
also essential to remember that the initial issue statement is often the "tip of the
iceberg" and that getting to the actual causes of and solutions to the problem takes
considerable time and effort. Causal frameworks (aka analytic framework; see
Chapter 8) are often useful in mapping out an issue.

Issue Components

The four key components of an issue statement include

1. Background/epidemiologic data
2. Questions about the program or policy
3. Solutions being considered
4. Potential outcomes

Initially, each of these four components should be framed succinctly, in a max-
imum of one paragraph each. As intervention approaches are later decided upon,
these brief initial statements will be refined and expanded into more complete
protocols.

An example of the four components of an issue statement, along with potential
data sources, is presented in Table 5-2. The section on *background and epidemiologic data* generally presents what is known of the descriptive epidemiology of a
public health issue. This includes data on person, place, and time that are often

	What & how much?	What & why?	How & how much?
Issue statement component	Background/ epidemiologic data	Questions about the program or policy	Solutions being considered
Sample questions to consider	What do the data show?	What might explain the data?	Which options are under active consideration?
	Are there time trends?	Why is the problem not being addressed?	How does one gather information from stakeholders?
	Are there high-risk populations?	Are there effective (and cost-effective) interventions?	What resources are needed for various options?
	Can the data be oriented by person, place, time?	What happens if we do nothing?	What resources are available for various options?
	Is public health action warranted?	Do we need more information?	

FIGURE 5-2. A sequential framework for understanding the key steps in developing an issue statement.

Table 5-2. Examples of an Initial Issue Statement for Breast Cancer Control

Component	Example Statement/Questions	Potential Data Sources
Background/ epidemiologic data	Based on data from the BRFSS, only 83% of California women aged 50 and older are receiving mammography screening each year. Rates of screening have remained constant over the past 5 years and are lowest among lower-income women.	CDC WONDER CDC BRFSS data State vital statistics State and local surveillance reports
Questions about the program or policy	Do we understand why screening rates are lower among lower-income women? Why is this a problem? Are there examples in the scientific literature of effective programs to increase the rate of mammography screening among women? Are there similar programs targeted to lower-income women? Are there cost-effectiveness studies of these interventions? Have policies been enacted and evaluated that have had a positive impact on mammography screening rates?	MEDLINE/PubMed Professional meetings Guidelines Legislative records
Solutions being considered	Numerous solutions have been proposed, including: (1) increased funding for mammography screening among low-income women; (2) a mass media campaign to promote screening; (3) education of health care providers on how to effectively counsel women for mammography screening; and (4) a peer support program that involves the target audience in the delivery of the intervention.	Program staff Policymakers Advisory groups or coalitions Women with breast cancer
Potential outcomes	Rate of breast cancer mortality Rate of breast cancer mortality among low-income women Rate of mammography screening Cost of breast cancer treatment Rate of counseling for mammography among primary care providers	CDC WONDER CDC BRFSS data HEDIS data Hospital discharge data Program records

presented as rates or percentage changes over time. It is often useful to present a visual display of the epidemiologic data. For example, Figure 5-3 shows time trends in heart disease mortality in five countries in Europe.[10] These data show large disparities by country, where more than a threefold difference is seen in rates in Ireland compared with those in Lithuania.[10] Large gender variations are noted for important risk factors such as cigarette smoking (Figure 5-4).[11] It is often useful to examine ethnic variations in a preventable risk factor over some time period. For example, Figure 5-5 shows the large disparities by race/ethnicity in

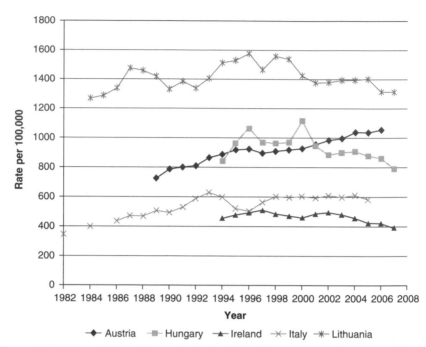

FIGURE 5-3. Ischemic heart disease deaths in selected European countries, 1982–2007.[10]

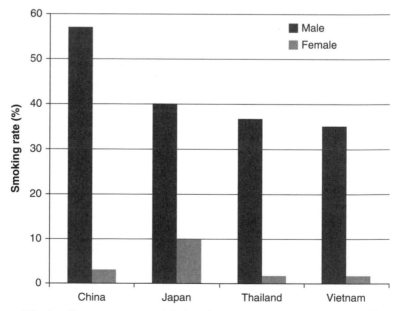

FIGURE 5-4. Smoking rates among adults in selected Asian countries, by gender.[11]

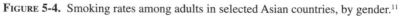

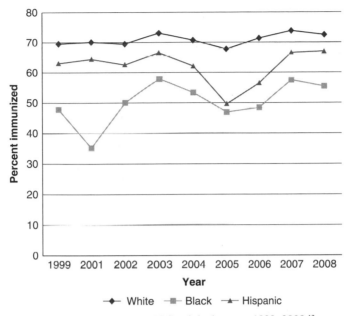

FIGURE 5-5. Immunization rates among U.S. adults by race, 1999–2008.[12]

immunization coverage in the United States.[12] If available, qualitative information may also be presented with the background statement. For example, focus group data may be available that demonstrate a particular attitude or belief toward a public health issue. The concepts presented earlier in this chapter related to community assessment are often useful in assembling background data. In all cases, it is important to specify the source of the data so that the presentation of the problem is credible.

In considering the *questions about the program or policy,* the search for effective intervention options (our Type 2 evidence) begins. You may want to undertake a strategic planning process in order to generate a set of potentially effective program options that could address the issue. The term *program* is defined broadly to encompass any organized public health action, including direct service interventions, community mobilization efforts, policy development and implementation, outbreak investigations, health communication campaigns, health promotion programs, and applied research initiatives.[9] The programmatic issue being considered may be best presented as a series of questions that a public health team will attempt to answer. It may be stated in the context of an intervention program, a health policy, cost-effectiveness, or managerial challenge. For an intervention, you might ask, "Are there effective intervention programs in the literature to address risk factor X among population Y?" A policy question would consider

"Can you document the positive effects of a health policy that was enacted and enforced in State X?" In the area of cost-effectiveness, it might be "What is the cost of intervention Z per year of life saved?"[13] And a managerial question would ask, "What are the resources needed to allow us to effectively initiate a program to address issue X?"

As the issue statement develops, it is often useful to consider *potential solutions*. However, several caveats are warranted at this early phase. First, solutions generated at this phase may or may not be evidence based, since all the information may not be in hand. Also, the program ultimately implemented is likely to differ from the potential solutions discussed at this stage. Finally, solutions noted in one population or region may or may not be generalizable to other populations (see discussion of external validity in Chapter 2). There is a natural tendency to jump too quickly to solutions before the background and programmatic focus of a particular issue is well defined. In Table 5-3, potential solutions are presented that are largely developed from the efforts of *The Guide to Community Preventive Services,* an evidence-based systematic review described in Chapter 3.[14]

When framing *potential solutions* of an issue statement, it is useful to consider whether a "high-risk" or population strategy is warranted. The high-risk strategy focuses on individuals who are most at risk for a particular disease or risk factor.[15,16] Focusing an early detection program on lower-income individuals who have the least access to screening, for example, is a high-risk approach. A population strategy is used when the risk being considered is widely disseminated across a population. A population strategy might involve conducting a mass media campaign to increase early detection among all persons at risk. In practice, these two approaches are not mutually exclusive. The *Healthy People 2020* health goals for the United States, for example, call for elimination of health disparities (a high-risk approach) and also target overall improvements in social and physical environments to promote health for all (a population approach).[17] Data and available resources can help in determining whether a population approach, a high-risk strategy, or both are warranted.

Although it may seem premature to consider *potential outcomes* before an intervention approach is decided upon, an initial scan of outcomes is often valuable at this stage. It is especially important to consider the answer to the questions, "What outcome do we want to achieve in addressing this issue? What would a good or acceptable outcome look like?" This process allows you to consider potential short- and longer-term outcomes. It also helps shape the choice of possible solutions and determines the level of resources that will be required to address the issue. For many U.S. public health issues (e.g., numerous environmental health exposures), data do not readily exist for community assessment and evaluation at a state or local level. Long-term outcomes (e.g., mortality rates) that are often available are not useful for planning and implementing programs with a time horizon of a few years.

Table 5-3. Example of an Initial Issue Statement for Influenza Vaccination among People Aged 65 Years and Older

Component	Example Statement/Questions	Potential Data Sources
Background/ epidemiologic data	Based on BRFSS data, rates of influenza immunization among people aged 65 years and older have increased nearly 16% among Blacks since 1999. Despite this increase, influenza immunization rates for Black and Hispanic adults aged 65 years and older are lower than those of Whites and below those recommended.	National Health Interview Survey US Administration on Aging State vital statistics State and local surveillance reports
Questions about the program or policy	How effective are vaccinations in reducing hospitalizations and deaths due to influenza? What are historical rates of influenza vaccination among people aged 65 years and older? Are all income and racial/ethnic groups affected equally? Are there public health interventions that have been documented to increase coverage of influenza vaccination among people aged 65 years and older?	MEDLINE Healthy People 2010, state health plans Professional meetings Guidelines Legislative records
Solutions being considered	Numerous solutions have been proposed, including: (1) educational programs for the target population; (2) client reminder/recall interventions delivered via telephone or letter; (3) home visits for socioeconomically disadvantaged populations; (4) community mass media programs; and (5) programs to expand vaccination access in health care settings.	Program staff Guidelines Policy makers Advisory groups (e.g., AARP)
Potential outcomes	Rates of immunization Rates of influenza incidence (a reportable disease) Rates of influenza vaccination among various Health Maintenance Organizations Rates of mortality due to influenza	CDC WONDER CDC BRFSS data HEDIS data Program records

A significant challenge to be discussed in later chapters is the need to identify valid and reliable intermediate outcomes for public health programs.

Importance of Stakeholder Input

As the issue definition stage continues, it is often critical to obtain the input of "stakeholders." Stakeholders, or key players, are individuals or agencies with a vested interest in the issue at hand.[18] When addressing a particular health policy, policy makers are especially important stakeholders. Stakeholders can also be individuals who would potentially receive, use, and benefit from the program or policy being considered. In particular, three groups of stakeholders are relevant[9]:

1. Those involved in program operations, such as sponsors, coalition partners, administrators, and staff
2. Those served or affected by the program, including clients, family members, neighborhood organizations, and elected officials
3. Primary users of the evaluation—people who are in a position to do or decide something regarding the program. (These individuals may overlap with the first two categories.)

Table 5-4 shows how the considerations and motivations of various stakeholders can vary.[19] These differences are important to take into account while garnering stakeholder input.

Table 5-4. Major Health Policy Considerations Among Stakeholders in the United States

Stakeholder	*Consideration*
Politicians	The cost of medical care is high and rising quickly.
	There are many uninsured Americans and many Americans are at risk for losing their insurance coverage.
	The increasing costs of the Medicaid and Medicare programs strain state and federal budgets.
	Health care providers charge too much.
	There are too many doctors (a rural politician might say the opposite) and too many specialists relative to primary care physicians.
Health-care professionals	There is an overutilization of medical services, especially in certain areas of the country; and an underutilization of some services in other areas.
	There is an increase in the "intensity" of health services, i.e., technology that results in increased costs.
	The effect of improved health services over time has been decreased death rates and increased life expectancy.
	More efficient health care delivery will reduce health care costs.
Public health advocates	The health of the American public has improved substantially as demonstrated by declining death rates and longer life expectancy.
	Major public health programs have been successful in reducing key risk factors such as cigarette smoking, control of hypertension, and dietary changes.
	There are millions of Americans who lack health care coverage.
	Environmental monitoring and control have helped decrease morbidity and mortality.
	Prevention is the cornerstone of effective health policy.
Consumers	Personal and out-of-pocket health care costs are too high.
	Quality medical care is often not provided.
	There are substantial risks to the public from "involuntary" environmental hazards such as radiation, chemicals, food additives, and occupational exposures.

Source: Adapted from Kuller.[19]

Box 5-1. Reducing Infant Mortality in Texas

For the newly hired director of the Maternal and Child Health Bureau at the U.S. Department of Health and Human Services, the issue of disparities in infant mortality rates is of high interest. You have been charged with developing a plan for reducing the rate of infant mortality. The plan must be developed within 12 months and implemented within 2 years. The data show that the infant mortality rate in the United States declined from 1995 to 2000, but the rate has not changed significantly since 2000. Furthermore, significant differences among infant mortality rates of different races continue. The rate among non-Hispanic blacks is currently 13.6% and the rate among non-Hispanic whites is currently 5.8%, a relative difference of 137%. Program staff, policy makers, and advisory groups (stakeholders) have proposed numerous intervention options, including (1) increased funding for family planning services; (2) a mass media campaign to encourage women to seek early prenatal care; and (3) global policies that are aimed at increasing health care access for pregnant women. Program personnel face a significant challenge in trying to obtain adequate stakeholder input within the time frame set by the governor. You have to decide on the method(s) for obtaining adequate and representative feedback from stakeholders in a short time frame. Some of the issues you need to consider include the following:

- The role of the government and the role of the private sector in reducing infant mortality
- The positions of various religious groups on family planning
- The key barriers facing women of various ethnic backgrounds when obtaining adequate prenatal care and
- The views of key policy makers in Texas who will decide the amount of public resources available for your program.

An example of the need for stakeholder input is given in Box 5-1. In this case, there are likely to be individuals and advocacy groups with strong feelings regarding how best to reduce infant mortality. Some of the approaches, such as increasing funding for family planning, may be controversial. As described in other parts of this book, there are several different mechanisms for gaining stakeholder input, including:

- Interviews with leaders of various voluntary and nonprofit agencies that have an interest in this issue
- Focus groups with clients who may be served by various interventions
- Newspaper content analysis of clippings that describe previous efforts to enhance health

SUMMARY

This chapter is a transition point to numerous other chapters in this book. It begins a sequential and systematic process for evidence-based decision making in public health. The extent to which a practitioner may undergo a full-fledged baseline community assessment is often dependent on time and resources (see Chapters 4 and 10). It should also be remembered that public health is a team sport, and review and refinement of an initial issue statement with one's team are essential.

Key Chapter Points

- There are multiple reasons to draft an issue statement early in an evidence-based process.
- An assessment of the external environment, based on strategic planning methods, will help in understanding the context for a program or policy.
- Breaking an issue into its component parts (background/epidemiologic data, questions about the program or policy, solutions being considered, and potential outcomes) will enhance the process.
- Input from all stakeholders is essential for informing the approaches to solving many public health problems. This can be obtained via a community assessment, which is described in the next chapter.

SUGGESTED READINGS AND SELECTED WEBSITES

Suggested Readings

Bryson JM. *Strategic Planning for Public and Nonprofit Organizations. A Guide to Strengthening and Sustaining Organizational Achievement.* San Francisco, CA: Jossey-Bass Publishers, 1995.
Fielding J, Kumanyika S. Recommendations for the concepts and form of Healthy People 2020. *Am J Prev Med.* 2009;37(3):255–257.
Rose G. *The Strategy of Preventive Medicine.* Oxford, UK: Oxford University Press, 1992.
Swayne LM, Duncan WJ, Ginter PM. *Strategic Management of Health Care Organizations.* 6th ed. West Sussex, UK: John Wiley & Sons Ltd; 2008.
Timmreck TC. *Planning, Program Development, and Evaluation. A Handbook for Health Promotion, Aging and Health Services.* 2nd ed. Boston, MA: Jones and Bartlett Publishers; 2003.

Selected Websites

Behavioral Risk Factor Surveillance System <http://www.cdc.gov/brfss/>. The Behavioral Risk Factor Surveillance System (BRFSS) is the world's largest ongoing telephone health survey system, tracking health conditions and risk behaviors in the United States yearly since 1984. Currently, data are collected in all 50 states, the District of Columbia, and three U.S. territories. The Centers for Disease Control and Prevention (CDC) has developed a standard core questionnaire so that data can be compared across various strata. The Selected Metropolitan/Micropolitan Area Risk Trends (SMART) project provides localized data for selected areas. BRFSS data are used to identify emerging health problems, establish and track health objectives, and develop and evaluate public health policies and programs.

CDC Wonder <http://wonder.cdc.gov>. CDC WONDER is an easy-to-use system that provides a single point of access to a wide variety of CDC reports, guidelines, and numeric public health data. It can be valuable in public health research, decision making, priority setting, program evaluation, and resource allocation.

The Community Health Status Indicators (CHSI) Project <http://community-health.hhs.gov/>. The Community Health Status Indicators (CHSI) Project includes 3141 county health status profiles representing each county in the United States excluding territories. Each CHSI report includes data on access and utilization of health care services, birth and death measures, *Healthy People 2010* targets, and U.S. birth and death rates, vulnerable populations, risk factors for premature deaths, communicable diseases, and environmental health. The goal of CHSI is to give local public health agencies another tool for improving their community's health by identifying resources and setting priorities.

European Health for All Database <http://www.euro.who.int/HFADB>. The European Health for All Database (HFA-DB) has been a key source of information on health in the European Region since the World Health Organization (WHO)/Europe launched it in the mid-1980s. It contains time series from 1970. HFA-DB is updated biannually and contains about 600 indicators for the 53 Member States in the Region. The indicators cover basic demographics, health status (mortality, morbidity), health determinants (such as lifestyle and environment), and health care (resources and utilization).

Partners in Information Access for the Public Health Workforce <http://phpartners.org/>. Partners in Information Access for the Public Health Workforce is a collaboration of U.S. government agencies, public health organizations, and health sciences libraries that provides timely, convenient access to selected public health resources on the Internet.

Partnership for Prevention <http://www.prevent.org/>. Working to emphasize disease prevention and health promotion in national policy and practice, Partnership for Prevention is a membership association of businesses, nonprofit organizations, and government agencies. The site includes action guides that translate several of the *Community Guide* recommendations into easy-to-follow implementation guidelines.

WHO Statistical Information System <http://www.who.int/whosis/en/>. WHOSIS, the WHO Statistical Information System, is an interactive database bringing together core health statistics for the 193 WHO Member States. It comprises more than 100 indicators, which can be accessed by way of a quick search, by major categories, or through user-defined tables. The data can be further filtered, tabulated, charted, and downloaded.

REFERENCES

1. Straus SE, Richardson WS, Glasziou P, et al. *Evidence-Based Medicine. How to Practice and Teach EBM.* 3rd ed. Edinburgh, UK: Churchill Livingstone; 2005.
2. Witkin BR, Altschuld JW. *Conducting and Planning Needs Assessments. A Practical Guide.* Thousand Oaks, CA: Sage Publications; 1995.
3. Wright J, Williams R, Wilkinson JR. Development and importance of health needs assessment. *BMJ.* 1998;316(7140):1310–1313.
4. Bryson JM. *Strategic Planning for Public and Nonprofit Organizations. A Guide to Strengthening and Sustaining Organizational Achievement.* San Francisco, CA: Jossey-Bass Publishers; 1995.
5. Ginter PM, Duncan WJ, Capper SA. Keeping strategic thinking in strategic planning: macro-environmental analysis in a state health department of public health. *Public Health.* 1992;106:253–269.
6. Hadridge P. Strategic approaches to planning health care. In: Pencheon D, Guest C, Melzer D, Muir Gray JA, eds. *Oxford Handbook of Public Health Practice.* Oxford, UK: Oxford University Press; 2001:342–347.
7. Swayne LM, Duncan WJ, Ginter PM. *Strategic Management of Health Care Organizations.* 6th ed. West Sussex, UK: John Wiley & Sons Ltd; 2008.
8. Timmreck TC. *Planning, Program Development, and Evaluation. A Handbook for Health Promotion, Aging and Health Services.* 2nd ed. Boston, MA: Jones and Bartlett Publishers; 2003.
9. Centers for Disease Control and Prevention. Framework for program evaluation in public health. *MMWR.* 1999;48(RR-11):1–40.
10. World Health Organization Regional Office for Europe. European Health for All database http://www.euro.who.int/HFADB.
11. World Health Organization. *WHO Report on the Global Tobacco Epidemic, 2009.* Geneva: WHO; 2009.
12. Centers for Disease Control and Prevention. Behavioral Risk Factor Surveillance System website. 2010. http://www.cdc.gov/nccdphp/brfss/
13. Tengs TO, Adams ME, Pliskin JS, et al. Five-hundred life-saving interventions and their cost-effectiveness. *Risk Anal.* 1995;15(3):369–390.
14. Zaza S, Briss PA, Harris KW, eds. *The Guide to Community Preventive Services: What Works to Promote Health?* New York, NY: Oxford University Press; 2005.
15. Rose G. Sick individuals and sick populations. *Int J Epidemiol.* 1985;14(1):32–38.
16. Rose G. *The Strategy of Preventive Medicine.* Oxford, UK: Oxford University Press; 1992.
17. Fielding J, Kumanyika S. Recommendations for the concepts and form of Healthy People 2020. *Am J Prev Med.* 2009;37(3):255–257.
18. Soriano FI. *Conducting Needs Assessments. A Multdisciplinary Approach.* Thousand Oaks, CA: Sage Publications; 1995.
19. Kuller LH. Epidemiology and health policy. *Am J Epidemiol.* 1988;127(1):2–16.

6

Quantifying the Issue

> Everything that can be counted does not necessarily count; everything that counts cannot necessarily be counted.
>
> —Albert Einstein

As discussed in Chapter 4, the community assessment should include the health condition or risk factor being considered, the population affected, the size and scope of the problem, prevention opportunities, and potential stakeholders. This task requires basic epidemiologic skills to obtain additional information about the frequency of the health condition or risk factor in an affected population. For example, if there is concern about *excess disease* (a term that will be used as a generic synonym for any health condition or risk factor in this chapter) in a population, we should determine the parameters that define the population at risk. Should we focus on the total population, or restrict the population to males or females of certain ages? Once the population is defined, we must estimate the frequency of disease present in the population. Can we determine the number of diseased persons from existing public health surveillance systems, or must we conduct a special survey of the defined population? Once disease rates are computed, do we see any patterns of disease that identify or confirm subgroups within the defined population that have the highest disease rates? Finally, can we use this information to develop and evaluate the effectiveness of new public health programs and policies?

This chapter provides an overview of the principles of epidemiology that relate to public health practice. It focuses primarily on methods used to measure and characterize disease frequency in defined populations. It includes information about public health surveillance systems and currently available data sources via the Internet. It also provides an overview of the methods used to evaluate the effectiveness of new public health programs that are designed to reduce the prevalence of risk factors and the disease burden in target populations.

OVERVIEW OF DESCRIPTIVE EPIDEMIOLOGY

Epidemiology is commonly defined as the study of the distribution and determinants of disease frequency in human populations and the application of this study to control health problems.[1] In a more comprehensive definition relevant to public health practice, Terris[2] stated that *epidemiology* is the study of the health of human populations for the following purposes:

1. To discover the agent, host, and environmental factors that affect health, in order to provide a scientific basis for the prevention of disease and injury and the promotion of health
2. To determine the relative importance of causes of illness, disability, and death, in order to establish priorities for research and action
3. To identify those sections of the population that have the greater risk from specific causes of ill health, in order to direct the indicated action appropriately
4. To evaluate the effectiveness of health programs and services in improving the health of the population

The first two functions provide etiologic (or Type 1) evidence to support causal associations between modifiable and nonmodifiable risk factors and specific diseases, as well as the relative importance of these risk factors when establishing priorities for public health interventions. The third function focuses on the frequency of disease in a defined population and the subgroups within the population to be targeted with public health programs. The last function provides experimental (or Type 2) evidence that supports the relative effectiveness of specific public health interventions to address a particular disease.

The terms *descriptive epidemiology* and *analytic epidemiology* are commonly used when presenting the principles of epidemiology. Descriptive epidemiology encompasses methods for measuring the frequency of disease in defined populations. These methods can be used to compare the frequency of disease within and between populations in order to identify subgroups with the highest frequency of disease and to observe any changes that have occurred over time. Analytic epidemiology focuses on identifying essential factors that influence the prevention, occurrence, control, and outcome of disease. Methods used in analytic epidemiology are necessary for identifying new risk factors for specific diseases and for evaluating the effectiveness of new public health programs designed to reduce the disease risk for target populations.

Estimating Disease Frequency

One way to measure disease frequency is to count the number of diseased persons in a defined population and to report that number of cases. Often newspaper articles from a city will compare the current year's number of cases of sexually transmitted diseases with the number from last year. Yet this case count is not informative for understanding the dynamics of disorder in a population. A much better method is to estimate the rate of disease in a defined population over time. The rate is computed by dividing the number of persons with the disease of interest by the number of persons at risk of developing the disease during a specified period. For example, 6,490 Texas residents were diagnosed with colon cancer. Thus, the colon cancer rate equals 6,490 cases divided by 22,928,508 people residing in Texas on July 1, 2005 (or the midpoint of the year). The rate is 0.00028 colon cancer per person, or 28 colon cancers per 100,000 people per year. Here, we use data from the Centers for Disease Control and Prevention (CDC) WONDER's cancer incidence database to identify colon cancers that occurred among people residing in Texas during 2005 and data from the U.S. Census Bureau to estimate the number of people residing in Texas on July 1, 2005.

Although a disease rate represents the number of cases of disease that occur in the population during a specified period, in estimating a denominator, it is very difficult to follow each person in the population for the same amount of time over long periods. Therefore, a more precise way of dealing with persons who move in or out of the population during the study period is to estimate "person-time" for the population at risk, or the amount of time that each person in the population is free from disease during the study period. In our example, every person residing in Texas from January 1 to December 31, 2005, contributes 1 person-year if she or he is not diagnosed with colon cancer during the study period. Each person diagnosed with colon cancer during the study period, who moves from the state, or whose colon cancer status is unknown contributes a fraction of a person-year, based on the amount of time that elapsed from January 1, 2005, to the date of diagnosis or departure from the study population, respectively. The sum of every person's person-time contribution equals the total number of person-years for this population during the 1-year study period. If we are unable to determine the amount of person-time for each person in the study population, the total person-years (22,928,508 person-years) can be estimated by multiplying the average size of the population at the mid-point of the study period by the duration of the study period. In our example just given, this is the number of people in the state at the midpoint of the year (22,928,508) multiplied by the duration of the study period (1 year). Disease rates calculated in this fashion measure the occurrence, or incidence, of disease in the population at risk.

This incidence rate should be contrasted with the prevalence rate, which captures the number of existing cases of disease among surviving members of the population. Prevalence provides essential information when planning health services for the total number of persons who are living with the disease in the community, whereas incidence reflects the true rate of disease occurrence in the same population.

Planning for public health services requires a good grasp of the prevalence of the condition in the population, to properly plan for needed personnel and supplies.

Although incidence rates are ideal for measuring the occurrence of disease in a population for a specified period, they are often not available. In this case, it may be prudent to use cause-specific mortality rates based on the number of deaths from the disease of interest that occurs in the population during the same study period. Mortality rates are often used in lieu of incidence rates but are only reasonable surrogate measures when the disease is highly fatal. Of course, mortality rates are more appropriate if the goal is to reduce mortality among populations where screening programs can identify early stages of diseases, such as breast cancer or HIV infection, or where public health programs can reduce the mortality risk for other conditions, such as sudden infant death syndrome or alcohol-related motor vehicle accidents.

Using Intermediate Endpoints

Although incidence or mortality rates can be used to evaluate the effectiveness of public health programs, it may not be feasible to wait years to see these effects. On a population basis, these end point outcomes actually may be somewhat rare. Instead, the focus should be on identifying and using intermediate or "upstream" measures as long as there is sufficient Type 1 evidence supporting the relationship between changes in behavior and disease reduction in target populations.[3] If the goal is to reduce breast cancer mortality, then an appropriate intermediate measure is the percentage of women 50 years of age or older who are screened annually for breast cancer. There is sufficient Type 1 evidence to show that mammography screening reduces the risk of breast cancer mortality among women 50 to 69 years of age, recently confirmed in a U.S. Preventive Services Task Force recommendation.[4] Hence, programs designed to increase annual mammography screening rates in a community should reduce breast cancer mortality rates in the long term by providing women, screened and diagnosed with early-stage breast cancer, with more effective treatment options.

Other examples of intermediate measures are the percentage of residents in a community who choose not to smoke cigarettes (to reduce lung cancer risk), who exercise regularly (to reduce cardiovascular disease risk), or who practice safer sex (to reduce HIV infection risk). Furthermore, such measures as changes in knowledge, attitudes, or intentions to change behavior may be very useful for determining the perceived health risk in the general population and whether perceptions differ within subgroups of the population.

Intermediate measures are not readily available for many populations. However, the Behavioral Risk Factor Surveillance System (BRFSS), which provides prevalence data for health behaviors at a national and a state level, is a data source that contains intermediate indicators. Most recently, the *MMWR (Morbidity and Mortality Weekly Report)* reported on county-level prevalence of diabetes and obesity, describing the most high-risk U.S. counties in 2007 as concentrated in the south and Appalachian regions.[5] These rates are based on random samples of residents from each state who complete telephone-based questionnaires each year. For example, we know from this survey that among those interviewed during 2008, 71% of Wyoming women 50 years of age or older reported having a mammogram within the past 2 years. This percentage alone, or combined with that of subsequent years, can be used to establish a baseline rate and to monitor the frequency of annual mammography screening for any new public health program designed to increase annual mammography screening rates in this population.

Estimating Disease Frequency for Smaller Populations

Disease rates can be estimated if all cases of disease can be enumerated for the population at risk during a specified period and the size of the population at risk (or amount of person-time) can be determined. In many countries, disease rates are routinely computed using birth and death certificate data because existing surveillance systems provide complete enumeration of these events. Although disease rates are commonly computed using national and state data, estimating similar rates for smaller geographically or demographically defined populations may be problematic. The main concern is the reliability of disease rates when there are too few cases of disease occurring in the population. As an example, the U.S. National Center for Health Statistics will not publish or release rates based on fewer than 20 observations. The rationale behind this practice can be illustrated by examining the relative standard error based on various sample sizes, with rates based on fewer than 20 cases or deaths being very unreliable (Figure 6-1). The relative standard error is the standard error as a percentage of the measure itself.

Several approaches may prove useful to achieve greater representation of "low-frequency populations" such as recent immigrants or minority populations.[6] These strategies may be related to sampling (e.g., expand the study or observation period by using multiple years to increase the number of cases of disease and person-time units for the target population). Analytic strategies may also be useful, such as aggregating data in a smaller geographical area over several years. Alternate field methods may also be useful (e.g., door-to-door surveys that might increase response rates). Sometimes "synthetic" estimates are useful. These estimates can be generated by using rates from larger geographic regions to estimate the number of cases of disease for smaller populations. For example, the number of cigarette smokers in a particular county can be estimated by multiplying the statewide

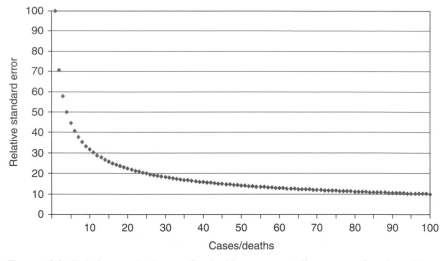

FIGURE 6-1. Relative standard error of an incidence or mortality rate as a function of the number of cases or deaths.
(*Source:* New York State Department of Health.)

smoking rate by the number of persons residing in the county. The CDC uses this approach in its smoking-attributable morbidity, mortality, and economic costs (SAMMEC) calculations. The methodology for calculating this statistic is provided by the CDC.[7] This approach was recently used in *MMWR* to characterize state-specific smoking-attributable mortality and years of life lost for the years 2000 through 2004.[8]

Rosen and colleagues[9] provided guidance for analyzing regional data that take into account seven factors: (1) when available, the importance of the health problem for a community; (2) the regional pattern of the descriptive data; (3) the (tested or anticipated) quality of the data; (4) the consistency of the data with other health indicators; (5) the consistency of the data with known risk factors; (6) trends in the data; and (7) the consistency of the data with other independent studies and with the experiences of local health personnel. Using several of these principles, researchers were able to analyze national data from Sweden over a 35-year time period to determine that patients with cancer have a greater risk for committing suicide than the general population.[10] The approach also showed that alcohol-related mortality among men in a specific county in Sweden was lower but increasing faster than the national rate. Their step-by-step analysis dealt with many problems that are crucial in regional health analysis by looking closely at the quality of the data for their analysis and by examining trends using other factors associated with alcohol-related mortality.

CHARACTERIZING THE ISSUE BY PERSON, PLACE, AND TIME

Stratifying Rates by Person

Rates are routinely computed for specific diseases using data from public health surveillance systems. These rates, if computed for the total population, such as state or county populations, are crude (or unadjusted) rates because they represent the actual frequency of disease in the defined population for a specified period. Category-specific rates, which are "crude rates" for subgroups of the defined population, provide more information than do crude rates about the patterns of disease. Category-specific rates are commonly used to characterize disease frequency by person, place, and time for a defined population (see example in Box 6-1[11,12]). In most public health surveillance systems, demographic variables (e.g., age, sex, and race/ethnicity) are routinely collected for all members of the defined population. Some surveillance systems (e.g., BRFSS) also collect other demographic characteristics, including years of formal education, income level, and health insurance status.

Using category-specific rates to look at disease patterns will identify subgroups within the population with the highest disease rates, permitting hypotheses about why the rates may be higher for some subgroups. For example, age-adjusted breast

---

Box 6-1. Suicide Rates by Person, Place, and Time

In 2006, suicide was the 11th leading cause of death in the United States. There were almost twice as many deaths due to suicide as homicide (33,300 versus 18,573 deaths).[11] Overall, the crude suicide rate was 11.1 deaths per 100,000 population. Suicide rates by person, place, and time revealed the following trends:

- Suicide rates were highest for people who were 45 to 54 years old (17.2/100,000) followed by those who were older than 75 years (15.9/100,000).
- Age-adjusted suicide rates were four times higher for males (18.0/100,000) than for females (4.5/100,000), although females are more likely to attempt suicide.
- Age-adjusted suicide rates for whites (12.1/100,000) and Native Americans (11.6/100,000) were twice as high as for other race/ethnicity groups.
- Age-adjusted suicide rates were highest in the Western census region (12.2/100,000) and lowest in the Northeastern census region (8.3/100,000).
- Age-adjusted suicide rates have been declining sporadically from 13.2 deaths per 100,000 in 1950 to 10.9 deaths per 100,000 in 2006.
- Over half of all suicides in 2005 were committed with a firearm.[12]

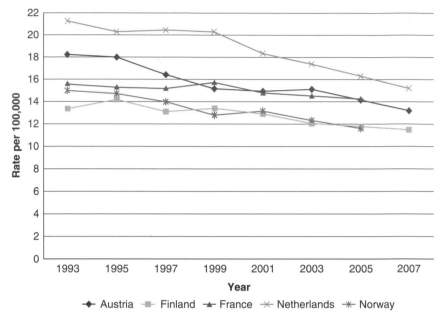

FIGURE 6-2. Age-adjusted breast cancer mortality rates for selected European countries.

cancer mortality rates for selected European countries are shown in Figure 6-2. Despite universal health care systems in all of these countries, they do show differences in mortality rates. All five countries show improvement in rates between 1993 and 2007, while Finland and Norway have achieved quite low rates. The Netherlands had a higher death rate at the beginning of the observational window and improved, and has the highest overall rate in 2007. Further uncovering of evidence may reveal differences in baseline demographic characteristics, prevention program differences, or health care access and organization of medical services.

Stratifying Rates by Place

Category-specific rates are often computed to show patterns of disease by place of residence for the defined population. This information is routinely collected in most public health surveillance systems and can be used to identify areas with the highest disease rates. Figure 6-3 shows breast cancer mortality rates by Missouri County, data that provide useful information for determining whether to implement new breast cancer mortality reduction programs statewide or selectively in those counties where the mortality rates are highest, rather than statewide. For larger metropolitan areas, ZIP codes, census tracts, and neighborhoods can be used to stratify disease rates geographically if the number of diseased persons and

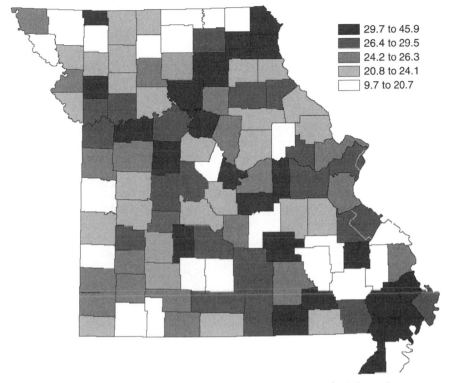

FIGURE 6-3. Age-adjusted breast cancer mortality rates by county for Missouri women, 1997–2007.
(*Source:* New York State Department of Health.)

the size of the defined population are large enough to provide precise rates. This may provide additional information to pinpoint areas where HIV infection, homicide, or infant mortality rates are highest for a community. Other important variables, such as population density and migration patterns, can also be used to stratify disease rates but are not usually collected in public health surveillance systems.

Stratifying Rates by Time

Category-specific rates, based on data from public health surveillance systems, are routinely reported each year. Looking at rates over time may reveal significant changes that have occurred in the population as the result of public health programs, changes in health care policies, or other events. Figure 6-4 shows age adjusted breast cancer incidence and mortality rates for white and African American women in the United States for 1975 through 2005.[13] An overall decrease in mortality in both groups of women is observed, with higher mortality

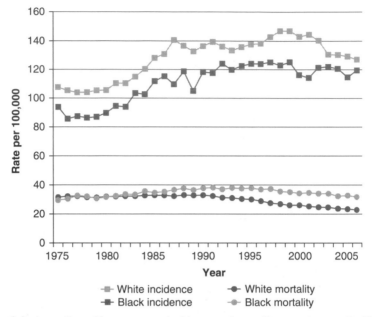

FIGURE 6-4. Age-adjusted breast cancer incidence and mortality rates by year for U.S. women, 1975–2006.

among African American women. Socioeconomic disparities have increased in mammography screening.[14]

Although not often computed, disease rates by birth cohort are another way of looking at patterns of disease over time. In Figure 6-5, the lung cancer mortality rate for all men in the United States appears to increase with age, except for those 85 years or older. However, age-specific lung cancer mortality rates are higher for younger birth cohorts. For example, the lung cancer mortality rate for 65- to 74-year-old men is approximately 200 deaths per 100,000 men for those born between 1896 and 1905. The mortality rate for the same age group continues to increase in subsequent birth cohorts, with the highest rate of approximately 430 deaths per 100,000 for the cohort born between 1916 and 1925. The most logical explanation for this pattern is differences in cumulative lifetime exposure to cigarette smoke seen in the birth cohorts that are represented in this population during 2000. In other words, members of the population born after 1905 were more likely to smoke cigarettes and to smoke for longer periods than were those born prior to 1905. Hence, the increasing age-specific lung cancer mortality rates reflect the increasing prevalence of cigarette smokers in the population for subsequent birth cohorts. An example of cohort effect is clearer for the generations shown because of the marked historic change in smoking patterns. At the present time, with increased

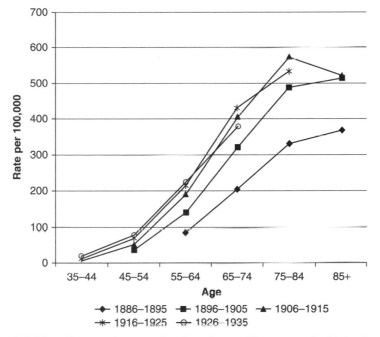

FIGURE 6-5. Mortality rates due to trachea, bronchus, and lung cancer by birth cohort for United States men. The heavy line represents age-specific mortality rates for 2000. Dashed lines represent age-specific rates for birth cohorts denoted by labels in boxes.

awareness of the dangers of smoking, the prevalence of smoking is declining, but these changes will not manifest themselves in present age cohorts for some time.

Adjusting Rates

Although category-specific rates are commonly used to characterize patterns of disease for defined populations, it is sometimes necessary to adjust rates. Crude rates are often adjusted when the objective is to compare the disease rates between populations or within the same population over time. Rate adjustment is a technique for "removing" the effects of age (or any other factor) from crude rates so as to allow meaningful comparisons across populations with different age structures or distributions. For example, comparing the crude bronchus and lung cancer mortality rate in Florida (70 deaths per 100,000 persons) with that of Alaska (32 deaths per 100,000 persons) for the years 1999 through 2006 is misleading, because the relatively older population in Florida will lead to a higher crude death rate, even if the age-specific bronchus and lung cancer mortality rates in Florida and Alaska are similar. For such a comparison, age-adjusted rates are preferable.

Table 6-1. Direct Adjustment of Lung Cancer Mortality Rates for Florida and Alaska Residents (1999–2006)

Age (yr)	FLORIDA			ALASKA		
	Lung Cancer Mortality Rate/ 100,000	2000 Standard U.S. Population	Expected Number of Deaths	Lung Cancer Mortality Rate/ 100,000	2000 Standard U.S. Population	Expected Number of Deaths
<5	0.0	110,589	0.0	0.0	110,589	0.0
5–14	0.0	145,565	0.0	0.0	145,565	0.0
15–24	0.1	138,646	0.1	0.0	138,646	0.0
25–34	0.4	135,573	5.4	0.0	135,573	0.0
35–44	6.6	162,613	10.7	3.7	162,613	6.0
45–54	36.9	134,834	49.8	23.4	134,834	31.6
55–64	119.8	87,247	104.5	90.1	87,247	78.6
65–74	259.6	66,037	171.4	277.7	66,037	183.4
75–84	354.1	44,842	158.8	414.2	44,842	185.7
85+	316.8	15,508	49.1	306.7	15,508	47.6
Total		1,000,000	549.8		1,000,000	532.9

Age-adjusted lung cancer mortality rate for Florida residents = 549.8 deaths/1,000,000 persons = 55 deaths/100,000 persons.

Age-adjusted lung cancer mortality rate for Alaska residents = 532.9 deaths/1,000,000 persons = 53 deaths/100,000 persons.

The calculations required to compute age-adjusted rates are reasonably straightforward (Table 6-1). First, age-specific bronchus/lung cancer mortality rates are generated for each state. Second, the age-specific bronchus/lung cancer mortality rates for each state are multiplied by the number of persons in the corresponding age groups from the 2000 U.S. standard population (which have been prorated to equal 1,000,000). This produces the number of "expected" deaths in each age group if the numbers of persons at risk of dying in each age group were the same for the state and U.S. populations. The total number of expected deaths in each state is then divided by the total number of persons in the United States standard population to compute the age-adjusted bronchus/lung cancer mortality rate for Florida (55 deaths per 100,000) and Alaska (53 deaths per 100,000) residents.

PUBLIC HEALTH SURVEILLANCE SYSTEMS

A tried and true public health adage is "what gets measured, gets done."[15] This measurement often begins with public health surveillance—the ongoing systematic collection, analysis, interpretation, and dissemination of health data for the purpose of preventing and controlling disease, injury, and other health problems.[16] Surveillance systems are maintained at federal, state, and local levels and can be used to estimate the frequency of diseases and other health conditions for defined populations. At least five major purposes for surveillance systems can be described: (1) assessing health and monitoring health status and health risks; (2) following disease-specific events and trends; (3) planning, implementing, monitoring, and evaluating health programs and policies; (4) conducting financial management and monitoring information; and (5) conducting public health research.[17] The few surveillance systems that currently exist can provide information on births, deaths, infectious diseases, cancers, birth defects, and health behaviors. Each system usually contains sufficient information to estimate prevalence or incidence rates and to describe the frequency of diseases or health condition by person, place, and time. Although data from surveillance systems can be used to obtain baseline and follow-up measurements for target populations, there may be limitations when using the data to evaluate intervention effectiveness for narrowly defined populations. In this case, it may be necessary to estimate the frequency of disease or other health condition for the target population by using special surveys or one of the study designs described later in this chapter.

Vital Statistics

Vital statistics are based on data from birth and death certificates and are used to monitor disease patterns within and across defined populations. Birth certificates include information about maternal/paternal/newborn demographics, lifestyle exposures during pregnancy, medical history, obstetric procedures, and labor/delivery complications for all live births. Fetal death certificates include the same data, in addition to the cause of death, for all fetal deaths that exceed a minimum gestational age and/or birth weight. The data collected on birth and fetal death certificates are similar for many states and territories since the design of the certificates were modified, based on standard federal recommendations issued in 1989. The reliability of the data has also improved since changing from a "write in" to a "check box" format, although some variables are more reliable than others. Birth-related outcomes—maternal smoking, preterm delivery, and fetal death rates—are routinely monitored, using data from birth and fetal death certificates.

Like birth certificates, death certificates provide complete enumeration of all events in a defined population. Death certificates include demographic and cause-of-death data that are used to compute disease and injury-specific mortality rates. Mortality rates can be estimated for local populations if the number of deaths and the size of the defined population are large enough to provide precise rates. Birth and death certificates are generated locally and maintained at state health departments. Data from birth and death certificates are analyzed at state and national levels and electronically stored at state health departments, and the National Center for Health Statistics. Country–specific mortality data are also available in data systems such as the European Health for All database, maintained by the World Health Organization.[18]

Reportable Diseases

In addition to vital statistics, all states and territories mandate the reporting of some diseases. Although the type of reportable diseases may differ by state or territory, they usually include specific childhood, food-borne, sexually transmitted, and other infectious diseases. These diseases are reported by physicians and other health care providers to local public health authorities and are monitored for early signs of epidemics in the community. The data are maintained by local and state health departments and are submitted weekly to the CDC for national surveillance and reporting. Disease frequencies are stratified by age, gender, race/ethnicity, and place of residence and reported routinely in *MMWR*. However, reporting is influenced by disease severity, availability of public health measures, public concern, ease of reporting, and physician appreciation of public health practice in the community.[17,19]

Registries

Disease registries routinely monitor defined populations, thereby providing very reliable estimates of disease frequency. All 50 states have active cancer registries supported by the state or federal government. These registries provide data that can be used to compute site-specific cancer incidence rates for a community, if the number of cancers and the size of the defined population are large enough to provide precise rates. Since 1973, the federally sponsored Cancer Surveillance, Epidemiology and End Results (SEER) program has provided estimates of national cancer rates based on 10% to 15% of the total population.[20] Along with state-based cancer registries, this surveillance system can provide rates for specific types of cancer, characterized by person, place, and time. All invasive cancers that occur among the state's residents are confirmed pathologically and recorded electronically for surveillance and research purposes. They are also linked with death certificates to provide additional information about disease-specific survival rates.

In 1998, the U.S. Congress passed the Birth Defects Prevention Act that authorized CDC to collect, analyze, and make available data on birth defects; operate regional centers for applied epidemiologic research on the prevention of birth defects; and inform and educate the public about the prevention of birth defects. Subsequently, CDC awarded cooperative agreements to specific states to address major problems that hinder the surveillance of birth defects and the use of data for prevention and intervention programs. The states were awarded funding to initiate new surveillance systems where none now exist, to support new systems, or to improve existing surveillance systems. Birth defects registries are either active or passive reporting surveillance systems designed to identify birth defects diagnosed for all stillborn and live-born infants. Active reporting surveillance systems provide more reliable estimates of the prevalence of specific birth defects, if staff and resources are available to search medical records from hospitals, laboratories, and other medical sources for all diagnosed birth defects in a defined population. Passive reporting surveillance systems are designed to estimate the prevalence of birth defects that can be identified using computer algorithms to link and search birth certificates, death certificates, patient abstract systems, and other readily available electronic databases.

Surveys

There are several federally sponsored surveys, including the National Health Interview Survey (NHIS), National Health and Nutrition Examination Survey (NHANES), and BRFSS, that have been designed to monitor the nation's health. These surveys are designed to measure numerous health indices, including acute and chronic diseases, injuries, disabilities, and other health-related outcomes. Some surveys are ongoing annual surveillance systems, while others are conducted periodically. These surveys usually provide prevalence estimates for specific diseases among adults and children in the United States. Although the surveys can also provide prevalence estimates for regions and individual states, they cannot currently be used to produce estimates for smaller geographically defined populations.

USE OF THE INTERNET AND OTHER READILY AVAILABLE TOOLS

Some data sources and tools are readily available on the Internet and can be used to estimate baseline and follow-up rates for needs assessment and for evaluating the effectiveness of new public health interventions. The data from some national and state-based public health surveillance systems can be obtained online or from reports from websites maintained by the sponsoring agencies. Examples are provided at the end of this chapter under "Selected Websites."

OVERVIEW OF DESIGNS IN ANALYTIC EPIDEMIOLOGY

As stated earlier, descriptive epidemiology provides information about the patterns of disease within defined populations that can be used to generate etiologic or intervention-based hypotheses. These hypotheses can be evaluated using study designs and analytic methods that encompass the principles of analytic epidemiology. Most study designs can be used to provide Type 1 evidence to support causal associations between modifiable (and nonmodifiable) risk factors and specific diseases. Once there is sufficient Type 1 evidence, additional work is needed to determine the effectiveness of public health programs designed to reduce the prevalence of these risk factors in the population. Experimental and quasi-experimental study designs are generally used, depending upon available resources and timing, to evaluate the effectiveness of new public health programs. Issues related to program and policy evaluation are also covered in Chapter 10.

Experimental Study Designs

Experimental study designs provide the most convincing evidence that new public health programs are effective. If study participants are randomized into groups (or arms), the study design is commonly called a randomized controlled trial. When two groups are created, the study participants allocated randomly to one group are given the new intervention (or treatment) and those allocated to the other group serve as controls. The study participants in both groups are followed prospectively, and disease (or health-related outcome) rates are computed for each group at the end of the observation period. Because both groups are identical in all aspects, except for the intervention, a lower disease rate in the intervention group implies that the intervention is effective.

The same study design can also be used to randomize groups instead of individuals to evaluate the effectiveness of health behavior interventions for communities. Referred to as a group-randomized trial, groups of study participants, such as schools within a school system or communities within a state, are randomized to receive the intervention or to serve as controls for the study. Initially, the groups may be paired, based on similar characteristics. Then, each group within each pair is allocated randomly to the intervention or control group. This helps to balance the distribution of characteristics of the study participants for both study groups and to reduce potential study bias. The intervention is applied to all individuals in the intervention group, and withheld or delayed for the control group. Measurements are taken at baseline and at the end of the observation period to determine if there are significant differences between the disease rates for the intervention and control groups. The group-randomized design has been used to evaluate the effectiveness of public health interventions designed to increase immunization coverage, reduce tobacco use, and increase physical activity.[21]

Quasi-Experimental Study Designs

Experimental study designs are considered the gold standard, because randomization of study participants reduces the potential for study bias. However, it is not always feasible to use this study design when evaluating new public health programs. This is particularly challenging for policy evaluation, where it is often impossible to randomize the exposure.[22] Often, quasi-experimental study designs are used to evaluate the effectiveness of new programs. Quasi-experimental studies are identical in design to experimental studies, except that the study participants are not allocated randomly to the intervention or control group. Study participants in each group are followed for a predetermined period, and outcomes (e.g., disease rates, behavioral risk factors) are computed for each group to determine if the intervention is effective. As is the case for experimental study designs, baseline (or preintervention) measurements are crucial because the investigator must determine how similar the intervention and control groups are prior to the intervention. Ideally, outcomes should be identical at baseline and for the period prior to the execution of the study. Examining the characteristics of the study groups by person, place, and time will reduce the probability of concluding that the intervention is effective when actually there are other factors historically affecting the risk factors in the community.

If a comparable control group is not available, quasi-experimental study designs can still be used to measure the impact of public health interventions on a particular health outcome in the same population. Actually, quasi-experimental study designs are commonly used when comparing new public health initiatives that affect the total population.

Reichardt and Mark[23] have described four prototypical quasi-experimental study designs: (1) before-after; (2) interrupted time-series; (3) nonequivalent group; and (4) regression-discontinuity designs. Each of these designs can be altered with a variety of design features to make them more complex (e.g., multiple control groups, variations in treatments, multiple outcome variables).[23,24] In a before-after design, a participant is measured before (pretest) and after a treatment (posttest) is introduced. The treatment effect is the difference between pretest and posttest. The interrupted time-series design is an extension of the before-after approach in that it adds further measurements over time. The outcome of interest is measured at multiple points before and after a treatment is introduced (see example in Box 6-2[25-27]and Figure 6-6). In nonequivalent group designs, comparisons are made among participants who receive different treatments but have

Box 6-2. *Back to Sleep* Campaign

Well before the American Academy of Pediatrics recommended in 1992 placing healthy infants
on their backs or sides for sleeping, there was a rich history of international research findings
to demonstrate that a change was necessary. In particular, case-control studies in the United
Kingdom in 1990 and in New Zealand in 1991 were strongly persuasive and broad consensus
was attained.[26] Following the Academy's recommendation, a nationwide public health
intervention was begun in 1994, referred to as the *Back to Sleep* campaign, aimed at changing
what were customary practices of having infants sleep on their stomachs. Further research in
Washington State showed that risk factors for patterns of high-risk sleep position could be
identified and revealed that programs aimed at changing behaviors needed to be tuned, for
example, to maternal race and ethnicity, country of residence and parity.[27] An annual national
telephone survey has monitored more recent trends and factors associated with sleeping position
from 1993 up to 2007 and reports that significant progress has been made. There has been a
highly significant decrease in prone sleep and a highly significant increase in supine sleep, with
race no longer a statistically significant predictor of sleep position. Since 1993, these authors
report that adjusted odds ratios of having infants sleep in the supine position have increased
over five-fold. Still, there are racial disparities in the adoption of supine sleep position with
whites adopting at the highest rates and African Americans adopting at lower rates.[25] The SIDS
death rates (shown in Figure 6-6) reflect these changes in infant sleep position, with the rate of
0.78 death per 1000 births in 1996 falling to 0.54 death per 1000 births in 2005.

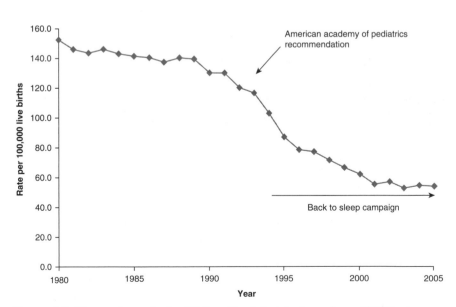

FIGURE 6-6. Time-series analysis of U.S. sudden infant death syndrome (SIDS) rates,
1980–2005.

been assigned to the treatments nonrandomly. This may arise when participants select a treatment condition based on personal preferences.[23] Therefore, the primary threat to internal validity involves selection bias among treatment groups. In the regression-discontinuity design, participants are ordered on a quantitative assignment variable (QAV) and allotted to a treatment condition according to a cutoff score on that variable.[23] Therefore, the treatment effect is estimated using a statistical technique (multiple regression) to relate the outcome of interest to the QAV in each treatment group. See Table 6-2 for a description of the strengths and weaknesses of these designs.

Observational Study Designs

Because it may not be ethical to use experimental or quasi-experimental study designs in all research settings, investigators can use observational study designs to evaluate hypotheses that prior exposures increase the risk of specific diseases. Generally, observational study designs are used to provide Type 1 evidence, for which the exposure has already occurred and disease patterns can be studied for those with and without the exposure of interest. A good historical example is the association between cigarette use and lung cancer. Because people choose whether to smoke cigarettes (one would not assign this exposure), we can evaluate the hypothesis that cigarette smokers are at increased risk of developing lung cancer by following smokers and nonsmokers over time to assess their lung cancer rates.

Cohort and case-control studies are two observational study designs that can be used to evaluate the strength of the association between prior exposure and risk of disease in the study population. Cohort studies compare the disease rates of exposed and unexposed study participants who are disease free at baseline and followed over time to estimate the disease rates in both groups. Cohort studies are often conducted when the exposure of interest is rare in the community, because all who have been exposed can be identified and followed to determine if the disease rate is significantly higher (or lower) than the rates for unexposed individuals from the same population. Studies that have focused on the effects of diet or exercise on specific diseases or health-related outcome[28] are good examples of cohort studies.

Case-control studies compare the frequency of prior exposures for study participants who have been diagnosed recently with the disease (cases) with those who have not developed the disease (controls). Case-control studies are the preferred study design when the disease is rare, and they are efficient when studying diseases with long latency. As is true for all study designs, selecting appropriate controls and obtaining reliable exposure estimates are crucial when evaluating any hypothesis that a prior exposure increases (or decreases) the risk of a specific disease. A recent study provides an example of an unusually large case-control study that examined lung cancer cases in Italy for differences in history of occupations.[29]

Table 6-2. Comparison of Quasi-Experimental Study Designs

Design	Schematic*	Strengths	Weaknesses
1. Before-after	O X O	Simplest measure; quick outcome; demonstrates feasibility of implementing intervention; may indicate value of a more systematic evaluation	Threats to validity: history, maturation, seasonality, testing, instrumentation, attrition, regression to mean
2. Interrupted time-series	O O O O O X O O O O O	Removes some threats to validity of No. 1 (maturation, seasonality, regression to mean) and inferentially stronger; no control group necessary; can use multiple interventions, groups, outcomes	Multiple observations requires resources; permutations of design can require sophisticated statistical procedures; autocorrelation must be addressed
3. Nonequivalent group	X O O	Easy to implement observations; little disruption to services; opportunistic natural experiments easy to capture; design permutations allow flexibility of measurement, comparisons, and interventions	Allocation to groups may be influenced by motivation; comparability of groups difficult to assess; pre- and post-test assessments of groups complex; complex statistical procedures necessary for assessing comparability
4. Regression-discontinuity		Split into groups accomplished by statistical criteria; group assignment relatively clean statistically with usual threats to validity removed; results statistically more credible	Requires almost 3 times the sample of an experimental design; may be useful when an experimental design not feasible

*0 = Observation; X = implementation of treatment.

Source: Reichardt and Mark.[23]

Public health professionals operating in typical settings may find much more modest case-control designs useful for exploring possible exposures for health issues encountered.

Cross-sectional studies, a third type of observational study design, can be completed relatively quickly and inexpensively to look at associations between exposure and disease. Because information regarding potential exposures and existing diseases for the study participants is measured simultaneously when the study is conducted, cross-sectional studies are unable to ascertain whether the exposure preceded the development of the disease among the study participants. Hence, cross-sectional studies are used primarily to generate hypotheses. Nevertheless, cross-sectional studies are used for public health planning and evaluation. For example, if a public health administrator wants to know how many women of reproductive age smoked cigarettes while pregnant, knowledge about the prevalence of maternal smoking in the community is important. Knowing the maternal smoking rates for subgroups of this population will help target interventions, if needed, for each subgroup. Cross-sectional studies are also used to help set research priorities based on consideration of the disease burden. A cross-sectional study in China was able to establish, for example, that a rapid screening test for detecting 14 high-risk types of human papillomavirus was effective in two county hospitals in rural China.[30]

SUMMARY

As they develop, implement, and evaluate new public health intervention programs, public health professionals need a core set of epidemiologic skills to quantify the frequency of disease in target populations.

Key Chapter Points

- Knowing the frequency of disease in the population before implementing any new public health program is crucial and can help focus efforts for reducing the disease burden by targeting high-risk groups in the population.
- Public health surveillance systems provide the necessary data to measure the frequency of some diseases, but special surveys are often needed to obtain baseline data for other diseases in defined populations.
- Public health surveillance data are currently available via the Internet for some diseases and can be used to look interactively at disease patterns by person, place, and time.
- Understanding the tradeoffs of various study designs will improve how we evaluate the effects of various public health programs and policies.

SUGGESTED READINGS AND SELECTED WEBSITES

Suggested Readings

Aschengrau A, Seage G. *Essentials of Epidemiology in Public Health*. 2nd ed. Sudbury, MA: Jones and Bartlett; 2008.

Bauman A, Keopsell T. Epidemiologic issues in community interventions. In: Brownson RC, Petitti DB, eds. *Applied Epidemiology: Theory to Practice*. 2nd ed. New York, NY: Oxford University Press; 2006:164–206.

Friis RH, Sellers TA. *Epidemiology for Public Health Practice*. 3rd ed. Gaithersburg, MD: Aspen Publishers; 2009.

Gordis L. Epidemiology. 4th ed. Philadelphia, PA: Saunders Elsevier; 2009.

Shadish W, Cook T, Campbell D. *Experimental and Quasi-Experimental Designs for Generalized Causal Inference*. Boston, MA: Houghton Mifflin; 2002.

Teutsch SM, Churchill RE, eds. *Principles and Practice of Public Health Surveillance* 2nd ed. New York, NY: Oxford University Press, 2000.

Wholey J, Hatry H, Newcomer K, eds. *Handbook of Practical Program Evaluation*. 2nd ed. San Francisco, CA: Jossey-Bass; 2004.

Selected Websites

CDC BRFSS <http://www.cdc.gov/nccdphp/brfss> The BRFSS, an ongoing data collection program conducted in all states, the District of Columbia, and three U.S. territories, and the world's largest telephone survey, tracks health risks in the United States. Information from the survey is used to improve the health of the American people. The CDC has developed a standard core questionnaire so that data can be compared across various strata.

CDC WONDER <http://wonder.cdc.gov> CDC WONDER is an easy-to-use system that provides a single point of access to a wide variety of CDC reports, guidelines, and numeric public health data. It can be valuable in public health research, decision making, priority setting, program evaluation, and resource allocation.

National Center for Health Statistics <http://www.cdc.gov/nchs/> National Center for Health Statistics is the principal vital and health statistics agency for the U.S. government. NCHS data systems include information on vital events as well as information on health status, lifestyle and exposure to unhealthy influences, the onset and diagnosis of illness and disability, and the use of health care. NCHS has two major types of data systems: systems based on populations, containing data collected through personal interviews or examinations (e.g., National Health Interview Survey and National Health and Nutrition Examination Survey), and systems based on records, containing data collected from vital and medical records. These data are used by policymakers in the U.S. Congress and the administration, by medical researchers and by others in the health community.

Epidemiology Supercourse <http://www.pitt.edu/~superl/> This course, coordinated by the University of Pittsburgh School of Public Health, is designed to provide an overview on epidemiology and the Internet for medical and health–related students around the world.

Kansas Information for Communities <http://kic.kdhe.state.ks.us/kic/> The Kansas Information for Communities (KIC) system gives data users the opportunity to prepare their own queries for vital event and other health care data. The queries designed into this system can fulfill many health data requests. As KIC is implemented, more data will be added. KIC programs will allow users to generate their own tables for specific characteristics, year of occurrence, age, rate, sex, and county.

Missouri Information for Community Assessment < http://www.dhss.mo.gov/MICA/> The Missouri Information for Community Assessment (MICA) system is an interactive system that allows anyone to create a table of specific data from various data files including births, deaths, hospital discharges, and others. The user can also produce a map with counties and/or cities shaded according to user-defined criteria.

County Health Rankings <http://www.countyhealthrankings.org/> The County Health Rankings are being developed by the University of Wisconsin Population Health Institute through a grant from the Robert Wood Johnson Foundation. This website serves as a focal point for information about the County Health Rankings, a project developed to increase awareness of the many factors—clinical care access and quality, health-promoting behaviors, social and economic factors, and the physical environment—that contribute to the health of communities; foster engagement among public and private decision makers to improve community health; and develop incentives to encourage coordination across sectors for community health improvement.

Texas Health Data <http://soupfin.tdh.state.tx.us/> Texas Health Data allows a user to generate a table showing frequencies, frequencies and rates, and frequencies and percents by column or row and a map showing frequencies or frequencies and rates by quartiles or quintiles. At present, the years of data available for births are 1990 through 1999. Population estimates and projections are available for 1990 through 2010.

REFERENCES

1. Porta M, ed. *A Dictionary of Epidemiology*. 5th ed. New York, NY: Oxford University Press; 2008.
2. Terris M. The Society for Epidemiologic Research (SER) and the future of epidemiology. *Am J Epidemiol*. 1992;136(8):909–915.

3. Brownson R, Seiler R, Eyler A. Measuring the impact of public health policy. *Prev Chronic Dis.* In press.
4. Screening for breast cancer: U.S. Preventive Services Task Force recommendation statement. *Ann Intern Med.* 2009;151(10):716–726, W-236.
5. Estimated county-level prevalence of diabetes and obesity: United States, 2007. *MMWR Morb Mortal Wkly Rep.* 2009;58(45):1259–1263.
6. Andresen EM, Diehr PH, Luke DA. Public health surveillance of low-frequency populations. *Annu Rev Public Health.* 2004;25:25–52.
7. Centers for Disease Control and Prevention. Smoking-Attributable Mortality, Morbidity, and Economic Costs (SAMMEC). http://apps.nccd.cdc.gov/sammec/methodology.asp
8. State-specific smoking-attributable mortality and years of potential life lost—United States, 2000–2004. *MMWR Morb Mortal Wkly Rep.* 2009;58(2):29–33.
9. Rosen M, Nystrom L, Wall S. Guidelines for regional mortality analysis: an epidemiological approach to health planning. *Int J Epidemiol.* 1985;14(2):293–299.
10. Bjorkenstam C, Edberg A, Ayoubi S, et al. Are cancer patients at higher suicide risk than the general population? *Scand J Public Health.* 2005;33(3):208–214.
11. Heron M, Hoyert D, Murphy S, et al. *Deaths: Final data for 2006. National vital statistics reports.* Hyattsville, MD: National Center for Health Statistics; 2009.
12. Miller M, Hemenway D. Guns and suicide in the United States. *N Engl J Med.* 2008;359(10):989–991.
13. Horner M, Ries L, Krapcho M, et al. *SEER Cancer Statistics Review, 1975–2006.* Bethesda, MD: National Cancer Institute; 2009.
14. Harper S, Lynch J, Meersman SC, et al. Trends in area-socioeconomic and race-ethnic disparities in breast cancer incidence, stage at diagnosis, screening, mortality, and survival among women ages 50 years and over (1987–2005). *Cancer Epidemiol Biomarkers Prev.* 2009;18(1):121–131.
15. Thacker SB. Public health surveillance and the prevention of injuries in sports: what gets measured gets done. *J Athl Train.* 2007;42(2):171–172.
16. Thacker S. Historical developments. In: Teutsch S, Churchill R, eds. *Principles and Practice of Public Health Surveillance.* 2nd ed. New York, NY: Oxford University Press; 2000:1–16.
17. Teutsch S, Churchill R, eds. *Principles and Practice of Public Health Surveillance.* 2nd ed. New York, NY: Oxford University Press; 2000.
18. World Health Organization Regional Office for Europe. European Health for All database. http://www.euro.who.int/HFADB
19. Thacker SB, Stroup DF. Future directions for comprehensive public health surveillance and health information systems in the United States. *Am J Epidemiol.* 1994;140(5):383–397.
20. Jemal A, Siegel R, Ward E, Murray T, Xu J, Thun MJ. Cancer statistics, 2007. *CA Cancer J Clin.* 2007;57(1):43–66.
21. Zaza S, Briss PA, Harris KW, eds. *The Guide to Community Preventive Services: What Works to Promote Health?* New York, NY: Oxford University Press; 2005.
22. Brownson RC, Royer C, Ewing R, McBride TD. Researchers and policymakers: travelers in parallel universes. *Am J Prev Med.* 2006;30(2):164–172.
23. Reichardt C, Mark M. Quasi-experimentation. In: Wholey J, Hatry H, Newcomer K, eds. *Handbook of Practical Program Evaluation.* 2nd ed. San Francisco, CA: Jossey-Bass; 2004:126–149.

24. Shadish W, Cook T, Campbell D. *Experimental and Quasi-Experimental Designs for Generalized Causal Inference*. Boston, MA: Houghton Mifflin; 2002.
25. Colson ER, Rybin D, Smith LA, Colton T, Lister G, Corwin MJ. Trends and factors associated with infant sleeping position: the national infant sleep position study, 1993–2007. *Arch Pediatr Adolesc Med*. 2009;163(12):1122–1128.
26. Dwyer T, Ponsonby AL. Sudden infant death syndrome and prone sleeping position. *Ann Epidemiol*. 2009;19(4):245–249.
27. McKinney CM, Holt VL, Cunningham ML, et al. Maternal and infant characteristics associated with prone and lateral infant sleep positioning in Washington state, 1996–2002. *J Pediatr*. 2008;153(2):194–198, e191–e193.
28. Hu FB, Manson JE, Stampfer MJ, et al. Diet, lifestyle, and the risk of type 2 diabetes mellitus in women. *N Engl J Med*. 2001;345(11):790–797.
29. Consonni D, De Matteis S, Lubin JH, et al. Lung cancer and occupation in a population-based case-control study. *Am J Epidemiol*.2010;171(3):323–333.
30. Qiao YL, Sellors JW, Eder PS, et al. A new HPV-DNA test for cervical-cancer screening in developing regions: a cross-sectional study of clinical accuracy in rural China. *Lancet Oncol*. 2008;9(10):929–936.

7

Searching the Scientific Literature and Organizing Information

> Where is the wisdom we have lost in knowledge? Where is the knowledge we have lost in information?
>
> —T.S. Eliot

As you develop an issue statement and begin to understand the epidemiologic nature of a particular public health issue along with the intervention options, the scientific literature is a crucial source of information. Because of the considerable growth in the amount of information available to public health practitioners, it is essential to follow a systematic approach to literature searching. The underpinnings of an evidence-based process rest largely on one's ability to find credible, high-quality evidence as efficiently and exhaustively as possible. A systematic searching process also helps ensure that others can replicate the same results. With modern information technologies, especially personal computers and the seemingly limitless reach of the Internet, spreading, virtually all public health workers have an excellent opportunity to find valuable information quickly. Published information resources are now increasingly available for anyone with an Internet connection, enabling professionals outside major institutions to perform professional and thorough searches for needed resources.

This chapter provides guidance on how to search the scientific literature. It focuses on the importance of a literature search, where to search, how to find evidence, and how to organize the results of a search. Evaluation of the quality of the evidence is covered in other chapters (primarily Chapters 2, 3, and 10).

BACKGROUND

As noted in Chapter 1, there are many types and sources of evidence on public health programs and policies. Scientific information (the "scientific literature") on

theory and practice can be found in textbooks, government reports, scientific journals, policy statements, and at scientific meetings. Three levels of reading the
scientific literature have been described: (1) browsing—flicking through actual
books and articles, looking for anything of interest, and browsing topic-related
sites on the Internet; (2) reading for information—approaching the literature in
search of an answer to a specific question; and (3) reading for research—reading
in order to obtain a comprehensive view of the existing state of knowledge on a
specific topic.[1] In practice, most of us obtain most of our information through
browsing.[2,3] However, to conduct a literature review for building evidence-based
programs efficiently, it is important to take a more structured approach. We focus
primarily on journal publications here because they have gone through a process
of peer review to enhance the quality of the information and are the closest thing
to a gold standard that is available (see Chapter 2).

When conducting a search of the scientific literature, there are four types of
publications to look for:

1. *Original research articles:* the papers written by the authors who conducted
   the research. These articles provide details on the methods used, results, and
   implications of results. A thorough and comprehensive summary of a body of
   literature will consist of careful reading of original research articles.
2. *Review articles:* a narrative summary of what is known on a particular topic.
   A review article presents a summary of original research articles. The *Annual
   Review of Public Health* is an excellent source of review articles on a variety
   of topics (http://arjournals.annualreviews.org/loi/publhealth). A limitation of
   review articles is that they do not always follow systematic approaches, a practice that sometimes leads to inconsistent results.[4]
3. *Review articles featuring a quantitative synthesis of results:* a quantitative synthesis involves a process such as meta-analysis—a quantitative approach that
   provides a systematic, organized, and structured way of integrating the findings
   of individual research studies.[5,6] This type of review is often called a systematic
   review (see Chapter 3). In meta-analysis, researchers produce a summary
   statistical estimate of the measure of association. For example, the Cochrane
   Collaboration, an international organization of clinicians, epidemiologists, and
   others, has produced quantitative reviews on the effectiveness of various health
   care interventions, and practices covering a wide range of subjects (www
   cochrane.org). Much information is available to all on this site, with membership through an organization required for downloading full reports.
4. *Guidelines:* Practice guidelines are formal statements that offer advice to clinicians, public health practitioners, managed-care organizations, and the public
   on how to improve the effectiveness and impact of clinical and public health
   interventions. Guidelines translate the findings of research and demonstration

projects into accessible and useable information for public health practice. There are several examples of useful guidelines.[7–9] The terminology used within them differs across the globe. Thus, in the European Community, directives are stronger than recommendations, which are stronger than guidelines.[10] No such hierarchy exists in North America.

Review articles and guidelines often present a useful short cut for many busy practitioners who do not have the time to master the literature on multiple public health topics.

In addition to the type of publication, timeliness of scientific information is an important consideration. To find the best quality evidence for medical decision making, Sackett and colleagues recommended that practitioners burn their (traditional) textbooks.[11] Although this approach may seem radical, it does bring to light the limitations of textbooks for providing information on the cause, diagnosis, prognosis, or treatment of a disorder. To stay up to date in clinical practice, a textbook may need to be revised on a yearly basis. However, research and publication of results in a journal is a deliberative process that often takes years from the germination of an idea, to obtaining funding, carrying out the study, analyzing data, writing up results, submitting to a journal, and waiting out the peer-review process and publication lag for a journal.

The number of scientific publications has increased dramatically since the 1940s.[12] There are an estimated 24,000 scientific journals in the world, publishing together approximately 1.4 million new research papers each year.[13] To assimilate even a fraction of this large body of evidence, the practitioner needs to find ways to take advantage of the vast amount of scientific information available, and to find information quickly. Of increasing interest to health professionals is the ease with which this literature may be accessed by those not directly supported by major library resources. Consequently there is interest in open access availability of scientific publications. A recent study reported that 4.6% of articles become immediately available, and that an additional 3.5% become available after an embargo period.[13] Further, 11.3% of articles are also available from subject-specific, institutional repositories or authors' websites. These authors suggest that the most powerful technique for obtaining access to articles is to search using Google Scholar. Therefore nearly 20% of articles may be readily accessible, and professionals may also use the PubMed author information to obtain the author's e-mail address, for direct requests of articles. With easy access to abstracts, and increasing ability to obtain research articles, public health professionals regardless of their institutional resources may be able to actively work with the scientific literature in their areas of concern.

Methods for searching the literature have changed dramatically. Thirty years ago, a practitioner wishing to find information on a particular topic would speak with a librarian and inform him or her of the type of information being sought, perhaps provide a sample article, and help in selecting some key words. The librarian would run the search, consult with the practitioner as to whether it captured the desired types of articles, modify the search as needed, rerun it, consult with the practitioner again, etc. This whole iterative process could take weeks. Current practitioners with an Internet connection can now search for relevant information from the world's scientific literature, and with training and experience, discern relevance and quality so as to improve the practice of public health. There also are online training modules on how to search the literature such as that at www.ebbp.org.

UNDERTAKING A SEARCH OF THE SCIENTIFIC LITERATURE

Although any search algorithm is imperfect, a systematic approach to literature searching can increase the chances of finding pertinent information. Figure 7-1 describes a process for searching the literature and organizing the findings of a search. The following topics provide a step-by-step breakdown of this process.[12]

We focus mainly on the use of PubMed because it is the largest and most widely available bibliographic database, with coverage of over 19 million articles from MEDLINE and life sciences journals. We also focus on the search for peer-reviewed evidence programs, studies, and data that have been reviewed by other researchers and practitioners.

Review the Issue Statement and Purpose of the Search

Based on the issue statement described in Chapter 4, the purpose of the search should be well outlined. Keep in mind that searching is an iterative process, and a key is the ability to ask one or more answerable questions. While the goal of a search is to identify all relevant material and nothing else, in practice, this is difficult to achieve.[6] The overarching questions include: "Which evidence is relevant to my questions?" and "What conclusions can be drawn regarding effective intervention approaches based on the literature assembled?"[14]

Select a Bibliographic Database

There are numerous bibliographic databases that are now available online (Table 7-1). We recommend that readers become familiar with one or more of them. Some of the databases in Table 7-1 require a fee, but if an individual has access to a library,

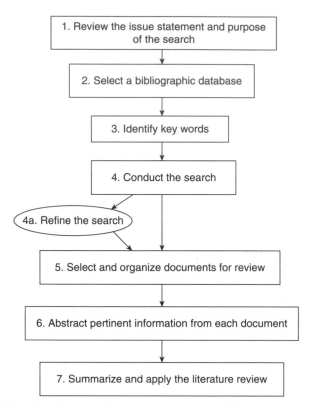

FIGURE 7-1. Flowchart for organizing a search of the scientific literature.
(The later stages [especially steps 5 and 6] of the process are based largely on the Matrix
Method, developed by Garrard.)[12]

a global fee may already cover the cost. These resources are available at PubMed
at http://www.ncbi.nlm.nih.gov/sites/entrez, make it a widely used database by
scholars and the public for searching the biomedical literature in the United States.
It is maintained by the National Library of Medicine and has several advantages
over other databases—it is free to users, updated frequently, and relatively user
friendly. MEDLINE does not provide the full text of articles, but rather lists the
title, authors, source of the publication, the authors' abstract (if one is available),
key word subject headings, and a number of other "tags" that provide information
about each publication. For some journals (e.g., the *British Medical Journal*), the
full text of articles can be accessed via a link on the search results page. Numerous
other evidence databases exist for a variety of health care specialties and subspe-
cialties. Subspecialty databases do not currently exist for public health, so it is
recommended that practitioners become familiar with MEDLINE and similar
databases in Table 7-1.

Table 7-1. Computer-Stored Bibliographic Databases

Database	Dates	Subjects Covered	Fee	Website
PubMed	1966–present	The premier source for bibliographic coverage of biomedical literature; includes references and abstracts from over 5200 journals	No	(www.ncbi.nlm.nih.gov/pubmed)
Current Contents® (subcategories: Clinical Medicine, Life Sciences, or Social and Behavioral Sciences)	Past year, updated weekly	Tables of contents and bibliographic data from current issues of the world's leading scholarly research journals; indexed and loaded within days of publication	Yes	http://science.thomsonreuters.com/ training/ccc/l>
PsycINFO®	1887–present	The world's most comprehensive source for bibliographic coverage of psychology and behavioral sciences literature; with special subset files ClinPSYC; databases contain more that 1.5 million records. Available to nonmembers of the American Psychological Association for a fee	Yes	http://www.apa.org/psycinfo/
Dissertation Abstracts Online	1861–present	American and Canadian doctoral dissertations	Yes	http://library.dialog.com/bluesheets/ html/bl0035.html
CANCERLIT®	1966–present	Cancer literature from journal articles, government and technical reports, meeting abstracts, special publications, and theses	No	http://cancernet.nci.nih.gov/search/ cancer_literature/
TOXLINE®	1980–present	Extensive array of references to literature on biochemical, pharmacologic, physiologic. and toxicologic effects of drugs and other chemicals	No	<http://toxnet.nlm.nih.gov/index.html>

Identify Key Words

Key words are terms that describe the characteristics of the subject being reviewed. A useful search strategy is dependent on the sensitivity and precision of the key words used. "Sensitivity" is the ability to identify all relevant material, and "precision" is the amount of relevant material among the information retrieved by the search.[6,15] Thus, *sensitivity* addresses the question "Will relevant articles be missed?" while *precision* addresses the question "Will irrelevant articles be included?" Most bibliographic databases require the use of standardized key words. These key words are often found in the list of Medical Subject Heading (MeSH) terms. There are a number of tutorials on the PubMed site about using the database, including information about identifying and selecting MeSH terms. There are two small screens on right of the search page of PubMed that are helpful. One, named "Titles with your search terms" will permit the user to consult other published articles similar to what is being searched in order to check the search terms used. Looking at these titles may suggest additional search terms to include. There is also a screen "Search details" which includes MeSH terms. This screen may be helpful when entering open text on a search, and noting that an indicated MeSH term may be a better choice. For a literature search in MEDLINE, these sources of key words are useful (Box 7-1):

1. Identify two scientific papers that cover the topic of interest—one more recent and one less recent.[6] These papers can be pulled up on PubMed. In the MEDLINE abstract, a list of MeSH terms will be provided. These can, in turn, be used in subsequent searches.
2. Key words can be found within the alphabetical list of MeSH terms, available online at <http://www.nlm.nih.gov/mesh/meshhome.html>.
3. MEDLINE and Current Contents do not require users to use standardized key words. Therefore, you can select your own key words—these are searched for in article titles and abstracts. Generally, using nonstandardized key words provides a less precise literature search than does using standardized terms. However, the MEDLINE interface between standardized and nonstandardized key words allows complete searching without a detailed knowledge of MeSH terms.

Conduct the Search

After the databases and initial key words are identified, it is time to run the search. Once the initial search is run, the number of publications returned will likely be large and include many irrelevant articles. Several features of PubMed can

Box 7-1. Searching for Evidence on the Effectiveness of Cardiovascular Health Programs

The state "healthy heart" coordinator within the Mississippi Department of Health is in charge of starting a new program in community-based intervention to promote cardiovascular health. She has completed an initial statement of the issue under consideration and now wishes to search the literature. She connects with PubMed via the Internet and begins a search. First, she uses nonstandardized key words, including "cardiovascular disease" and "community intervention." The first run of a search yields 1786 citations. Next, she limits the search to literature published in the past ten years; using the same key words, this results in 1133 citations. In the third iteration, the same key words are used, literature is limited to the past 10 years, and only review articles are selected. This results in 162 citations for which abstracts can be scanned. While this is a large number of articles, they scan to about nine screens of references to look at, a reasonable task. After scanning these abstracts, the program coordinator obtains copies of the most essential articles.

The coordinator next conducted a second round of searching on the same topic using the standard McSH terms "Cardiovascular Diseases" and "Health Education." The initial search using these words yielded 14,538 citations, the next search was limited to the past 10 years, resulting in 8272 articles. Finally, the procedure, limited to review articles, yielded 1616 citations. A further refinement to a limit of publication within the last 5 years still produced a listing of 905 articles, too long for practical literature searching. In this case, further refinement of the disease MeSH term might be indicated.

In this example, the use of nonstandardized key words appeared to better identify the types of articles needed by the coordinator.

---

assist searchers in limiting the scope of the search to the most relevant articles. Figure 7-2 shows a partial listing from a PubMed search using the key words "evidence-based public health."

- Searches can also be limited to English-language publications, to a certain date of publication, or to certain demographics of the participants, such as age and gender. These tags are found by clicking the "Limits" icon.
- Specific designations such as "editorial," "letter," or "comment" can be excluded, or the search can be limited to "journal article." An initial search can focus on review articles by selecting the publication type. This allows a search of the citation list of review articles in order to identify original research articles of particular interest.
- PubMed will allow you to link to other "related articles" by simply clicking an icon on the right side of each citation.
- If a particularly useful article is found, the author's name can be searched for other similar studies. The same author will often have multiple publications on

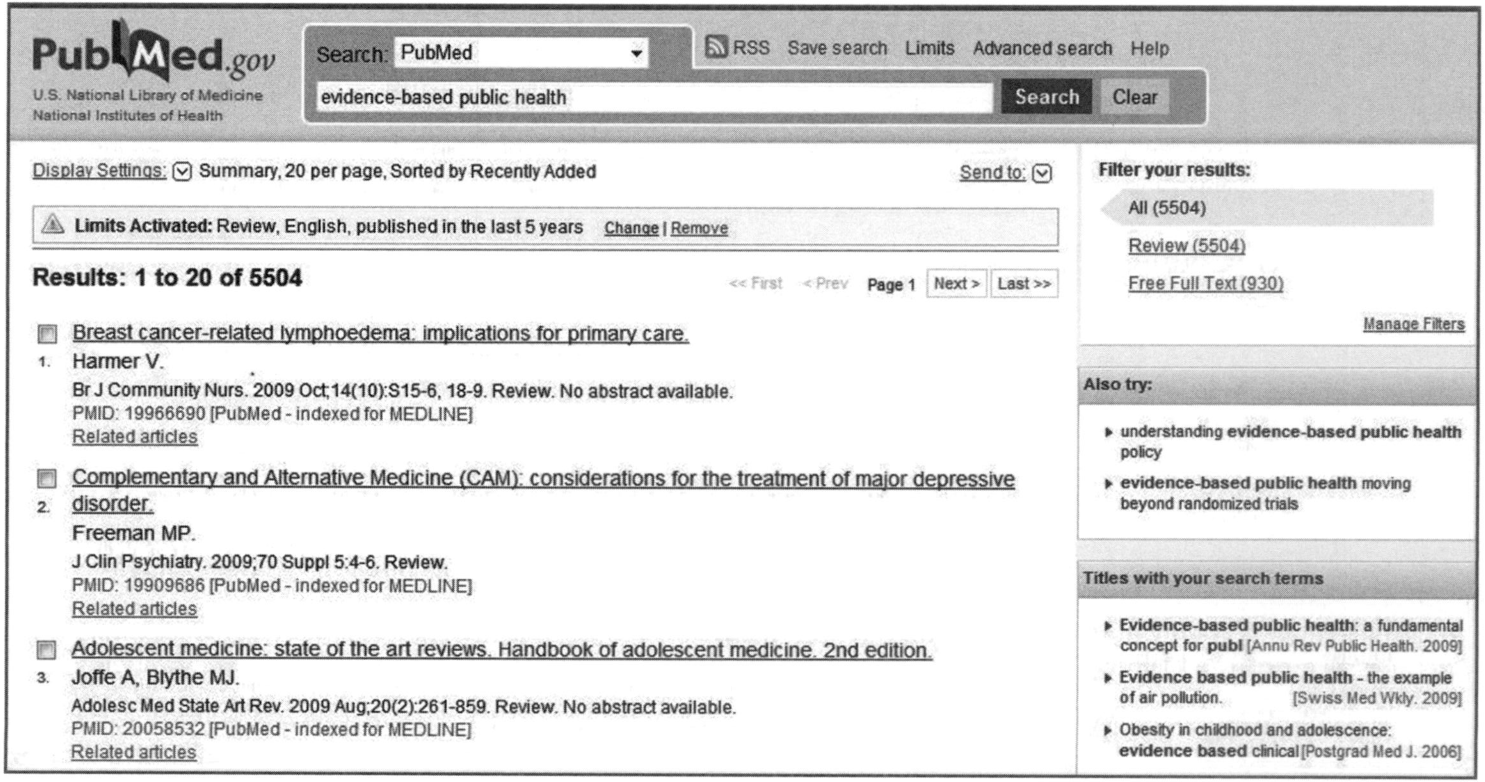
PubMed.gov
U.S. National Library of Medicine
National Institutes of Health
Search: PubMed
RSS Save search Limits Advanced search Help
evidence-based public health
Search
Clear
Display Settings: Summary, 20 per page, Sorted by Recently Added
Send to:
Limits Activated: Review, English, published in the last 5 years
Change | Remove
Results: 1 to 20 of 5504
<< First < Prev Page 1 Next > Last >>
Breast cancer-related lymphoedema: implications for primary care.
1.
Harmer V.
Br J Community Nurs. 2009 Oct;14(10):S15-6, 18-9. Review. No abstract available.
PMID: 19966690 [PubMed - indexed for MEDLINE]
Related articles
Complementary and Alternative Medicine (CAM): considerations for the treatment of major depressive disorder.
2.
Freeman MP.
J Clin Psychiatry. 2009;70 Suppl 5:4-6. Review.
PMID: 19909686 [PubMed - indexed for MEDLINE]
Related articles
Adolescent medicine: state of the art reviews. Handbook of adolescent medicine. 2nd edition.
3.
Joffe A, Blythe MJ.
Adolesc Med State Art Rev. 2009 Aug;20(2):261-859. Review. No abstract available.
PMID: 20058532 [PubMed - indexed for MEDLINE]
Related articles
Filter your results:
All (5504)
Review (5504)
Free Full Text (930)
Manage Filters
Also try:
understanding evidence-based public health policy
evidence-based public health moving beyond randomized trials
Titles with your search terms
Evidence-based public health: a fundamental concept for publ [Annu Rev Public Health. 2009]
Evidence based public health - the example of air pollution. [Swiss Med Wkly. 2009]
Obesity in childhood and adolescence: evidence based clinical [Postgrad Med J. 2006]

FIGURE 7-2. Web page for a PubMed literature search (<http://www.nlm.nih.gov>).

the same subject. To avoid irrelevant retrievals, you should use the author's last name and first and middle initials in the search.

- In nearly every case, it is necessary to refine the search approach. As articles are identified, the key word and search strategy will be refined and improved through a "snowballing" technique that allows users to gain familiarity with the literature and gather more useful articles.[12] Articles that may be useful can be saved during each session by clicking "send to" within PubMed.

- Searches may be refined using Boolean Operators, words that relate search terms to each other, thus increasing the reach of the search. Help screens of different data bases will provide more information, but the most common Boolean operators are (used in CAPS): AND, NOT, OR, NEAR, and ( ). The word AND used in this way combines the search terms so that the yield includes articles including both. An example would be: breast neoplasms AND adolescents, which when further limited by "review articles" yield about 700 articles in PUBMED. An example of the operator NOT would be: accidents NOT automobile. The operator OR permits coupling two search terms that may tap a similar domain. The operator NEAR will define two search terms that must appear within 10 words of each other in order select an article. Use of parentheses will define a search term that must appear as listed. For example, the search terms (school clinic) must appear as that phrase to be identified, rather than search "school" and "clinic" separately. Boolean terms are highly useful in specifying a search and can be used to facilitate a search more efficiently.

Select and Organize Documents for Review

Once a set of articles has been located, it is time to organize the documents.[12] This will set the stage for abstracting the pertinent information. Generally, it is helpful to organize the documents by the type of study (original research, review article, review article with quantitative synthesis, guideline). It is often useful to enter documents into a reference management database such as EndNote® (http://www.endnote.com). These software applications allow users to switch from one reference format to another when producing reports and grant applications and to download journal citations directly from the Internet, eliminating the chance for typing errors. They also have helpful search and sort capabilities. A systematic method of organizing the articles themselves is essential. A limited number of articles on a certain topic can be kept in a three-ring binder, but larger bodies of evidence may be entered in a reference management database such as EndNote® by key word; articles can then be filed alphabetically by the last name of the first author of each article or simply with an identification number. This allows users to search a database by key word later in the research process.

Abstract Pertinent Information from Each Document

When a group of articles has been assembled, the next step is to create an evidence matrix—a spreadsheet with rows and columns that allows users to abstract the key information from each article.[12] Creating a matrix provides a structure for putting the information in order. In developing a matrix, the choice of column topics is a key consideration. It is often useful to consider both methodological characteristics and content-specific results as column headings. A sample review matrix is shown in Table 7-2. In this example, studies were also organized within rows by an ecologic framework, described in detail in Chapter 8. The Community Guide provides excellent evaluation about programs designed to address a number of areas of strong public health concern, based upon an evidence-based review of the supporting literature assessing interventions. For example, one topic is "Preventing Excessive Alcohol Use" and a subtopic is "Regulation of Alcohol Outlet Density." For that section, the task force presents an excellent Summary Evidence Table demonstrating the utility of systematically categorizing the literature:

www.thecommunityguide.org/alcohol/supportingmaterials/SETAlcoholOutletDensity.pdf

Summarize and Apply the Literature Review

Once a body of studies has been abstracted into a matrix, the literature may be summarized for various purposes. For example, you may need to provide background information for a new budget item that is being presented to the administrator of an agency. Knowing the best intervention science should increase the chances of convincing key policy makers of the need for a particular program or policy. You may also need to summarize the literature in order to build the case for a grant application that seeks external support for a particular program.

SEEKING SOURCES OUTSIDE THE SEARCHABLE LITERATURE

A great deal of important evidence on public health topics is not found in published journal articles and books.[6,16] Reasons for the limitations of searching the published literature include the following: (1) many researchers and practitioners fail to write up their research because of competing projects and other time demands; (2) journal editors are faced with difficult decisions on what to publish and there is a tendency toward publishing studies showing a significant effect of an intervention (publication bias), and (3) in some areas of the world, lack of resources precludes systematic empirical research. The following approaches should prove useful in finding evidence beyond the scientific literature.

Table 7-2. Example Evidence Matrix for Literature on Physical Activity Promotion at Various Levels of an Ecologic Framework

		METHODOLOGICAL CHARACTERISTICS			CONTENT-SPECIFIC FINDINGS		
Lead author, article title, journal citation	Year	Study Design	Study Population	Sample Size	Intervention Characteristics	Results	Conclusions	Other Comments

Individual Level

Brownson et al. Patterns and correlates of physical activity among women aged 40 years and older, United States. *Am J Public Health* 2000:90: 264–270	2000	Cross-sectional	Ethnically diverse U.S. women, aged 40 years and older	2912	N/A—not an intervention	Physical activity lowest among African American and American Indian women (odds ratios = 1.35 and 1.65);72% of women were active based on a composite definition;Rural women were less active than urban dwellers	Minority women are among the least active subgroups in America	Cross-sectional nature limits causal inferences; Telephone survey data may not be entirely representative

(continued)

Table 7-2. (Continued)

		METHODOLOGICAL CHARACTERISTICS			CONTENT-SPECIFIC FINDINGS		
Lead author, article title, journal citation	Year	Study Design	Study Population	Sample Size	Intervention Characteristics	Results	Conclusions	Other Comments

Interpersonal Level

Simons et al. A pilot urban church-based program to reduce risk factors for diabetes among Western Samoans in New Zealand. *Diabetic Med* 1998;15: 136–142	1998	Prospective; nonrandomized	Western Samoan church members, South Auckland, New Zealand; 34% male, 66% female	Intervention = 78; control = 144	Social support, health education, supervised and structured exercise	Weight remained stable n the intervention church but increased in the control church (p = 0.05). In the intervention church, there was an associated reduction in waist circumference, p < 0.001), an increase in diabetes knowledge, p < 0.001) and an increase in the proportion exercising regularly, p < 0.05).	Diabetes risk reduction programs based upon lifestyle change, diabetes awareness, and empowerment of high-risk communities can significantly reduce risk factors for future type 2 diabetes	Participation rates: Introductory talk = 93%; Video session = 18%; Exercise session = 84%

Organizational Level

Sharpe et al. Exercise beliefs and behaviors among older employees: a health promotion trial. *Gerontologist* 1992;32: 444–449.	1992	Group randomized by worksite unit	University employees, ages 50–69, 53% male, 91% white, 5% black	250 Initially, 121 used for analysis	Health counseling and exercise	The change in walking or other exercise from baseline to 1-year follow-up was not significantly different between intervention and control groups.	Baseline exercise frequency was the only predictor of exercise behavior 1 year later.

Community Level

King et al. Increasing exercise among blue-collar employees: the tailoring of worksite programs to meet specific needs. *Prev Med* 1988;17(3): 357–365.	1988	Prospective; quasi-experimental	Employees at Stanford Univ. skilled trade division, Palo Alto, CA; 100% men; mean age, 45 years	22	16-Week exercise program using an on-site parcourse, and incorporating such motivational strategies as public monitoring, intershop competition, and activity-based incentives	Participants showed increases in fitness levels ($p < 0.0001$) and decreases in weight ($p < 0.05$) compared with nonparticipants; Attendees also showed greater confidence about the ability to exercise	Low cost program appears to influence fitness and weight Long-term program adherence needs to be studied

(continued)

Table 7-2. (Continued)

| Lead author, article title, journal citation | Year | METHODOLOGICAL CHARACTERISTICS | | | | CONTENT-SPECIFIC FINDINGS | | |
		Study Design	Study Population	Sample Size	Intervention Characteristics	Results	Conclusions	Other Comments
Health Policy Level								
Linenger et al. Physical fitness gains following simple environmental change. *Am J Prev Med* 1991 7(5):298–310	1991	Nonrandomized group trial	San Diego naval air station community members (intervention) and two control communities; 85% male in intervention site	2372	Modification of physical environment (e.g., bike paths, new equipment, athletic events); organizational policy intervention (release time encouraged)	Significant improvement in physical readiness test (PRT) and 1.5 mile run in intervention community compared with either control community or a Navy-wide sample; 12.4% failed the PRT in 1987 compared with 5.1% in 1988 in the intervention site;	A relatively simple program improved fitness performance	The generalizability to a nonmilitary population should be considered.

The "Fugitive" Literature

The "fugitive" or "grey" literature includes government reports, book chapters, conference proceedings, and other materials that are not found in online databases such as MEDLINE. These are particularly important in attempting a summary of the literature involving meta-analysis or cost-effectiveness analysis (see Chapter 3). It can be difficult to locate the fugitive literature. Experts on the topic of interest are probably the best source of information—you can write or e-mail key informants asking them to provide information on relevant published literature that would not be identified through database searching. More broad-based searches can be conducted of the Internet using search engines such as Google (www.google.com), or MetaCrawler (www.metacrawler.com). The advantage of these search engines is their ability to find a large number of sources. The main disadvantage is the user's lack of control over the quality of the information returned. Information collected from a wide search of the Internet must be viewed with a critical eye.[17] The RePORTER (Research Portfolio Online Reporting Tool) database, maintained by the U.S. National Institutes of Health, provides summaries of funded research projects that can be useful in finding information prior to its appearance in the peer-reviewed literature (http://projectreporter.nih.gov/reporter.cfm).

Key Informant Interviews

Often a public health practitioner wants to understand not only the outcomes of a program or policy but also the process of developing and carrying out an intervention (see Chapter 9). Many process issues are difficult to glean from the scientific literature because the methods sections in published articles may not be comprehensive enough to show all aspects of the intervention. A program may evolve over time and what is in the published literature may differ from what is currently being done. In addition, many good program and policy evaluations go unpublished.

In these cases, key informant interviews may be useful. Key informants are experts on a certain topic and may include a university researcher who has years of experience in a particular intervention area or a local program manager who has the field experience to know what works when it comes to designing and implementing effective interventions. There are several steps in carrying out a "key informant" process:

1. Identify the key informants who might be useful for gathering information. They can be found in the literature, via professional networks, and increasingly, on the Internet (see <http://www.profnct.com>, a site that puts journalists and

interested persons in touch with scientific experts who are willing to share their expertise).

2. Determine the types of information needed. It is often helpful to write out a short list of open-ended questions that are of particular interest. This can help in framing a conversation and making the most efficient use of time. Prior to a conversation with an expert, it is useful to e-mail him or her questions to allow thinking about replies.

3. Collect the data. This often can be accomplished via a 15- to 30-minute telephone conversation if the questions of interest are well framed ahead of time.

4. Summarize the data collected. Conversations can be recorded and transcribed using formative research techniques. More often, good notes are taken and conversations recorded to end up with a series of bullet points from each key informant conversation.

5. Conduct follow-up, as needed. As with literature searching, key informant interviews often result in a snowballing effect in which one expert identifies another who is also knowledgeable. As information becomes repetitious, the data collector can decide when enough information has been collected.

Professional Meetings

Annually, there are dozens of relevant and helpful professional meetings in public health, ranging from large conventions such as that of the American Public Health Association to smaller, specialty meetings such as the annual meeting on diabetes prevention and control. Important intervention research is often presented at these meetings. There are regional public health associations that hold meetings and are a rich source for networking and developing resources. The smaller venues allow one to talk informally with the researcher to learn details of his or her work and how it might apply in a particular setting. Practitioners should seek out meetings that use a peer-review process for abstract review, helping to ensure that high-quality research is presented. Meetings generally provide a list of presenters and abstracts of presentations prior to or during the meeting. The main limitation for many practitioners is the inability to attend a variety of professional meetings because of limited travel funds.

SUMMARY

Literature searching can be an inexact science because of the wide scope of public health and inconsistencies in search strategies,[18] but a systematic search of the literature is a key for evidence-based decision making.

Key Chapter Points

- It is important to understand the various uses of different types professional literature i.e., original research articles, review articles, reviews with quantitative synthesis, and guidelines.
- A step-by-step approach to literature searching will improve the sensitivity and precision of the process.
- Other valuable sources of scientific information can include the fugitive literature, key informant interviews, and professional meetings.

Although this chapter attempts to provide the essential information for locating scientific information quickly, there is no substitute for trying out these approaches and customizing procedures to your own needs.

SUGGESTED READINGS AND SELECTED WEBSITES

Suggested Readings

Galvan, Jose L. Writing Literature Reviews. Third Edition. Glendale CA: Pryczak Publishing. 2006.
Garrard J. *Health Sciences Literature Review Made Easy. The Matrix Method.* 2nd ed. Sudbury, MA: Jones and Bartlett Publishers; 2006.
Greenhalgh T. How to read a paper. Getting your bearings (deciding what the paper is about). British Medical Journal. 1997;315:243–246.
Pan, M. Ling. Preparing Literature Reviews: Qualitative and Quantitative Approaches. 3rd Edition. Glendale, CA:. Pryczak Publishing. 2008.

Selected Websites

The Agency for Healthcare Research and Quality <http://www.ahrq.gov/>. The Agency for Healthcare Research and Quality's (AHRQ) mission is to improve the quality, safety, efficiency, and effectiveness of health care for all Americans. Information from AHRQ's research helps people make more informed decisions and improve the quality of health care services.

Annual Review of Public Health <http://publhealth.annualreviews.org/>. The mission of Annual Reviews is to provide systematic, periodic examinations of scholarly advances in a number of scientific fields through critical authoritative reviews. The comprehensive critical review not only summarizes a topic but also roots out errors of fact or concept and provokes discussion that will lead to new research activity. The critical review is an essential part of the scientific method.

The Cochrane Collaboration <http://www.cochrane.org/>. The Cochrane Collaboration is an international not-for-profit and independent organization, dedicated to making up-to-date, accurate information about the effects of health care readily available worldwide. It produces and disseminates systematic reviews of health care interventions and promotes the search for evidence in the form of clinical trials and other studies of interventions. The major product of the Collaboration is the *Cochrane Database of Systematic Reviews,* which is published quarterly as part of *The Cochrane Library.*

Evidence-based behavioral practice <http://www.ebbp.org/>. The EBBP.org project creates training resources to bridge the gap between behavioral health research and practice. An interactive website offers modules covering topics such as the EBBP process, systematic reviews, searching for evidence, critical appraisal, and randomized controlled trials. This site is ideal for practitioners, researchers and educators.

Google Scholar <http://scholar.google.com/>. Google Scholar provides a simple way to broadly search for scholarly literature. From one place, you can search across many disciplines and sources: articles, theses, books, abstracts and court opinions, from academic publishers, professional societies, online repositories, universities and other web sites. Google Scholar helps locate relevant work across the world of scholarly research.

National Academy of Sciences: Institute of Medicine <http://www.iom.edu/>. The Institute of Medicine (IOM) is an independent, nonprofit organization that works outside of government to provide unbiased and authoritative advice to government, the private sector, and the public. This site includes IOM reports published after 1998. All reports from the IOM and the National Academies, including those published before 1998, are available from the National Academies Press.

Partners in Information Access for the Public Health Workforce <http://phpartners.org/>. Partners in Information Access for the Public Health Workforce is a collaboration of U.S. government agencies, public health organizations, and health sciences libraries which provides timely, convenient access to selected public health resources on the Internet.

PubMed <http://www.ncbi.nlm.nih.gov/pubmed/>. PubMed comprises more than 19 million citations for biomedical articles from MEDLINE and life science journals. Citations may include links to full-text articles from PubMed Central or publisher web sites.

The Research Portfolio Online Reporting Tool <http://report.nih.gov/index.aspx>. The Research Portfolio Online Reporting Tool (RePORT) provides access to reports, data, and analyses of NIH research activities. The RePORT Expenditures and Results (RePORTER) query tool provides details on NIH-supported research projects.

REFERENCES

1. Jones R, Kinmonth A-L. *Critical Reading for Primary Care.* Oxford, UK: Oxford University Press; 1995.
2. Greenhalgh T. How to read a paper. Getting your bearings (deciding what the paper is about). *Br Med J.* 1997;315:243–246.
3. Makela M, Witt K. How to read a paper: critical appraisal of studies for application in healthcare. *Singapore Med J.* 2005;46(3):108–114; quiz 115.
4. Breslow RA, Ross SA, Weed DL. Quality of reviews in epidemiology. *Am J Public Health.* 1998;88(3):475–477.
5. Glass GV. Primary, secondary and meta-analysis of research. *Educ Res.* 1976;5:3–8.
6. Petitti DB. *Meta-analysis, Decision Analysis, and Cost-Effectiveness Analysis: Methods for Quantitative Synthesis in Medicine.* 2nd ed. New York, NY: Oxford University Press; 2000.
7. Canadian Task Force on the Periodic Health Examination. The periodic health examination. Canadian Task Force on the Periodic Health Examination. *Can Med Assoc J.* 1979;121(9):1193–1254.
8. US Preventive Services Task Force. *Guide to Clinical Preventive Services.* 2nd ed. Baltimore, MD: Williams & Wilkins; 1996.
9. Zaza S, Briss PA, Harris KW, eds. *The Guide to Community Preventive Services: What Works to Promote Health?* New York, NY: Oxford University Press; 2005.
10. Porta M, ed. *A Dictionary of Epidemiology.* 5th ed. New York, NY: Oxford University Press; 2008.
11. Straus SE, Richardson WS, Glasziou P, Haynes R. *Evidence-Based Medicine. How to Practice and Teach EBM.* 3rd ed. Edinburgh, UK: Churchill Livingston; 2005.
12. Garrard J. *Health Sciences Literature Review Made Easy. The Matrix Method.* 2nd ed. Sudbury, MA: Jones and Bartlett Publishers; 2006.
13. Bjork B, Roos A, Lauri M. Scientific journal publishing: yearly volume and open access availability. Paper 391. *Inform Res.* 2009;14(1).
14. Bartholomew LK, Parcel GS, Kok G, Gottlieb NH. *Planning Health Promotion Programs: Intervention Mapping.* 2nd ed. San Francisco, CA: Jossey Bass; 2006.
15. Dickersin K, Scherer R, Lefebvre C. Identifying relevant studies for systematic reviews. *BMJ.* 1994;309(6964):1286–1291.
16. Muir Gray JA. *Evidence-Based Healthcare: How to Make Health Policy and Management Decisions.* New York, NY/Edinburgh, UK: Churchill Livingstone; 1997.
17. Schindler JV, Middleton C. Conducting public health research on the World Wide Web. *Int Elect J Health Educ.* 2001;4:308–317.
18. Rimer BK, Glanz DK, Rasband G. Searching for evidence about health education and health behavior interventions. *Health Educ Behav.* 2001;28(2):231–248.

8

Developing and Prioritizing Intervention Options

> For every complex problem, there is a solution that is simple, neat, and wrong.
> —H. L. Mencken

A central challenge for public health is to articulate and act upon a broad definition of public health—one that incorporates a multidisciplinary approach to the underlying causes of premature death and disability.[1] To implement an evidence-based process within this framework, numerous program and policy options become apparent. Identifying and choosing among these options are not simple, straightforward tasks. The preceding chapters were designed to help readers define a problem and develop a broad array of choices. For example, methods from descriptive epidemiology and public health surveillance can be used to characterize the magnitude of a particular issue and tools such as economic evaluation are useful in assessing the benefits of an intervention compared with the costs.

After options are identified, priorities need to be set among various alternatives. In general, methods for setting priorities are better developed for clinical interventions than for community approaches, in part because there is a larger body of evidence on the effectiveness of clinical interventions than on that of community-based studies. There is also a larger base of cost-effectiveness studies of clinical interventions. However, it is unlikely that even the most conscientious and well-intentioned clinician will incorporate all recommended preventive services during each visit by a patient, given competing demands.[2,3] Decisions about which clinical services to deliver are driven in part by patient demands, recent news stories, medical education, and adequacy of reimbursement.[4] A patient in a clinical setting might have several health issues so part of the evidence-based medicine process is deciding which to address first. Similarly, communities have many public health challenges and a systematic process helps to prioritize these. In community settings, many of the tools and approaches for identifying and prioritizing interventions are still being developed and tested.

This chapter is divided into four main sections. The first describes some broad-based considerations to take into account when examining options and priorities. The next section outlines analytic methods and models that have been applied when setting clinical and community priorities in health promotion and disease prevention. The third part is an overview of the concepts of innovation and creativity in option selection. And the final portion describes the development and uses of analytic frameworks in developing and prioritizing options. This chapter primarily focuses on Type 1 evidence (etiology, burden) and its role in identifying and prioritizing public health issues. Details on Types 2 and 3 evidence (selecting and applying specific interventions) are provided in other chapters.

BACKGROUND

Resources are always limited in public health; in many ways programs in public health represent a "zero-sum game." That is, the total available resources for public health programs and services are not likely to increase substantially from year to year. Only rarely are there exceptions to this scenario, such as the investments several U.S. states have made in tobacco control, resulting in substantial public health benefits.[5] Therefore, careful, evidence-based examination of program options is necessary to ensure that the most effective approaches to improving the public's health are taken. The key is to follow a process that is systematic, objective, and time efficient, combining science with the realities of the environment.[6]

At a macrolevel, part of the goal in setting priorities carefully is to shift from resource-based decision making to a population-based process. To varying degrees this occurred in the United States during the twentieth century. In the resource-based planning cycle, the spiral of increased resources and increased demand for resources helped to drive the cost of health care services continually higher, even as the health status of some population groups declined.[7] In contrast, the population-based planning cycle gives greater attention to population needs and outcomes, including quality of life, and has been described as the starting point in decision making.[7] On a global scale, the Millennium Development Goals[8] offer insights into the need to set a broad range of priorities and the need to involve many sectors (e.g., economics, education) outside of health to achieve progress (Table 8-1). The population-based, intersectoral planning cycle is the desired framework and is either implicitly or explicitly followed throughout this chapter.

When one is examining options, there are at least six different sources of information, including several that have been discussed in earlier chapters. These sources can be grouped in two broad categories: scientific information and "other expert" information. Among scientific sources, the practitioner might seek program options derived from peer-reviewed sources; this might include journal

Table 8-1. Health in the Millennium Development Goals

Goal	Focus
1	Eradicate extreme poverty and hunger
2	Achieve universal primary education
3	Promote gender equality and empower women
4	Reduce child mortality
5	Improve maternal health
6	Combat HIV/AIDS, malaria, and other diseases
7	Ensure environmental sustainability
8	Develop a global partnership for development

articles or evidence-based summary documents such as clinical or community guidelines. Within the broad group of "other expert" information, one might seek input from professional colleagues in the workplace, at professional meetings, or via key stakeholders (see Chapters 4 and 5). Overarching all of these categories is the mechanism for identifying options. Electronic mechanisms such as the Internet can be especially promising in this regard for busy practitioners. Using the Internet, program options can be rapidly scanned from a desktop computer. Some excellent examples of useful Internet sites are provided at the end of this chapter.

As options are being considered and a course of action determined, it is important to distinguish decision making from problem solving. Problem solving involves the determination of one correct solution; it is like solving a mathematical problem. In contrast, decision making in organizations is the process of making a choice from among a set of rational alternatives. In choosing a public health approach, there is often not one "correct" answer but rather a set of options to be identified and prioritized.[9,10] Decision making in public health settings occurs in the context of uncertainty. Epidemiologic uncertainty in study design and interpretation was discussed in Chapters 2 and 6. Other influences on the decision-making process include politics, legal issues, economic forces, and societal values. Modern decision-making theory also recognizes that individual decision makers are influenced by their values, unconscious reflexes, skills, and habits.[11] Key elements for effective decision making in the context of uncertainty include

- Acquiring sufficient evidence on all alternatives
- Approaching the problem in a rational and systematic fashion
- Relying on experience, intuition, and judgment.

It is also important to understand that decision making often involves some element of risk and that these risks can occur at various levels. At the program level, the program option chosen may not be the optimal choice or may not be implemented properly, thus limiting the ability to reach objectives. Within an organization, program staff may be hesitant to provide objective data on various options, especially when a negative outcome could lead to program discontinuation (and loss of jobs). But an organization and leaders who support creativity and innovation will encourage new ideas even when risk is present.

ANALYTIC METHODS FOR PRIORITIZING HEALTH ISSUES AND PROGRAM OPTIONS

There are many different ways of prioritizing program and policy issues in public health practice. Although it is unlikely that "one size fits all," several tools and resources have proved useful for practitioners in a variety of settings. In addition to using various analytic methods, priority setting will occur at different geographic and political levels. An entire country may establish broad health priorities. In the Netherlands, a comprehensive approach was applied to health services delivery that included an investment in health technology assessment, use of guidelines, and development of criteria to determine priority on waiting lists. Underlying this approach was the belief that excluding certain health care services was necessary to ensure access of all citizens to essential health care.[12] In Croatia, a participatory, "bottom up" approach combined quantitative and qualitative approaches to allow each county to set its priorities based on local population health needs.[13] The Croatian example also provides an example of how a country can avoid a centralized, "one-size-fits-all" approach that may be ineffective.

In other instances, an individual state or province may conduct a priority-setting process. Based on the recommendations of an 11-member group of consumers and health care professionals, the state of Oregon ranked public health services covered under its Medicaid program, using cost-effectiveness analysis and various qualitative measures, to extend coverage for high priority services to a greater number of the state's poor residents.[14,15] These approaches often need to take community values into account. In Oregon, for example, a series of 47 community meetings resulted in a grouping of 13 key values into three categories: value to society, value to an individual in need of a service, and attributes that are essential to basic health care (e.g., prevention, quality of life).[16,17] The Oregon Health Services Commission ranks medical services from most to least important to low-income populations and the state legislature defines the health care package benefits from this list.[16]

Experience in New Zealand and Australia shows that stakeholder input can be valuable in priority setting and developing community action plans[18,19] (Box 8-1). Many of the same approaches that have been applied at a macrolevel can be used to prioritize programs or policies within a public health or voluntary health agency, within a health care organization, or at a city or county level.

Box 8-1. Prioritizing Environmental Interventions to Prevent Obesity

Obesity is increasing at such a rate that some now consider it a pandemic. Researchers from New Zealand and Australia proposed an ecological framework for understanding obesity that included influences of biology, individual behavior, and the environment.[18] With this framework, they developed the ANGELO (Analysis Grid for Elements Linked to Obesity) model that has been used to prioritize the settings and sectors for interventions to address obesity. The ANGELO method utilizes a grid that includes two sizes of environments on one axis (i.e., microsettings, such as neighborhoods and schools, and macrosectors such as transportation systems and health care systems). On the other axis, four types of environments (physical, economic, political, and sociocultural) are mapped. This framework has been used in six diverse obesity prevention projects in Australia, New Zealand, Fiji, and Tonga, where data were collected from group and individual (stakeholder) interviews among local residents and health workers.[19] Stakeholders generated a long list of potential "obesogenic" elements and ranked each according to the perceived relevance to their community and their potential changeability. The ANGELO framework has proven to be a flexible and efficient tool for action planning and setting priorities that is responsive to community needs and the latest scientific knowledge.[18]

Prioritizing Clinical Preventive Services

There have been few systematic attempts to develop and apply objective criteria for prioritizing clinical preventive services. As noted in Chapter 3, prioritization of clinical interventions tends to benefit from the development of guidelines for primary care providers. These include the efforts of the Canadian Task Force on the Periodic Health Examination[20] and the U.S. Preventive Services Task Force.[21]

An approach to prioritizing clinical preventive services was first proposed by Coffield and colleagues.[4,22,23] This approach was developed in conjunction with the publication of the third edition of *The Guide to Clinical Preventive Services.* With analytic methods, clinical interventions were ranked according to two dimensions: burden of disease prevented by each service and average cost-effectiveness. Burden was described by the clinically preventable burden (CPB): the amount of disease that would be prevented by a particular service in usual practice if the service were delivered to 100% of the target population. CPB was measured in quality-adjusted life years (QALYs), as defined in Chapter 3. Cost-effectiveness (CE) was the ratio of net costs to burden of disease prevented, that is (costs of prevention-costs averted)/QALYs saved. Each service was assigned CPB and CE scores from 1 to 5 (according to quintile), with 5 being the best possible score. The rankings were added so that each service ended up with a final score from 1 to 10 (Table 8-2). It is worth noting that scores are not proportionate, for example, a total score of 8 is

Table 8-2. Ranking of Clinical Preventive Services for the US Population

Clinical preventive service	CPB	CE	Total
Discuss daily aspirin use: men 40+, women 50+	5	5	10
Childhood immunizations	5	5	10
Smoking cessation advice and help to quit: adults	5	5	10
Alcohol screening and brief counseling: adults	4	5	9
Colorectal cancer screening: adults 50+	4	4	8
Hypertension screening and treatment: adults 18+	5	3	8
Influenza immunization: adults 50+	4	4	8
Vision screening: adults 65+	3	5	8
Cervical cancer screening: women	4	3	7
Cholesterol screening and treatment: men 35+, women 45+	5	2	7
Pneumococcal immunization: adults 65+	3	4	7
Breast cancer screening: women 40+	4	2	6
Chlamydia screening: sexually active women under 25	2	4	6
Discuss calcium supplementation: women	3	3	6
Vision screening: preschool children	2	4	6
Folic acid chemoprophylaxis: women of childbearing age	2	3	5
Obesity screening: adults	3	2	5
Depression screening: adults	3	1	4
Hearing screening: adults 65+	2	2	4
Injury-prevention counseling: parents of child 0–4	1	3	4
Osteoporosis screening: women 65+	2	2	4
Cholesterol screening: men <35, women <45 at high risk	1	1	2
Diabetes screening: adults at risk	1	1	2
Diet counseling: adults at risk	1	1	2
Tetanus-diphtheria booster: adults	1	1	2

Sources: Maciosek et al.[23] and Maciosek et al.[4]

more valuable but not necessarily twice as valuable as a total score of 4.[24] With this method, the three interventions with the highest priority rankings were discussion of daily aspirin use with men 40 years and older and women 50 years and older, vaccination of children to prevent a variety of infectious diseases, and smoking cessation advice for adults.

There have also been attempts to develop and apply criteria for prioritizing health behaviors for populations, using the epidemiologic concept of risk and, in some cases, applying it to economic costs. One such model is the Health Risk Appraisal (HRA). HRA evolved from a counseling tool that physicians and health educators used with their patients into a simulation model that projects results of behavior change programs targeted at particular populations. The HRA contains three essential features: (1) an assessment of personal health habits and risk factors based on questionnaire responses from the patient or client; (2) a quantitative or qualitative assessment of an individual's future risk of death or adverse health outcomes; and (3) the provision of educational messages on ways of reducing health risks.[25] Outcome results can be assessed as savings attributed to medical costs for numerous health behaviors.[26]

Prioritizing Public Health Issues at the Community Level

There are both qualitative and quantitative approaches to setting public health priorities for communities. Although many and diverse definitions of "community" have been offered, we define it as a group of individuals that shares attributes of place, social interaction, and social and political responsibility.[27] In practice, many data systems are organized geographically and therefore communities are often defined by place. A sound priority-setting process can help generate widespread support for public health issues when it is well documented and endorsed by communities.[28]

The prioritization approach, based on comparison of a population health problem with the "ideal" or "achievable" population health status, is sometimes used to advance the policy decision-making process by singling out an objective, limited set of health problems. It usually involves identifying desirable or achievable levels for an epidemiologic measure such as mortality, incidence, or prevalence. One such approach used the lowest achieved mortality rate, calculated from mortality rates that actually have been achieved by some population or population segment at some time and place, and risk-eliminated mortality rates, estimated by mortality levels that would have been achieved with elimination of known risk factors.[29] A variation of this approach can be used to identify disparities related to race/ethnicity, gender, or other groupings of populations. Similar approaches have been applied in states in the United States,[30,31] in Japan,[32] and in Spain.[33]

Multiple groups of researchers and practitioners have proposed standardized criteria for prioritizing public health issues at the community level.[6,13,28,34–38] Each of these methods differs, but they have at least three common elements. First, each relies on some measure of burden, whether measured in mortality, morbidity, or years of potential life lost. Each method also attempts to quantify preventability (i.e., the potential effects of intervention). And finally, resource issues are often addressed in the decision making process, in terms of both costs of intervention and the resources of an organization to carry out a particular program or policy. Two analytical methods frequently used as auxiliary in the prioritization process are economic appraisal and an approach based on comparison with "ideal" or "achievable" population health status.[29] Several approaches to categorizing and prioritizing various interventions that use the three common elements will be discussed briefly here as well as one example each of the approaches based on economic data and achievable population health status.

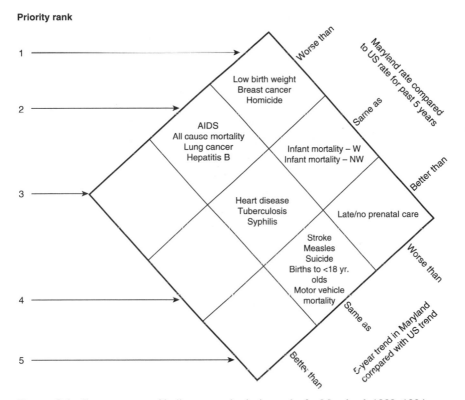

Figure 8-1. Consensus set of indicators and priority ranks for Maryland, 1989–1994.

Using a different process, the Maryland Department of Health in cooperation with 24 local jurisdictions established a prioritization process based on consensus indicators and comparisons with U.S. rates and trends[28] (Figure 8-1). They refer to their model as the "golden diamond." It permitted state and local comparisons of various endpoints, based on morbidity and mortality rates. Ranks were used to help decide where state and local resources should be focused. This initial prioritization was based solely on data and did not include qualitative factors. One of its major advantages is that it is based on existing data sets and is therefore relatively easy to carry out.

Another approach to prioritization, largely based on quantitative methods, was proposed by Hanlon and Pickett[34] and further elaborated by Vilnius and Dandoy[6] and Simoes and colleagues.[37] The model, the Basic Priority Rating (BPR), is based on the following formula:

$$BPR = [(A + B) C]/3 \times D$$

where A is the size of the problem, B is the seriousness of the problem, C is the effectiveness of intervention, and D is propriety, economics, acceptability, resources, and legality (known as PEARL). Values for each part of the formula are converted from rates and ratings to scores. Finer details of these quantitative rating systems are available in the original publications.[6,34,37]

As an illustration, the Missouri Department of Health and Senior Services applied a prioritization method using surveillance-derived data (the Priority MICA).[37] The Priority MICA extends the work of Vilnius and Dandoy by adding to the earlier criteria (magnitude, severity, urgency, preventability), a new criterion of community support, two additional measures of severity (disability, number of hospital days of care), two additional measures of urgency (incidence and prevalence trends), a criterion of racial disparity, another measure of magnitude (prevalence of risk factors, measured from two sources), and a new measure of preventability. The ranking of a final score, from highest to lowest priority, identified the counties with significantly higher morbidity and mortality than the state. This information can be displayed in maps to identify each of the priority diseases and conditions and to prioritize by geographical area (county). For each condition, map colors reflected the three possible classifications of mortality and morbidity in each county in relation to the state: significantly higher than state, higher than state, same/less than state. These data show how the outcome selected (e.g., disability, racial disparity in deaths) can have a large impact on the relative importance of different diseases[37] (Table 8-3). These data are available online at http:// www.dhss.mo.gov/PriorityMICA/.

A relatively straightforward and more qualitative way of categorizing program and policy options has been presented by Green and Kreuter[39] (Table 8-4). Within this 2 × 2 framework, options can be categorized according to their importance and changeability. Importance might be based on burden of disease, injury, impairment, or exposure. Changeability is synonymous with preventability. Within this framework, options in the upper left and lower right cells are relatively easy to prioritize. Those in the lower left and upper right are more difficult to assess. A highly important issue but one about which little is known from a preventive standpoint should be the focus of innovation in program development. A strong focus on evaluation should be maintained in this category so that new programs can be assessed for effectiveness. A program or policy in the upper right corner might be initiated for political, social, or cultural reasons.

Regardless of the method used, the first major stage in setting community priorities is to decide upon the criteria. The framework might include one of those described earlier or may be a composite of various approaches. After criteria are determined, the next steps include forming a working team and/or advisory group, assembling the necessary data to conduct the prioritization process, establishing a

Table 8-3. Ranking of Diseases on the Basis of Different Criteria, Missouri, 2002

		SPECIFIC CRITERIA		
Ranking	All Measures	Deaths for People Younger Than 65 Years	Disability	Racial Disparity for Deaths
1	Diabetes	Heart disease	Affective disorder	Sickle cell anemia
2	Alcohol- and substance-related diseases	Lung cancer	Alcohol- and substance-related diseases	Assaults/ homicides
3	Heart disease	Motor vehicle accidents	Arthritis/lupus	Tuberculosis
4	COPD*	Suicides/self-inflicted injuries	Alzheimer's disease/dementia/ senility	HIV/AIDS
5	Arthritis/lupus	Alcohol- and substance-related diseases	COPD	Dental health problems
6	Pneumonia and influenza	Infant health problems	Diabetes	Pregnancy complications
7	Motor vehicle accidents	Assaults/homicides	Asthma	Asthma
8	Assaults/ homicides	Stroke/other cerebrovascular disease	Anxiety-related mental disorder	Burns (fire and flames)
9	Stroke/other cerebrovascular disease	COPD	Lead poisoning	Abuse/neglect
10	Infant health problems	Breast cancer	Stroke/other cerebrovascular disease	Cervical cancer

*COPD denotes chronic obstructive pulmonary disease.

Source: Simoes et al.[37]

Table 8-4. Considerations in Setting Program Priorities

	More Important	Less Important
More changeable	Highest priority for program focus	Low priority except to demonstrate change for political or other purpose
	Example: interventions to improve vaccination coverage in children, adolescents, and adults	*Example:* programs to prevent work-related pneumoconiosis
Less changeable	Priority for innovative program with evaluation essential	No intervention program
	Example: programs to prevent mental impairment and disability	*Example:* programs to prevent Hodgkin's Disease

Source: Adapted from Green and Kreuter.[39]

To use	Sample criteria	Measure	Score	Weight[b]	Weighted score	Priority score
✓	(tailor to ensure criteria can be applied to all health issues being weighed)	(cite specific measure and data source if available)	(score data, assign points, or rank using identified method)	(assign value to criteria if desired)	(score multiplied by weight)	(sum of weighted scores for each criterion used)
	Prevalence					
	Mortality rate					
	Community concern					
	Lost productivity (e.g., bed-disability days)					
	Premature mortality (e.g., years of potential life lost)					
	Medical costs to treat (or community economic costs)					
	Feasibility to prevent					
	Other					

FIGURE 8-2. Generic worksheet for priority setting. *Source: Healthy People 2010* Toolkit.[28] *Note:* A weight ensures that certain characteristics have a greater influence than others have in the final priority ranking. A sample formula might be: 2(Prevalence Score) + Community Concern Score + 3(Medical Cost Score) = Priority Score. In this example, the weight for prevalence is 2 and medical cost is 3. Users might enter data or assign scores (such as 1-5) for each criterion and use the formula to calculate a total score for the health event.

process for stakeholder input and review, and determining a process for revisiting priorities at regular intervals. Vilnius and Dandoy[6] recommend that a six-to-eight member group be assembled to guide the BPR process. This group should include members within and outside the agency. A generic priority-setting worksheet is provided in Figure 8-2.[28] This worksheet provides some guidance on the types of information that would typically need to be collected and summarized before a work group begins its activity.

Other Considerations and Caveats

In setting priorities within public health, it important to consider several issues related to leadership and measurement. No determination of public health priorities should be reduced solely to numbers; values, social justice, and the political climate all play roles. Changes in public health leadership present a unique challenge. The median tenure for a state public health officer is only about 2 years,[40] whereas for city and county health officers the median tenure is longer (about 6 years).[41] This turnover in leadership may lead to a lack of long-term focus on public health priorities. Each analytic method for prioritization has particular strengths and weaknesses. Some methods rely heavily on quantitative data, but valid and usable data can be difficult to come by, especially for smaller geographic areas such as cities or neighborhoods. It can also be difficult to identify the proper metrics for comparison of various health conditions. For example, using mortality alone would ignore the disabling burden of arthritis when it is compared to other chronic diseases. Utility-based measures (e.g., QALYs) are advantageous as they are comparable across diseases and risk factors. Rankings, especially close ranks, should be assessed with caution. One useful approach is to divide a distribution of health issues into quartiles or quintiles and compare the extremes of a distribution. In addition, some key stakeholders may find that quantitative methods of prioritization fail to present a full picture, suggesting the need to use methods that combine quantitative and qualitative approaches.

INNOVATION AND CREATIVITY
IN PROGRAM DEVELOPMENT

Another factor to consider in program development is innovation. Innovation has been defined as "a new method, idea, or product."[42] In many instances, there is a trade-off between the level to which a program is evidence based, via the scientific literature, and the degree to which it is innovative. Consider, for example, the evidence from a review of programs that promote seat belt use to prevent motor vehicle injuries. From these, there is strong evidence that enforcement programs are effective in promoting seat belt use and hence, reducing motor vehicle injuries.[43] If you were planning to set up a program, would you follow what has already been done or try a new (and perhaps more innovative) approach? In practice, it is crucial to search for existing and new program approaches for several reasons. First, there is no guarantee that a program proven to work in one population or geographic area will yield the same results in another locality (see discussion of external validity in Chapter 2). Second, since the evidence base in many areas of public health intervention is relatively weak, a continual discovery of new and innovative approaches is crucial.

And third, the development of innovative programs can be motivating for the people carrying out programs and the community members with whom they work.

Creativity in Developing Alternatives

Creativity and its role in effective decision making are not fully understood. Creativity is the process of developing original, imaginative, and innovative options.[42] To understand the role of creativity in decision-making, it is helpful to know about its nature and process and the techniques for nurturing it.

Researchers have sought to understand the characteristics of creative people. Above a threshold in the intelligence quotient, there does not appear to be a strong correlation between creativity and intelligence.[44] There also seem to be few differences in creativity between men and women.[45] Several other characteristics that have been consistently associated with creativity. The typical period in the life cycle of greatest creativity appears to be between the ages of 30 and 40. It also seems that more creative people are less susceptible to social influences than those who are less creative.

The creative process has been described in four stages: preparation, incubation, insight, and verification.[46] The preparation phase is highly dependent on the education and training of the individual embarking on the creative process. Incubation usually involves a period of relaxation after a period of preparation. The human mind gathers and sorts data, and then needs time for ideas to jell. In the incubation period, it is often useful to direct energies toward some other pursuits before returning to the task at hand. In the insight phase, one gradually or rapidly, becomes aware of a new idea or approach. And finally, in the verification phase, the individual verifies the appropriateness of the idea or solution. In the business setting, this would include consumer surveys or focus groups to test the acceptance of a new product.

Within an organizational setting, a number of processes can enhance creativity in decision-making. It is important to identify ways to create a trusting work environment and to reward creativity within an organization and to encourage the appropriate level of risk taking among employees, ensuring that individual freedom and autonomy are not unduly constrained. The risks of creativity were summarized by a manager:

"With creativity comes uncertainty. Whenever you have uncertainty people feel uncomfortable and insecure. If [a creative decision] is not successful, the negative things that can happen to you are ten times greater than the positive things" (pp. 723–724).[47]

Group Processes for Enhancing Creativity

In most areas of public health, important and creative decisions are enhanced by group decision-making processes. Often in a group process, a consensus is reached

Table 8-5. Advantages and Disadvantages of Group Decision Making

Advantages	Disadvantages
More information and knowledge are available	The process takes longer and may be costlier
More alternatives are likely to be generated	Compromise decisions resulting from indecisiveness may emerge
Better acceptance of the final decision is likely, often among those who will carry out the decision	One person may dominate the group
Enhanced communication of the decision may result	"Groupthink" may occur
More accurate and creative decisions often emerge	

Source: Griffin.[48]

on some topics. There are advantages and disadvantages to group decision-making processes (Table 8-5), but the former generally outweigh the latter.[48] Probably, the greatest advantage is that more and better information is available to inform a decision when a group is used. Additional advantages include better acceptance of the final decision, enhanced communication, and more accurate decisions. The biggest disadvantage of group decision making is that the process takes longer. However, the management literature shows that, in general, the more "person-hours" that go into a decision, the more likely it will be that the correct one emerges, and the more likely that the decision will be implemented.[49] Other potential disadvantages include the potential for indecisiveness, compromise decisions, and domination by one individual. In addition, an outcome known as "group-think" may result, in which the group's desire for consensus and cohesiveness overwhelms its desire to reach the best possible decision.[49,50] One way to offset groupthink is the rotation of new members into a decision-making group.

The following sections briefly outline three popular brainstorming techniques that are useful in developing and managing an effective group process: the Delphi method, the nominal group technique, and scenario planning. Other techniques for gathering information from groups and individuals (e.g., focus groups, key informant interviews) are described in Chapters 4 and 10.

The Delphi Method.   The Delphi method was developed by the Rand Corporation in the 1950s. It is named after the oracle of Delphi from Ancient Greece, who could offer advice on the right course of action in many situations.[51] It is a judgment tool for prediction and forecast, involving a panel of anonymous experts to whom intensive questionnaires and feedback were given in order to obtain consensus on a particular topic.[52,53] Although the method has been modified and used in various ways over the years, it remains a useful way to solicit and refine expert opinion. The Delphi method is most appropriate for broad, long-range issues such as strategic planning and environmental assessments. It is not feasible for routine decisions. It can be especially useful for a geographically dispersed group of experts. There are three types of Delphi: classic, policy, and decision.[54] The decision Delphi is most relevant here as it provides a forum for decisions. Panel members are not anonymous (although responses are), and the goal is a defined and supported outcome. Another important characteristic of the Delphi method is that it is iterative and responses are refined over rounds of sampling.

The first step in a Delphi process involves the selection of an expert panel. This panel should generally include a range of experts across the public health field, including practitioners, researchers, and funders. A panel of 30 or fewer members is often used.[55] The Delphi method may involve a series of questionnaires (by mail or e-mail) that begin more generally and, through iteration, become more specific over several weeks or months. Open-ended questions may be used in early drafts with multiple-choice responses in later versions. A flow chart for a typical Delphi process is shown in Figure 8-3,[56] Definitions of consensus within a Delphi method vary—from full consensus to majority rule—and should be specified at the outset. The critical elements of a successful Delphi process include identifying an appropriate panel of experts, designing a useful set of questions, and summarizing individual input.[56]

Nominal Group Technique. Another useful method is the nominal group technique (NGT).[57] Unlike the Delphi methods where panel members do not see each other, the NGT involves in-person interactions in the same room. However, 6 to 10 members represent a group in name only and may not always interact as a group in a typical work setting. The NGT can be useful in generating creative and innovative alternatives and is more feasible than a Delphi method for routine decisions. A key to a successful NGT is an experienced and competent facilitator, who assembles the group and outlines the problem to them. It is also important to outline the specific rules that the NGT will follow.[55] Often data and information, such as data from a community assessment, will have been provided to the group in advance of the meeting. Group members are asked to write down as many alternatives as they can think of. They then take turns stating these ideas, which are recorded on a flipchart or blackboard. Discussion is limited to simple clarification. After all alternatives have been listed, each is discussed in more detail. When discussion is completed, sometimes after a series of meetings, the various alternatives are generally voted on and rank-ordered. The primary advantage of NGT is that it can identify a large number of alternatives while minimizing the impact of group or individual opinions on the responses of individuals. The main disadvantage is that the team leader or administrator may not support the highest-ranked alternative, dampening group enthusiasm if his or her work is rejected.

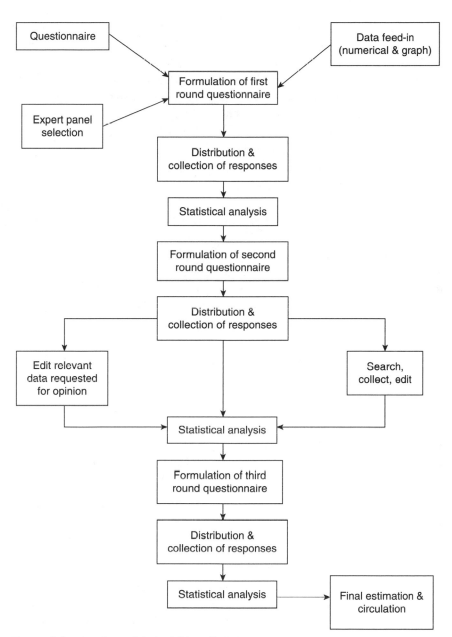

FIGURE 8-3. Flowchart of the Delphi methods.
(*Source:* Krueger and Casey[56])

Scenario Planning.   Often used in the corporate sector, scenario planning is a third useful group process for generating information for decision making. In this method, future-oriented scenarios are developed, based on how an event or system will look at some target time horizon. Scenario planning is particularly useful in an environment where there are numerous uncertainties and no clear map for the future.[58] The goal is to make decisions that are sound for all plausible futures.[59] Many characteristics and stages of scenario planning are similar to the process of environmental assessment, discussed in Chapter 5 in the context of strategic planning.

Although there are relatively few guidelines for writing scenarios, eight major stages of scenario planning have been proposed[55]:

1. Define the general area of interest or system for the scenario in operational terms.
2. Establish a concrete time horizon for the scenario.
3. Identify external constraints or factors that will affect the area or system of interest (e.g., social, economic, political, technological issues).
4. Describe the factors within the system that are likely to increase or decrease its chances of achieving desired goals and objectives.
5. Specify the likelihood of the occurrence of facilitators to or barriers to success.
6. Create one or more (often three) scenarios based on various assumptions arising in stages 3 to 5.
7. Subject the scenarios to testing and review by others.
8. Use the scenario for defining policy and future directions for action.

Although scenarios can be very useful in planning, they can also be difficult to write. It is advisable for newcomers to scenario writing to consult someone who is experienced.

DEVELOPING AND USING ANALYTIC FRAMEWORKS

Analytic frameworks (also called logic models or causal frameworks) have benefited numerous areas of public health practice, particularly in developing and implementing clinical and community-based guidelines.[60-62] An analytic framework is a diagram that depicts the interrelationships between program resources, intervention activities, outputs, shorter-term intervention outcomes, and longer-term public health outcomes. The major purpose of an analytic framework is to map out the linkages on which to base conclusions about intervention effectiveness. An underlying assumption is that various linkages represent "causal pathways," some of which are mutable and can be intervened upon. Numerous types of analytic frameworks are described in Battista and Fletcher.[63]

People designing public health interventions often have in mind an analytic framework that leads from program inputs to health outputs if the program works as intended. It is important for planning and evaluation purposes that what Lipsey has termed this "small theory" of the intervention be made explicit early, often in the form of a diagram.[64] In attempting to map inputs, mediators, and outputs, it important to determine whether mediators, or constructs, lie "upstream" or "downstream" from a particular intervention.[65] As an analytic framework develops, the diagram also identifies key outcomes to be considered when formulating a data collection plan is formulated. These are then translated into public health indicators (i.e., measures of the extent to which targets in health programs are being reached). Besides helping to identify key information to be collected, an analytic framework can also be viewed as a set of hypotheses about program action, including the time sequence in which program-related changes should occur; these can later guide data analysis. If the program is subsequently successful in influencing outcomes at the end of this causal chain, having measures of the intermediate steps available aids interpretation by clarifying how those effects came about. Conversely, if little change in ultimate outcomes is observed, having measures of intermediate steps can help to diagnose where the causal chain was broken.[66]

Analytic frameworks can be relatively simple or complicated, with every possible relationship between risk factors, interventions, and health outcomes. A generic analytic framework is shown in Figure 8-4.[63] A more comprehensive approach may describe potential relationships between an intervention, intermediate outcomes, physical activity, and long-term health outcomes, as described in Figure 8-5. An analytic framework (logic model) for program planning for oral health is shown in Figure 8-6.[67] By developing this and related diagrams, researchers and practitioners were able to (1) describe the inputs needed for a particular intervention, (2) indicate intervention options for changing relevant outcomes; (3) indicate categories of relevant interventions, (4) describe the outputs and outcomes that the interventions attempt to influence; and (5) indicate the types of intervention activities that were included in a program and those that were not.[68,69]

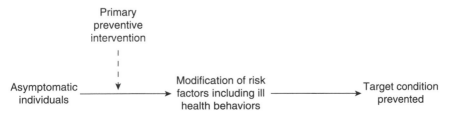

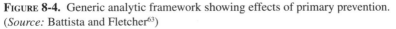

FIGURE 8-4. Generic analytic framework showing effects of primary prevention. (*Source:* Battista and Fletcher[63])

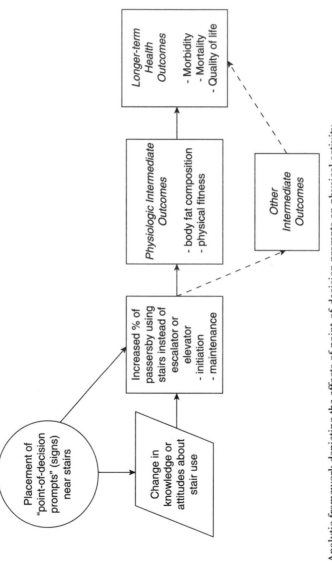

Figure 8-5. Analytic framework depicting the effects of point-of-decision prompts on physical activity.

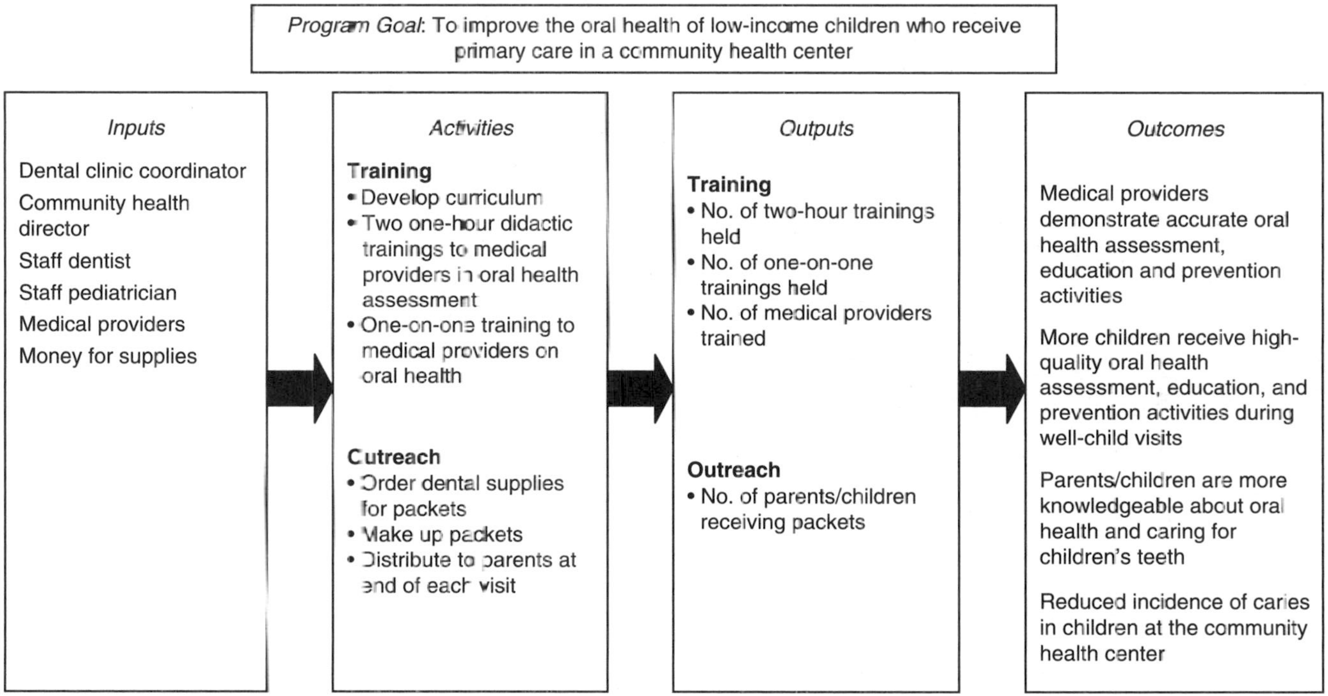

Program Goal: To improve the oral health of low-income children who receive primary care in a community health center

Inputs

Dental clinic coordinator
Community health director
Staff dentist
Staff pediatrician
Medical providers
Money for supplies

Activities

Training
- Develop curriculum
- Two one-hour didactic trainings to medical providers in oral health assessment
- One-on-one training to medical providers on oral health

Outreach
- Order dental supplies for packets
- Make up packets
- Distribute to parents at end of each visit

Outputs

Training
- No. of two-hour trainings held
- No. of one-on-one trainings held
- No. of medical providers trained

Outreach
- No. of parents/children receiving packets

Outcomes

Medical providers demonstrate accurate oral health assessment, education and prevention activities

More children receive high-quality oral health assessment, education, and prevention activities during well-child visits

Parents/children are more knowledgeable about oral health and caring for children's teeth

Reduced incidence of caries in children at the community health center

FIGURE 8-6. Analytic framework (logic model) depicting a program to improve oral health among low income children. (*Source:* Horsch[67])

Many other examples of analytic frameworks can be found in the literature. Some of these focus on programmatic areas such as promotion of physical activity,[70] drug abuse prevention,[71] and breast cancer screening.[72] Others look at mapping causal pathways in the context of program planning[38,73] or program evaluation.[61,74]

Constructing Analytic Frameworks

Several approaches and sources of information are beneficial as one begins to construct an analytic framework that will map intervention options related to a particular health issue. First, a comprehensive search of the scientific literature is essential. The methods outlined in Chapter 7 form the basis for such a search. Following this search, it is likely that the practitioner will find articles that show analytic frameworks, although these are likely to vary in completeness and sophistication. Another important part in developing a framework is the identification of mutable and immutable factors along the causal pathway. A mutable factor might relate to "exposure" to a mass media campaign on a particular health issue. Conversely, an immutable factor would be a person's gender.

It is helpful to construct analytic frameworks in a professional working group. The advantages to a group process are twofold: (1) after the literature is assembled, several members of the group can independently draft initial analytic frameworks on the same topic, and (2) once initial frameworks are available, review by a small group is likely to improve the modeling. It is important to note that the construction of an analytic framework should not be viewed as a static process. As more literature and the intervention process proceeds, the framework should be modified to fit advancing knowledge of determinants. If a work group finds it too difficult to construct an analytic framework, it may indicate that the program is too complex or that its basis is not well documented.

Considering the Broad Environment

One key component in developing analytic frameworks and subsequent interventions is consideration of the "upstream" causes of poor health status.[75,76] These factors are increasingly being recognized in the context of social epidemiology, that is, the socioenvironmental determinants of health, such as poverty and social isolation.[77] As shown in Table 8-6, the larger environment, including physical, social, legal, and cultural factors, needs to be fully considered as an intervention target.[78] Focus on environmental and policy factors is increasingly being recognized as an efficient and effective means for public health interventions.[78–80]

Even though the ultimate goal is individual behavior change, environmental programs can be designed at several different levels. Social support may be built for behavior change within a worksite, and community-wide policies may be

Table 8-6. Contrasting Approaches to Disease Prevention

Health Area	Individual	Environmental and Policy[a]
Smoking	Smoking cessation classes Hypnosis Nicotine patch	Cigarette taxation Clean indoor air laws Regulation of cigarette advertising
Stress	Stress reduction classes	Reduced work demands Affordable child care Crime prevention programs
Diet/weight loss	Exercise programs Cooking classes How-to-read food labels	Public transportation Affordable housing near workplace Urban public recreation areas Food security programs Funding for farmers' markets

[a]Includes the physical, legal, social, and cultural environments.

Source: Adapted from Yen and Syme.[78]

enacted to support the same health-promoting behavior. These so-called ecologic interventions are discussed in more detail in Chapters 4 and 9.

SUMMARY

The public health practitioner has many tools at his or her fingertips for identifying and prioritizing program and policy options. This chapter has summarized several approaches that have proven useful for public health practitioners. As one proceeds through this process, several key points should be kept in mind.

Key Chapter Points

- In public health decision making, there is often not one "correct" answer.
- Although decisions are made in the context of uncertainty and risk, classic decision theory suggests that when managers have complete information, they behave rationally.
- Group decision making has advantages and disadvantages, but in most instances, the former outweighs the latter.
- Priorities should not be set on quantitative factors alone.
- It is often useful to apply a prioritization process on a smaller scale initially when stakes are lower.
- Analytic frameworks can enhance decision making, reviews of evidence, program planning, and program evaluation.

SUGGESTED READINGS AND WEBSITES

Readings

Battista RN, Fletcher SW. Making recommendations on preventive practices: methodological issues. *Am J Prev Med* 1988;4(sSuppl):53–67.

Griffin RW. *Management.* Boston, MA: Houghton Mifflin Company, 2001.

Krueger RA, Casey MA. *Focus Groups: A Practical Guide for Applied Research.* 3rd ed. Thousand Oaks, CA: Sage Publications, 2000.

Simoes EJ, Land G, Metzger R, Mokdad A. Prioritization MICA: a Web-based application to prioritize public health resources. *J Public Health Manag Pract.* 2006;12(2):161–169.

Vilnius D, Dandoy S. A priority rating system for public health programs. *Public Health Reports.* 1990;105(5):463–470.

Selected Websites

The CDC Working Group on Evaluation <http://www.cdc.gov/eval/resources. htm>. The CDC Working Group on Evaluation has developed a comprehensive list of evaluation documents, tools, and links to other websites. These materials include documents that describe principles and standards, organizations and foundations that support evaluation, a list of journals and online publications, and access to step-by-step manuals.

Disease Control Priorities Project <http://www.dcp2.org>. The Disease Control Priorities Project (DCPP) is an ongoing effort to assess disease control priorities and produce evidence-based analysis and resource materials to inform health policymaking in developing countries. DCPP has produced three volumes providing technical resources that can assist developing countries in improving their health systems and, ultimately, the health of their people.

The Guide to Community Preventive Services (the *Community Guide*) <http:// www.thecommunityguide.org/index.html>. *The Guide to Community Preventive Services* (the *Community Guide*) provides guidance in choosing evidence-based programs and policies to improve health and prevent disease at the community level. The Task Force on Community Preventive Services, an independent, non-federal, volunteer body of public health and prevention experts appointed by the director of the CDC, has systematically reviewed more than 200 interventions to produce the recommendations and findings available at this site. The topics covered in the *Community Guide* currently include adolescent health, alcohol, asthma, birth defects, cancer, diabetes, HIV/AIDS, STIs and pregnancy, mental health, motor vehicle, nutrition, obesity, oral health, physical activity, social environment, tobacco, vaccines, violence, and worksite.

Healthy People <http://www.healthypeople.gov/>. *Healthy People* provides science-based, 10-year national objectives for promoting health and preventing disease in the United States. Since 1979, *Healthy People* has set and monitored national health objectives to meet a broad range of health needs, encourage collaborations across sectors, guide individuals toward making informed health decisions, and measure the impact of prevention activity.

Millennium Development Goals <http://www.un.org/millenniumgoals/>. This site provides information and resources on the Millennium Development Goals established by 189 world leaders at the United Nations Millennium Summit in 2000.

Partners in Information Access for the Public Health Workforce <http://phpartners. org/>. Partners in Information Access for the Public Health Workforce is a collaboration of U.S. government agencies, public health organizations, and health sciences libraries that provides timely, convenient access to selected public health resources on the Internet.

REFERENCES

1. Beaglehole R, Bonita R. *Public Health at the Crossroads: Achievements and Prospects*. Cambridge, UK: Cambridge University Press; 1997.
2. Jaen CR, Stange KC, Nutting PA. The competing demands of primary care: a model for the delivery of clinical preventive services. *J Fam Pract.* 1994;38:166–171.
3. Stange KC, Flocke SA, Goodwin MA, et al. Direct observation of rates of preventive service delivery in community family practice. *Prev Med.* 2000;31(2 Pt 1):167–176.
4. Maciosek MV, Coffield AB, Edwards NM, et al. Prioritizing clinical preventive services: a review and framework with implications for community preventive services. *Annu Rev Public Health.* Apr 29 2009;30:341–355.
5. Siegel M. The effectiveness of state-level tobacco control interventions: a review of program implementation and behavioral outcomes. *Annu Rev Public Health.* 2002;23:45–71.
6. Vilnius D, Dandoy S. A priority rating system for public health programs. *Public Health Reports.* 1990;105(5):463–470.
7. Green LW. Health education's contribution to public health in the twentieth century: a glimpse through health promotion's rear-view mirror. *Annu Rev Public Health.* 1999;20:67–88.
8. World Health Organization. *Health in the Millennium Development Goals*. Geneva: World Health Organization; 2004.
9. Savitz DA. *Interpretting Epidemiologic Evidence. Strategies for Study Design and Analysis*. New York, NY: Oxford University Press; 2003.
10. Savitz DA, Poole C, Miller WC. Reassessing the role of epidemiology in public health. *Am J Public Health.* 1999;89(8):1158–1161.
11. Simon HA. *Administrative Behavior: A Study of Decision-Making Processes in Administrative Organizations*. 4th ed. New York: Free Press; 1997.
12. Ham C. Priority setting in health care: learning from international experience. *Health Policy.* 1997;42:49–66.

13. Sogoric S, Rukavina TV, Brborovic O, et al. Counties selecting public health priorities—a "bottom-up" approach (Croatian experience). *Coll Antropol.* 2005;29(1): 111–119.
14. Eddy DM. Oregon's methods. Did cost-effectiveness analysis fail? *JAMA.* 1991; 266(3):417–420.
15. Klevit HD, Bates AC, Castanares T, et al. Prioritization of health care services: a progress report by the Oregon health services commission. *Arch Internal Med.* 1991;151:912–916.
16. Oregon Department of Human Services. *Oregon Health Plan. An Historical Overview.* Portland, OR; 2006.
17. Oregon Health Services Commission. *Prioritization of Health Services. A Report to the Governor and Legislature.* Portland, OR: Oregon Health Services Commission; 1995.
18. Swinburn B, Egger G, Raza F. Dissecting obesogenic environments: the development and application of a framework for identifying and prioritizing environmental interventions for obesity. *Prev Med.* 1999;29(6 Pt 1):563–570.
19. Simmons A, Mavoa HM, Bell AC, et al. Creating community action plans for obesity prevention using the ANGELO (Analysis Grid for Elements Linked to Obesity) Framework. *Health Promot Int.* Dec 2009;24(4):311–324.
20. Canadian Task Force on the Periodic Health Examination. The periodic health examination. Canadian Task Force on the Periodic Health Examination. *Can Med Assoc J.* 1979;121(9):1193–1254.
21. US Preventive Services Task Force. *Guide to Clinical Preventive Services: An Assessment of the Effectiveness of 169 Interventions.* Baltimore: Williams & Wilkins; 1989.
22. Coffield AB, Maciosek MV, McGinnis JM, et al. Priorities among recommended clinical preventive services (1). *Am J Prev Med.* 2001;21(1):1–9.
23. Maciosek MV, Coffield AB, Edwards NM, et al. Priorities among effective clinical preventive services: results of a systematic review and analysis. *Am J Prev Med.* 2006;31(1):52–61.
24. Maciosek MV, Coffield AB, McGinnis JM, et al. Methods for priority setting among clinical preventive services. *Am J Prev Med.* 2001;21(1):10–19.
25. DeFriese GH, Fielding JE. Health risk appraisal in the 1990s: opportunities, challenges, and expectations. *Annu Rev Public Health.* 1990;11:401–418.
26. Yen LT, Edington DW, Witting P. Associations between health risk appraisal scores and employee medical claims costs in a manufacturing company. *Am J Health Promot.* 1991;6(1):46–54.
27. Patrick DL, Wickizer TM. Community and health. In: Amick BCI, Levine S, Tarlov AR, Chapman Walsh D, eds. Society and Health. New York: Oxford University Press; 1995:46–92.
28. US Department of Health and Human Services. *Healthy People 2010 Toolkit.* Washington, DC: US Department of Health and Human Services; 2001.
29. Hahn RA, Teutsch SM, Rothenberg RB, Marks JS. Excess deaths from nine chronic diseases in the United States, 1986. *JAMA.* 1990;264(20):2654–2659.
30. Carvette ME, Hayes EB, Schwartz RH, et al. Chronic disease mortality in Maine: assessing the targets for prevention. *J Public Health Manag Pract.* 1996;2(3):25–31.
31. Hoffarth S, Brownson RC, Gibson BB, et al. Preventable mortality in Missouri: excess deaths from nine chronic diseases, 1979–1991. *Mo Med.* 1993;90(6): 279–282.

32. Fukuda Y, Nakamura K, Takano T. Increased excess deaths in urban areas: quantification of geographical variation in mortality in Japan, 1973–1998. *Health Policy.* 2004;68(2):233–244.
33. Regidor F, Inigo J, Sendra JM, Gutierrez-Fisac JL. [Evolution of mortality from principal chronic diseases in Spain 1975–1988]. *Med Clin (Barc*1992;99(19):725–728.
34. Hanlon J, Pickett G. *Public Health Administration and Practice.* Santa Clara, CA: Times Mirror/Mosby College Publishing; 1982.
35. Meltzer M, Teutsch SM. Setting priorities for health needs and managing resources. In: Stroup DF, Teutsch SM, eds. Statistics in Public Health. Quantitative Approaches to Public Health Problems. New York: Oxford University Press; 1998:123–149.
36. Murray CJ, Frenk J. Health metrics and evaluation: strengthening the science. *Lancet.* 2008;371(9619):1191–1199.
37. Simoes EJ, Land G, Metzger R, Mokdad A. Prioritization MICA: a Web-based application to prioritize public health resources. *J Public Health Manag Pract.* 2006;12(2):161–169.
38. Simons-Morton BG, Greene WH, Gottlieb NH. *Introduction to Health Education and Health Promotion.* Second ed. Prospect Heights, IL: Waveland Press; 1995.
39. Green LW, Kreuter MW. Commentary on the emerging Guide to Community Preventive Services from a health promotion perspective. *Am J Prev Med.* 2000;18(1S):7–9.
40. Gilbert B, Moos MK, Miller CA. State level decision-making for public health: the status of boards of health. *J Public Health Policy.* 1982;March:51–61.
41. Turnock BJ. *Public Health: What it is and How it Works.* 3rd ed. Gaithersburg, MD: Aspen Publishers, Inc.; 2004.
42. McKean E, ed. *The New Oxford American Dictionary.* 2nd ed. New York, NY: Oxford University Press; 2005.
43. Centers for Disease Control and Prevention. Motor-vehicle occupant injury: Strategies for increasing use of child safety seats, increasing use of safety belts, and reducing alcohol-impaired driving. A report of the Task Force on Community Preventive Services. *MMWR.* 2001;50(RR-7):1–16.
44. Cicirelli V. Form of the relationship between creativity, IQ, and academic achievement. *J Educ Psych.* 1965;56(6):303–308
45. Anastasi A, Schaefer CE. Note on the concepts of creativity and intelligence. *Jf Creative Behav.* 1971;5(2):113 116.
46. Busse TV, Mansfield RS. Theories of the creative process: a review and a perspective. *J Creative Behav.* 1980;4(2):91–103.
47. Ford C, Gioia D. Factors influencing creativity in the domain of managerial decision making. *J Manag.* 2000;26(4):705–732.
48. Griffin RW. *Management.* 7th ed. Boston, MA: Houghton Mifflin Company; 2001.
49. Von Bergen CW, Kirk R. Groupthink. When too many heads spoil the decision. *Manage Rev.* 1978;67(3):44–49.
50. Janis IL. *Groupthink.* Boston, MA: Houghton Mifflin; 1982.
51. Last JM. *A Dictionary of Public Health.* New York: Oxford University Press; 2007.
52. Crisp J, Pelletier D, Duffield C, Adams A, Nagy S. The Delphi Method? *Nursing Res.* 1997;46(2):116–118.
53. Dalkey N, Helmer O. An experimental application of the Delphi method to the use of experts. *Management Science.* 1963;9:458–467.
54. Rauch W. The decision Delphi. *Technological Forecasting and Social Change.* 1979;15:159–169.

55. Witkin BR, Altschuld JW. *Conducting and Planning Needs Assessments. A Practical Guide*. Thousand Oaks, CA: Sage Publications; 1995.
56. Krueger RA, Casey MA. *Focus Groups: A Practical Guide for Applied Research*. 3rd ed. Thousand Oaks, CA: Sage Publications; 2000.
57. Delbecq AL, Van de Ven AH. *Group Techniques for Program Planning*. Glenview, IL: Scott, Foresman; 1975.
58. Ginter PM, Swayne LM, Duncan WJ. *Strategic Management of Health Care Organizations*. 4th ed. Malden, MA: Blackwell Publishers Inc.; 2002.
59. Schwartz P. *The Art of the Long View. Paths to Strategic Insight for Yourself and Your Company*. New York, NY: Currency Doubleday; 1991.
60. Woolf SH, DiGuiseppi CG, Atkins D, Kamerow DB. Developing evidence-based clinical practice guidelines: lessons learned by the US Preventive Services Task Force. *Annu Rev Public Health*. 1996;17:511–538.
61. McLaughlin JJ, GB. Logic models: A tool for telling your program's performance story. *Eval ProgrPlan*. 1999;22:65–72.
62. Zaza S, Briss PA, Harris KW, eds. *The Guide to Community Preventive Services: What Works to Promote Health?* New York, NY: Oxford University Press; 2005.
63. Battista RN, Fletcher SW. Making recommendations on preventive practices: methodological issues. *Am J Prev Medicine*. 1988;4 Suppl:53–67.
64. Lipsey M. Theory as method: small theories of treatments. *New Direct Eval*. 2007;114:30–62.
65. MacKinnon DP, Dwyer JH. Estimating mediated effects in prevention studies. *Evaluation Research*. 1993;12:144–158.
66. Koepsell TD, Wagner EH, Cheadle AC, et al. Selected methodological issues in evaluating community-based health promotion and disease prevention programs. *Annu Rev Public Health*. 1992;13:31–57.
67. Horsch K. Using Logic Models for Program Planning and Evaluation. *Place-Based Education Evaluation Collaborative*. Richmond, VT 2008.
68. Briss PA, Brownson RC, Fielding JE, Zaza S. Developing and using the Guide to Community Preventive Services: lessons learned About evidence-based public health. *Annu Rev Public Health*. Jan 2004;25:281–302.
69. Briss PA, Zaza S, Pappaioanou M, et al. Developing an evidence-based Guide to Community Preventive Services—methods. The Task Force on Community Preventive Services. *Am J Prev Med*. 2000;18(1 suppl):35–43.
70. Dwyer JJ, Hansen B, Barrera M, et al. Maximizing children's physical activity: an evaluability assessment to plan a community-based, multi-strategy approach in an ethno-racially and socio-economically diverse city. *Health Promot Int*. 2003;18(3):199–208.
71. Pentz MA, Dwyer JH, MacKinnon DP, et al. A multicommunity trial for primary prevention of adolescent drug abuse. Effects on drug use prevalence. *JAMA*. 1989;261:3259–3266.
72. Worden JK, Mickey RM, Flynn BS, et al. Development of a community breast screening promotion program using baseline data. *Prev Med*. 1994;23:267–275.
73. Green LW, Kreuter MW. *Health Promotion Planning: An Educational and Ecological Approach*. 4th ed. New York, NY: McGraw Hill; 2005.
74. Centers for Disease Control and Prevention. Framework for program evaluation in public health. *MMWR*. 1999;48(RR-11):1–40.

75. McKinlay JB. Paradigmatic obstacles to improving the health of populations—implications for health policy. *Salud Publica Mex.* 1998;40(4):369–379.
76. McKinlay JB, Marceau LD. Upstream healthy public policy: lessons from the battle of tobacco. *Int J Health Serv.* 2000;30(1):49–69.
77. Berkman LF. Social epidemiology: social determinants of health in the United States: are we losing ground? *Annu Rev Public Health.* 2009;30:27–41.
78. Yen IH, Syme SL. The social environment and health: a discussion of the epidemiologic literature. *Annu Rev Public Health.* 1999;20:287–308.
79. McKinlay JB. The promotion of health through planned sociopolitical change: Challenges for research and policy. *Soc Sci Med.* 1993;36(2):109–117.
80. McKinlay JB, Marceau LD. To boldly go. *Am J Public Health.* 2000;90(1):25–33.

9

Developing an Action Plan and Implementing Interventions

> Even if you're on the right track, you'll get run over if you just sit there.
> —Will Rogers

Once a particular intervention—a program or policy—has been identified, sound planning techniques can ensure that the program is implemented effectively. It can be argued that planning is the most fundamental and most important administrative function.[1] In the context of community change, sound action planning is one of the key factors predicting success.[2] The focus of this chapter is on *action planning*—that is, planning for a defined program or policy with specific, time-dependent outcomes compared with ongoing planning that is a regular function within an organization.

Effective action plans have several key characteristics.[1-3] First, they have clear aims and objectives. Second, the roles and responsibilities of important stakeholders are clarified and respected. Third, there are clear mechanisms for accountability. Fourth, the plans are comprehensive in that they describe specific steps, timelines, as well as roles and responsibilities. While it is recognized that it is important to utilize multiple intervention tactics (e.g., communication, behavioral, policy, regulatory, environmental) to create change, each tactic should have a specific comprehensive plan for its implementation. Such comprehensiveness includes a listing of all possible action steps and anticipated changes. This is an area where a sound analytic framework (see Chapter 8) can be especially useful in describing potential interventions and their effects. The plan must also have mechanisms for evaluation. Finally, the intervention tactics laid out within an action plan need to be based on sound scientific evidence.

In simple terms, intervention (program or policy) development consists of planning, implementation, and evaluation (Figure 9-1). The earlier chapters in this book described the tools, strategies, and steps needed to determine which issue(s) should be addressed via a public health intervention. In this chapter, our attention

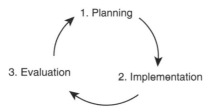

Figure 9-1. A simple planning cycle for program development and implementation.

turns to the matter of implementation: "What specific actions can we take that are most likely to yield the change in health and/or health behaviors we seek?"

To cover some essential issues for successful action planning, this chapter is organized in five main sections, designed to highlight ecologic frameworks, give examples of behavioral science theories that can increase the likelihood of carrying out effective interventions, review key principles of planning, outline steps in action planning, and describe important aspects of coalition-based interventions.

BACKGROUND

Solid action planning takes into account essentially all of the issues and approaches covered elsewhere in this book. For example, let's assume one is broadly concerned with the public health needs of a community. Early on, a partnership would have been established through which multiple stakeholders and community members are engaged in defining the main issues of concern and developing and implementing our intervention. The process would begin with a community assessment. This would start by examining epidemiologic data and conducting prioritization to select which health issue(s) to address. Once the quantitative data describing the main health issues had been established, additional community assessments (quantitative and qualitative) can be conducted to determine the specific needs and assets of the population of interest and the context (social, political, economic) within which the health problem exists. Through this process one would have identified the specific population and contextual issues that help to interpret and utilize a wide range of local data sets to guide the decision-making process.[4,5] Factors should be examined across the ecologic framework (as described in Chapter 4). In addition to a full community assessment, systematic reviews of the literature and cost-effectiveness studies would have assisted program planners in determining possible intervention approaches. Once a small set of possible interventions is identified, one would then examine the readiness of the community to engage in the specified interventions.

Table 9-1. Questions to Consider About Community Readiness

• Is there a common understanding among community members and leaders regarding the nature of the problem and its determinants?
• Are community-based organizations capable of engaging in the desired intervention (staff, resources, leadership support)?
• Does the intervention require that organizations work together? If so, what is the capacity of these organizations to work together (communication patterns, history, trust, group process skills)?
• Are the skills needed to implement the intervention available?
• What has been done before in this community and other similar communities?
• Can the intervention be modified to fit the community of interest? In terms of culture, geography, educational level, other important factors?
• Do leaders (elected, appointed, and lay) support the intervention?
• Is the community supportive of the approach?
• Are there resources to implement the approach?
• Can the existing community infrastructures support the intervention? If not, can the infrastructures be enhanced or built?

Source: Adapted from Plested et al.,[6] Baker et al.,[7] and Robinson et al.[8]

One aspect of readiness is the community/organizational capacity to conduct a specific intervention. Previous work has identified a number of issues to consider when determining which intervention to conduct in a particular community and/ or readiness of a community to engage in a particular intervention[6-8] (Table 9-1).

As described in Chapter 4, these data can be collected as part of a complete community assessment of the most important issues, and the fit of the intervention to the community of interest can assist in gaining community, organizational political support for a program. All of these steps are needed to determine the intervention (program, environmental change, or policy) that is most appropriate for a specific community and to determine the specific content and processes used for implementing the intervention. In addition, these are critical to consider for intervention monitoring and evaluation (see Chapter 10).

In addition to determining the readiness of a community to engage in an intervention, it is important to consider how to adapt the intervention to the population, culture, and context of interest.[9] This requires that community members and existing community-based organizations have an active role in the research process including initial assessments and the development, implementation, and evaluation of interventions. This type of approach is consistent with community-based participatory research (CBPR). Israel and colleagues[10] define CBPR as a collaborative approach to research that equitably involves, for example, community members, organizational representatives, and researchers in all aspects of the research process. The partners contribute unique strengths and shared responsibilities to enhance understanding of a given phenomenon and the social and cultural dynamics of the community. This can improve the ability to integrate the knowledge gained with action to improve the health and well-being of community members.[10] Driven by values of social or environmental justice,[11] CBPR creates the structures needed for all partners to engage in the research process. These structures are co-created by all partners and provide the opportunity for all partners to learn from each other (co-learning).[12,13]

One of the challenges that a program often encounters when adapting an intervention is the tension between fidelity, or keeping the key ingredients of an intervention that made it successful, and adaptation to fit the community of interest. Adapting interventions from one country to another requires considerations regarding the extent to which the determinants of the issue are comparable in both locations and differences in political and health care systems.[14] Even adapting an intervention from one location to another within a country requires the consideration of a number of factors.[15] Lee and colleagues[16] developed a useful approach for planned adaptation that includes four steps: (1) examining the evidence-based theory of change, (2) identifying population differences, (3) adapting the program content, and (4) adapting evaluation strategies.

There are several issues to consider in adapting an intervention that has been effective in one setting and with one population into another setting and population. Among these are attributes of applicability (whether the intervention process can be implemented in the local setting) such as the political environment, public acceptance of the intervention, cultural norms regarding the issue and the intervention

Table 9-2. Rating of the Attributes of Applicability and Transferability by the Type of Behavioral Intervention for the Prevention of HIV/AIDS in Men Having Sex With Men in the Chinese Setting

Attributes	TYPE OF BEHAVIORAL INTERVENTION		
	Individual	*Small Group*	*Community*
Applicability			
Political environment	++	++	++
Social acceptability	+	--	+
Cultural adaptability	++	++	++
Resource implications	++	++	++
Educational level of target population	++	++	++
Organizational structure and skills of local interventionists	+	+	+
Transferability			
Baseline prevalence of risk behaviors or HIV infection	±		±
The characteristics of the target population	+		±
The capacity to implement the intervention	+		±

Rating: ++, very favorable; +, favorable; ±, uncertain; --, very unfavorable.
Source: Adapted from Wang et al.[15]

proposed, history of the relationship between the community and the organization implementiation of the intervention, engagement of the community in the intervention development and implementation, and resources available for program. Other factors relate to transferability (whether the intervention effectiveness is similar in the local setting and the original study), baseline risk factors, target population characteristics, and the capacity to implement the intervention.[15,17] As an example, Wang and colleagues[15] analyzed a number of attributes of applicability and transferability when applying interventions to prevent HIV/AIDS in Chinese populations (Table 9-2). This illustration takes into account the literature on behavioral interventions (across ecological levels) to prevent HIV/AIDS among Chinese men.

ECOLOGIC FRAMEWORKS FOR ACTION PLANNING

As with community assessments, ecologic frameworks are important to consider in developing intervention action plans. Ecologic frameworks suggest the importance of individual, interpersonal, organizational, community (social and economic), and health policy factors because of the effect these variables have on individual behavior change and because of their direct effect on health.[18] At the extremes, an ecologic framework suggests intervening in two main areas: changing people or changing the environment.[19] In fact, the most effective interventions probably act at multiple levels because communities are made up of individuals who interact in a variety of social networks and within a particular context. The assessment of needs and resources, literature review, and evaluation of available data sets should guide which level (or levels) of the ecologic framework is the appropriate level for intervention.

An ecologic framework is a useful way to organize objectives and intervention approaches (Table 9-3). Programs focused on changing *individual* behavior may provide information and teach skills to enable individuals to change their behaviors. These programs may focus on changing knowledge, attitudes, beliefs, and behaviors. Various theories can be useful in directing practitioners to specific strategies that are appropriate to use in changing individual behavior (as described later in this chapter). Some theories, such as the stages-of-change theory, suggest that different approaches are likely to be more or less useful, depending on the individual's readiness for change.[20-22]

To address *interpersonal* factors, many programs include strategies to strengthen social support. As described by Israel,[23] these programs may act in various ways. For example, programs may attempt to strengthen existing networks by working with families and friends. Alternatively, programs may develop new network ties through social support groups or may enhance the capacity of natural helpers, such

Table 9-3. Summary of Objectives and Intervention Approaches Across Levels of an Ecologic Framework

	Individual	*Interpersonal*	*Organizational*	*Community*	*Health Policy*
Objectives address	Knowledge	Programs	Programs	Programs	Ordinances
	Attitudes	Practices	Practices	Practices	Regulations
	Behavior	Social support	Policies	Policies	Laws
		Social networks	Built environment	Built environment	Policies
Approaches	Information	Develop new social ties	Organizational change	Social change	Political action
	Education	Lay health advisors	Networking	Media advocacy	Lobbying
	Training	Peer support groups	Organizational development	Coalition building	Media advocacy
	Counseling		Environmental changes	Community evelopment	Policy advocacy
				Environmental changes	Coalition building

Source: Adapted from Simons-Morton et al.[39]

as people in positions of respect in a community, to provide health-related information and assistance. A program aimed at strengthening existing social networks to enhance individual behavior change might invite family members to join exercise facilities or take cooking classes together. Programs may also seek to enhance the total network through lay health advisors.[23] Lay health advisors are lay people to whom others normally turn to for advice, emotional support, and tangible aid.[24] Lay health advisors may provide information on specific health risks or behaviors or on services available to address various health needs. They may also assist clients in improving their communication skills or establish linkages with health and human service agencies for efficient and appropriate referral.[25] In some instances, building social ties may be a secondary aim of programs that primarily focus on other types of community-based activities.

At the *organizational* level, characteristics of an organization can be used to support positive behavior change. One may attempt to change the organization itself, and organizations may be an ideal setting for diffusion of interventions that have proved useful in other settings. Organizations such as day care facilities, schools, and worksites are particularly important for enhancing public health because people spend one-third to one-half of their lives in such settings.

Public health interventions may also attempt to create changes in *community* and *health policy* factors. These efforts often focus on creating changes in community structures, processes, and policies. Changes in community structures or processes could include development of community parks, libraries, or educational facilities and may also involve changes in decision-making structures to incorporate points of view that were previously unheard. In terms of policy changes, these programs may, for example, focus on creating smoke-free public places to support changes in individual smoking behavior and attempt to alter community norms around smoking. Alternately, efforts may be focused on creating policy and environmental changes in other social, community, or economic factors such as housing, jobs, wages, education, and physical structures that influence health and health behaviors.[26,27] For example, an intervention may succeed in changing attitudes and intentions to increase consumption of fruits and vegetables, but there are no jobs—and therefore no money—to allow purchase of the produce or the jobs that are available do not pay a wage that allows for purchase of produce or maintenance of utilities required for refrigeration and heating of food. Interventions aimed at encouraging economic development and living wages can alter capacity to change behavior.

Ecologic frameworks suggest that individual, interpersonal, organizational, community, and health policy factors are interrelated, and programs that address one level are likely to enhance outcomes at the other levels.[28] Levels of the ecologic framework are overlapping. A new health policy might be implemented in a worksite that employs a significant proportion of a town's population, and this might result in a change in social norms throughout a community. It is also important to note that ecologic frameworks are important to consider whether the program is categorical (focused on a particular disease process) or a broadly defined community program like community development. For example, programs that focus on a disease category such as breast cancer and receive categorical funding to change individual behavior (e.g., getting mammograms) will be more effective if the impact of interpersonal and organizational factors are also considered and interventions are modified accordingly.[28,29] This may entail providing low- or no-cost mammograms, changing the policy in the state so that more women are eligible for low- or no-cost mammograms, developing a lay health advisor approach to enhance breast cancer screening, or changing transportation systems to give women better access to screening and treatment services. These activities may occur simultaneously or sequentially.

In general, the use of ecologic models has outpaced evaluation studies in the attempt to document the effectiveness of these frameworks and the mechanisms by which changes in health behaviors occur.[28] As shown in Box 9-1, an ecologic framework can be modified and adapted for complex issues such as HIV prevention.[30,31] A study of 44 health promotion programs in Canada found that most programs (68%) were limited to one intervention setting, such as an organization, and only 2 of 44 programs occurred in four settings.[32] More recently, a

---

Box 9-1. An Ecologic Approach to HIV Prevention Among Asian and Pacific Islander American Men

In the United States, the incidence of AIDS is increasing at a higher rate among Asian and Pacific Islander men who have sex with men (MSM) than among Caucasian MSM.[30] To work out an approach that would be more effective in preventing HIV among Asian and Pacific Islander American men, Choi and colleagues[31] reviewed five major models of health behavior change: the Health Belief Model, the Theory of Reasoned Action, Social Learning Theory, Diffusion Theory, and the AIDS Risk Reduction Model. The authors concluded that these five models did not adequately address environmental influences on HIV transmission. Recent empirical evidence suggests that interventions need to target both individuals and environmental determinants of HIV transmission. To reach multiple levels of HIV prevention, Choi et al. proposed an ecologic framework of three levels as a potentially useful method of organizing interventions:

- Individual: programs to enhance the ability to accept his ethnic or sexual identity
- Interpersonal: interventions to target families, enhancing communication about sex in families with gay children
- Community: mass media campaigns to educate the community about sexual diversity and to promote positive images of ethnically diverse men in the gay community

Clear evaluation strategies must be used to examine the effects of HIV prevention programs that target multiple levels of an ecological framework.

---

study of 47 programs in the United States and the Netherlands found that ecologic interventions targeted a mean of 2.15 levels, with the most common targeting the organizational level.[33] Developing literature shows that action planning will be improved if it is based on an ecologic framework.

THE ROLE OF LOGIC MODELS AND THEORY IN CREATING PROGRAMS AND POLICIES

The effectiveness of public health interventions can be enhanced by the use of systematic planning frameworks (described later), logic models, and theory (e.g., the "transtheoretical model," social learning theory, policy development theories).[19,34]

Logic models, or analytic frameworks, were described in Chapter 8. When used in program planning, a logic model outlines specific activities and explains how they will lead to the accomplishment of objectives and how these objectives will enhance the likelihood of accomplishing program goals.[35,36] For example, a logic model lays out what the program participants will do (attend an educational session on breast cancer screening at their church), what it will lead to (increased knowledge regarding risk factors for breast cancer and specific methods of breast cancer screening), which will in turn will have an impact (increase breast cancer screening rates), with the intention that this will therefore produce a long-term outcome (decreased morbidity due to breast cancer). Several authors have conceptualized this process somewhat differently, yet the overall intent is that the program or policy be laid out with specific activities intended to achieve certain objectives that in turn are expected to have an impact on clearly delineated outcomes, both in the near and long term.

The specific program or policy activities to be developed should be determined by their ability to meet the objectives outlined in the logic model and should be based on sound theories or models of behavior and community change. The specific activities should be developed with attention to the frameworks and planning tools described later. Whereas theory helps practitioners ask the right questions and understand why people are not living more health-promoting lifestyles or following medical advice, planning frameworks describe what needs to be done before developing and organizing a program or policy, and both help to identify what should be monitored or measured during evaluation.[19]

Theory

A theory is a set of interrelated concepts, definitions, and propositions that presents a systematic view of events or situations by specifying relations among variables in order to explain and predict events or situations.[19] Theories and models explain behavior and suggest ways to achieve behavior change.[19] As noted by Bandura,[37] in advanced disciplines like mathematics, theories integrate laws, whereas in newer fields such as public health or behavioral science, theories describe or specify the determinants influencing the phenomena of interest. Moreover, in terms of action planning, theory can point to important intervention strategies. For example, if perceptions are considered important in maintaining behavior, then it will be crucial to include some strategies to alter perceptions, whereas if skills are considered important to change behavior, then some strategy to alter skills must be included in the intervention. If laws and rules influence health and behavior, policies need to be enacted and enforced to support health. While it is not possible to provide a summary of all of the theories that might be used in developing intervention strategies, some discussion of how theory can be translated to practice is important. Therefore, a brief overview of two individual-level theories is presented next with a focus on how the constructs in the theories guide specific action strategies.

Individual-Level Theories

Based on reviews conducted by Glanz and colleagues of journals in health education, medicine, and behavioral sciences, the most commonly used theories of how to change individual behavior are the Health Belief Model (HBM), the Social Cognitive Theory/Social Learning Theory, self-efficacy, the Theory of Reasoned Action/Theory of Planned Behavior, and the Stages-of-Change/Transtheoretical Model.[19,38] It is important to note that many of the constructs of the various theories overlap, sometimes with slightly differing terminology. For example, outcome expectations within the Social Learning Theory relate to an individual's belief about the likelihood that a specific behavior will lead to a particular outcome.[37] This relates closely to behavioral beliefs within the Theory of Reasoned Action/Theory of Planned Behavior. The following sections briefly describe two common behavior-change theories: the HBM and the Transtheoretical Model. Readers are referred elsewhere[19,35–37] for more detailed descriptions of various theories.

The Health Belief Model. The HBM may be the most widely used and best known of theoretical frameworks in health behavior change.[39,40] This model was developed in the 1950s, based on experience in a screening program for tuberculosis. The HBM is a "value expectancy theory" (i.e., in the context of health-related behavior, individuals hold both the desire to avoid illness or to get well [a value] and the belief that a specific health action will prevent illness [expectancy]). The expectancy can be further defined in terms of an individual's estimate of personal susceptibility to and severity of an illness and perceived benefits and barriers to action. The HBM also emphasized the role of perception in behavior change.[39] According to the HBM, an individual's cognitions or perceptions determine behavior.

The HBM recognizes four important categories of beliefs that are important in health behavior change:

1. Perceived susceptibility—an individual's opinion of the likelihood of getting a certain health condition
2. Perceived severity—an individual's opinion of the seriousness of a condition and its sequelae
3. Perceived benefits—an individual's opinion of the advantages of the advised action to reduce risk
4. Perceived barriers—an individual's opinion of the tangible and psychological costs of the advised action

Two more recently described constructs include cues to action (strategies to activate one's readiness) and self-efficacy (one's confidence in one's ability to take action).[40] The HBM can be useful in action planning,[41] because it provides an outline of some essential factors involved in individual behavior change and suggests that cognitions and perceptions are important in helping individuals to change their behavior. For example, based on the HBM one might decide to provide information to help to change perceptions regarding susceptibility or severity of a particular health condition (e.g., cardiovascular disease) or information on the benefits and barriers to taking action (e.g., benefits of increasing fruit and vegetable and lowering fat consumption). The addition of cues to action suggests that interventions might include grocery store and restaurant labeling regarding nutritional content of various foods.

The Transtheoretical Model (Stages of Change).   The Transtheoretical Model was developed to integrate principles across major theories of health behavior change, hence the name transtheoretical.[21,22] It suggests that people move through one of five "stages" and that health behavior change is an evolving process that can be more effectively achieved if the intervention of choice matches the stage of readiness to change behavior. In the following descriptions, the time frame has been defined for some behaviors such as smoking cessation but is less established for others such as beginning a physical activity program. The five stages are as follows:

1. Precontemplation—No intention to change behavior in the foreseeable future (usually measured as the next 6 months); unaware of the risk; deny the consequences of risk behavior
2. Contemplation—Aware that a problem exists; seriously thinking about overcoming it, but have not yet made a commitment to take action; anticipated that he or she will take action in the next 6 months
3. Preparation—Intend to take action in the near future and may have taken some inconsistent action in the past; time frame for taking action usually measured as within the next month
4. Action—Modify behavior, experiences, or environment to overcome problems; behavior change is relatively recent (generally, within the past 6 months)
5. Maintenance—Work to prevent relapse and maintain the behavior over a long period of time (usually from 6 months to 5 years)

[In addition, a sixth stage (Termination) applies to some addictive behaviors. In Termination, the individual is certain that he or she will not return (relapse) to the unhealthy behavior, even in times of stress as a way of coping.[22]]

Numerous studies have examined the effectiveness of staged materials in health education interventions. In general, studies find that stage-tailored materials are

Box 9-2. Stages of Change Intervention for Promoting Fruit and Vegetable Consumption in Worksites

The *5-a-Day for Better Health* program originally developed by the California Department of Health Services was designed to increase fruit and vegetable consumption in line with year 2010 and 2020 health objectives. A related project, *Seattle 5-a-Day*, was carried out at a total of 28 worksites that were randomized to either intervention or control.[42] The intervention occurred at the individual and organizational levels and was developed around the stages-of-change behavioral model. The project emphasized employee involvement in order to build ownership for the project. To move participants from precontemplation to contemplation, early-phase activities focused on raising general awareness and motivating thinking about change. A "teaser" campaign was used to alert employees that something new was coming soon to the worksite. In the second phase, events were held to move participants from contemplation to preparation. In the final phase, the goal was movement from preparation to action via skill building and worksite changes in the cafeteria, such as point-of-purchase displays. Based on data collected via a food frequency questionnaire at baseline and a 2-year follow-up, a net intervention effect of 0.3 daily serving of fruits and vegetables was shown. It appears that the stages-of-change model formed a useful framework for this intervention. This relatively simple intervention approach could be applied in worksites with cafeterias. This research also contributed to a systematic review of 11 worksite nutrition interventions where positive effects were seen in eight studies.[43]

more effective than generic materials in moving individuals through the various stages. In other words, at the early stages, cognitive change strategies are more likely to be helpful in moving individuals to the next stage, while in later stages, skill building may be useful. An example of a stage-based intervention for dietary change is shown in Box 9-2.[42,43] Researchers are also studying the utility of the Transtheoretical Model beyond the individual level. Their research is focusing on such issues as the potential interactions between social support and stages of change, the staging of organizations in the change process, and attempts to match health policy initiatives with the readiness to change in a community.[22]

COMMON PRINCIPLES ACROSS PLANNING FRAMEWORKS

Numerous frameworks for planning have been proposed over the past few decades. Among the earliest approaches was a simple program evaluation and review technique (PERT) chart. As described by Breckon and colleagues,[44] this was a graphically displayed time line for the tasks necessary in the development and implementation of a public health program. Subsequent approaches have divided program development into various phases, including needs assessment, goal setting, problem definition, plan design, implementation, and evaluation. There are numerous other planning frameworks that have proved useful for various intervention settings and approaches. Among them are

- The Planned Approach to Community Health (PATCH)[34]
- Predisposing, Reinforcing and Enabling Constructs in Educational/environmental Diagnosis and Evaluation, with its implementation phase: Policy, Regulatory and Organizational Constructs in Educational and Environmental Development (PRECEDE-PROCEED)[45]
- Intervention Mapping[46]
- Multilevel Approach to Community Health (MATCH)[39]

Each of these frameworks has been used to plan and implement successful programs. The PRECEDE-PROCEED model alone has generated thousands of documented health promotion applications in a variety of settings and across multiple health problems. Rather than providing a review of each of these planning frameworks, key planning principles have been abstracted that appear to be crucial to the success of interventions in community settings and are common to each framework. Those principles include the following:

1. Data should guide the development of programs. Elsewhere in this book, many types and sources of data are described that are useful in summarizing a community's health status, needs, and assets in the community to make changes.
2. Community members should participate in the process. As discussed in Chapter 4, active participation by a range of community members in setting priorities, planning interventions, and making decisions enhances the viability and staying power of many public health programs.
3. Participants should develop an intervention strategy that addresses more than one level of the ecological framework. Based on a participatory process, community members are encouraged to develop intervention strategies across multiple sectors, including mass media, schools, and health care facilities.
4. The community capacity for health promotion should be increased. A systematic planning process can be repeated to address various health priorities. Such an approach aims to increase capacity to improve public health by enhancing the community's skills in health planning and health promotion.
5. Evaluation should emphasize feedback and program improvement. Sound evaluation improves program delivery and for such, timely feedback to the community is essential.

Table 9-4. Steps in Designing a Successful Public Health Intervention

1. Develop partnership with appropriate organizations, agencies, and community members.
2. Review health data; determine contributing factors.
3. Conduct full community assessment.
4. Systematic reviews of the literature and cost-effectiveness studies to identify existing programs and policies.
5. Assess feasibility and potential for adaptation with organizational partners and those affected by the intervention...determine potential barriers and solutions.
6. Select and adapt specific intervention–program, environmental change, and/or policy.
7. Obtain support in the setting for intervention (e.g., community, health care, schools).
8. Develop logic model specifying specific goal, objectives, and action steps for the intervention selected.
9. Develop the evaluation plan for activities, objectives, and goal.
10. Develop work plan and timetables.
11. Assess resource needs.
12. Identify, train, and supervise workers.
13. Pilot test intervention and evaluation.
14. Monitor and evaluate program or policy.
15. Use evaluation results to modify intervention as appropriate.

Source: Adapted from the Planned Approach to Community Health (PATCH)[37] and Davis et al.[48]

A STEPWISE APPROACH TO SUCCESSFUL ACTION PLANNING

The preceding frameworks and keys to intervention success help to form a stepwise framework for successful action planning[47,48] (Table 9-4). Within this 15-step approach, previous chapters have dealt with a number of these issues; Chapter 10 addresses evaluation issues in detail. This section will highlight some of the key issues to consider including management, developing action plans, assessing resource needs, and identifying and training staff. While it is beyond the scope of this chapter or book to review each management or implementation issue in detail, several key issues will be briefly covered that are essential for any successful intervention.

Making the Correct Managerial Decisions

Developing and implementing effective programs and policies require sound management skills. Public health management is the process of constructing, implementing, and evaluating organized responses to a health problem or a series of interrelated health problems.[49] One of the goals of an evidence-based process is to make rational and well-grounded decisions—a management function. Important decisions always carry some element of risk. Sound management and planning are iterative, generally do not lead to a single option, and do not eliminate the risk of making poor judgments.[49] In addition, complex public health problems are rarely resolved by implementing a single program or policy. Rather, change often requires a set of actions. The goal of action planning is, therefore, to maximize the chances of efficient use of resources and effective delivery of specific programs and policies that are part of an overall strategic plan. Previous chapters provide data to help guide the managerial decisions regarding *which* programs or policies to implement. This chapter deals with implementation—the process of putting a program or policy into effect. In implementation, one seeks to accomplish the setting up, management, and execution of the program.[1]

Developing Action Plans

Developing action plans requires developing program objectives and specific activities to achieve these objectives. To develop program objectives, it is essential to understand the components of sound program objectives.[1,49] This is of paramount importance because sound planning and evaluation are based on a series of objectives. A rigorous commitment to setting and monitoring objectives builds quality control into a program or policy and allows for mid-course corrections via process evaluation (see Chapter 10). An intervention objective should include a clear identification of the health issue or risk factor being addressed, the at-risk population being addressed, the current status of the health issue or risk factor in the at-risk population, and the desired outcome of the intervention. A clearly defined objective can guide both the development of intervention content and the selection of appropriate communication channels. It also facilitates the development of quantitative evaluation measures that can be used to monitor the success of the intervention and to identify opportunities for improvement. Importantly, a clearly defined objective will improve the coordination of activities among the various partners participating in the intervention.

Several aspects of sound objective-setting have been described[1,50]:

- There should be sound scientific evidence to support the objectives.
- The result to be achieved should be important and understandable to a broad audience.
- Objectives should be prevention-oriented and should address health improvements that can be achieved through population-based and/or health-service interventions.
- Objectives should drive action and suggest a set of interim steps (intermediate indicators) that will achieve the proposed targets within the specified time frame.
- The language of objectives should be precise, avoiding use of general or vague verbs.
- Objectives should be measurable and may include a range of measures—health outcomes, behavioral risk factors, health service indicators, or assessments of

Table 9-5. Examples of Objectives and their Linkages to Action Strategies

Level/Organization	Objective	Action Strategies
National/U.S. Department of Health and Human Services	Increase the proportion of persons aged 2 years and older who consume at least two daily servings of fruit. Increase the proportion of persons aged 2 years and older who consume at least three daily servings of vegetables, with at least one-third being dark green or orange vegetables.	Convene a national steering committee that develops and implements a multipronged National Strategic Plan that uses social marketing tools; is integrated across state, regional, and local levels; and employs a public/private partnership approach at all levels.
State/Minnesota Department of Health (Obesity Plan)	Increase fruit and vegetable consumption.	Disseminate evidence-based nutrition information; increase marketing messages for health eating; collaborate with organizations to develop action strategies; support additional research.

community capacity. They should count assets and achievements and look to the positive.
- Specific timetables for completion of objectives should be described.

Table 9-5 presents examples of sound objectives from national and state government sectors. These are drawn from the strategic plans and other planning materials of the programs noted.

Developing the Work Plan and Timetables

A detailed action plan that includes the development of a work plan and a specific timeline for completion will enhance the chances of a successful program. Defining lines of authority and communication is crucial for a community-based intervention in which numerous activities may occur simultaneously. In conjunction, the time frame for the program or policy should be carefully mapped in the form of a timeline. For externally funded projects like grants and contracts, this timeline corresponds to the funding period. A timeline is a graphic presentation of information, including a list of all activities (or milestones) and designating when they are to be accomplished. Basic timeline construction includes the following[1]:

- A complete listing of activities, grouped by major categories
- Ascertaining which activities need to be done first

- Determining how long each activity will take
- Determining when each and every activity is to begin and finish
- Establishing the time units that are most appropriate (weeks, months, years)

A sample timeline is shown in Figure 9-2. Although there are many ways to organize a timeline, this example groups activities into four main categories: (1) administration, (2) intervention development and implementation, (3) data collection and evaluation, and (4) analysis and dissemination. For internal purposes, it is useful to add another component to this timeline—that of the personnel intended to carry out each task. Doing this in conjunction with the timeline will allow for assessment of workload and personnel needs at various times throughout the proposed project. Another important component of program delivery is the assessment of program implementation: How well was the program delivered[51]? These issues are covered in more detail in Chapter 10 within the context of process evaluation.

Assessing Resource Needs

A manager needs to determine the resources required to implement a particular program or policy. Resources can be grouped into five general areas:

1. Available funds: How many direct funds are available? What are the sources? Are there limitations on how and when funds can be spent? Are funds internal or external to a program or agency? Are there "in-kind" funds?
2. Personnel: How many and what types of personnel are needed? What type of training will be needed for program staff? What personnel do collaborating organizations bring to the project?
3. Equipment and materials: What types of equipment and supplies are needed for the program? Are there certain pieces of equipment that can be obtained "in-kind" from participating partners?
4. Facilities: For some types of interventions, is significant infrastructure needed (such as clinics, hospitals, or mobile vans)?
5. Travel: Is there travel directly related to carrying out the project? Are there related travel expenses for other meetings or presentations in professional settings?
6. A generic budget planning worksheet is provided in Figure 9-3.

Identifying and Training Staff

As an intervention develops, adequate staff and/or volunteer training is essential for smooth implementation of interventions. Formal training should be provided

Activity	Month											
	1	2	3	4	5	6	7	8	9	10	11	12
Administration												
• Hire and train staff	x	x										
• Assemble research team	x	x										
• Conduct staff meetings	x	x	x	x	x	x	x	x	x	x	x	x
• Oversee and manage budget	x	x	x	x	x	x	x	x	x	x	x	x
Intervention Development & Implementation												
• Conduct focus groups to refine interventions			x	x								
• Pilot test interventions					x	x						
• Finalize interventions and begin delivery							x	x	x			
Data collection & evaluation												
• Test and finalize questionnaires					x	x						
• Review pilot data and refine data collection approaches						x	x					
• Conduct process evaluation									x	x	x	x
• Conduct impact evaluation									x	x	x	x
Analysis and Dissemination (all year two or year three activities)												
• Edit data and conduct data entry												
• Refine and conduct analyzes												
• Write rough draft and final project report												
• Present findings at regional and national meetings												

FIGURE 9-2. Example time line for implementation of a public health intervention. (Only 1 year is displayed as an example.)

Line item	Internal resources (new budget allocation)	Internal in-kind (reallocation of existing resources)	External resources (grants, contracts, other public or private sources)	External in-kind (donated services or non-financial resources)
Personnel (staff or contractors) *Examples*: Coordinator Data manager Health educator Evaluator Administrative support staff Technical support/consultants Subject matter experts Meeting facilitators Graphic designer Marketing/public relations specialist Copy writer/editor Web site designer Fringe benefits				
Equipment and materials *Examples*: Office supplies Meeting supplies Computer supplies Graphic design software Data software Audio equipment Presentation equipment Other equipment purchase Computer/copier Maintenance				
Facilities *Examples*: Clinical space Space for group meetings Conference and meeting rooms				
Travel *Examples*: Staff meeting travel, lodging, and per diem Steering group travel and lodging Mileage associated with program implementation				
Other non-personnel service costs *Examples*: Conference call services Long distance services Web site service Transcription costs for focus group tapes				
Indirect/overhead costs				
Total costs				

FIGURE 9-3. Generic budget planning worksheet.

for staff members who have a limited background in specific intervention areas such as policy advocacy, health behavior change, evaluation, media communications, or coalition building. Special attention should also be given to basic skills such as planning, budgeting, personnel management, written and verbal communication, and cultural appropriateness. When a program involves local citizens, their training also becomes essential.[52] In the early phases, training of partners is often started by ensuring that all members of a partnership (academic, practice, and community) have the level of information and skills needed to take part in the evidence-based planning and decision-making process. Additional training may then take place to provide the specific information and skills required for the chosen intervention. Other types of training may focus on leadership development or strategic planning. The training should be included as a necessary first step in the work plan, and the person(s) responsible for training should be listed in the work plan.

When addressing training needs, several key questions come to mind:

- In which areas does each staff member need training?
- Who should conduct the training?
- Do some people have unused skills that could be useful to a program?
- How best should community members be oriented and trained regarding a program?
- How can training be time efficient?

Pilot Testing the Intervention and Evaluation

Pilot testing is an important part of intervention development. A pilot test is a "mini-study" carried out with a small number of individuals (often 20 or fewer) to detect any problems with intervention and evaluation strategies. Carefully examining the results of a pilot test can obviate problems before a large-scale intervention—where the stakes are higher—is undertaken. A pilot test allows one to:

1. Refine the original hypotheses and/or research questions
2. Produce information that will help improve evaluation approaches
3. Improve curriculum materials or evaluation instruments
4. Test approaches for data imputation and analysis
5. Uncover politically sensitive issues, allowing program planners to better anticipate difficulties
6. Estimate costs for people, equipment, materials, and time
7. Ascertain the cultural appropriateness of interventions in diverse populations by inclusion in program development
8. Enhance the marketability of an intervention with senior agency administrators when a pilot test is successful

To the extent possible, a pilot test should be conducted in the same manner as that intended for the full program. In some cases, a pilot study may use qualitative methods, such as focus groups or individual interviews, which are not part of the main project. However, pilot tests can also provide an opportunity to examine the utility and appropriateness of quantitative instruments. Pilot test subjects should be similar to those who will be in the actual project. Generally, pilot test subjects should not be enrolled in the main project; therefore, it is sometimes useful to recruit pilot subjects from a separate geographic region.[53] Complete notes should be taken during the pilot test so that the project team can debrief with all needed information.

SUMMARY

This chapter provides an overview of various approaches to action planning along with several related issues. An important caveat should be kept in mind when planning an intervention. It has been suggested that sometimes a disproportionate amount of effort and resources goes into the planning process compared with the actual intervention.[54] The diagnostic phases are often resource intensive in order to avoid action planning that leads to weak interventions. The key is to expend enough resources during the assessment and planning processes to be sure a problem is potentially solvable and the right interventions are chosen, while ensuring that adequate resources are available for actual implementation. It is also crucial that well-trained practitioners are available for intervention delivery.

Key Chapter Points

- Theories are especially useful in identifying mechanisms of changes and therefore specific interventions needed to create meaningful changes.
- Ecologic frameworks encourage the use of comprehensive, multilevel interventions.
- A stepwise and systematic approach to action planning can enhance the chances of intervention success.

SUGGESTED READINGS AND SELECTED WEBSITES

Suggested Readings

Bartholomew LK, Parcel GS, Kok G, Gottlieb NH. *Planning Health Promotion Programs: Intervention Mapping.* 2nd ed. San Francisco, CA: Jossey-Bass; 2006.

Glanz K, Rimer BK, Viswanath K. *Health Behavior and Health Education. Theory, Research, and Practice*. 4th ed. San Francisco, CA: Jossey-Bass Publishers; 2008.

Green LW, Kreuter MW. *Health Promotion Planning: An Educational and Ecological Approach*. 4th ed. New York, NY: McGraw-Hill; 2005.

McLeroy KR, Bibeau D, Sleekier A, Glanz K. An ecological perspective on health promotion programs. *Health Educ Q*. 1988;15:351–377.

Timmreck TC. *Planning, Program Development, and Evaluation. A Handbook for Health Promotion, Aging and Health Services*. 2nd ed. Boston, MA: Jones and Bartlett Publishers; 2003.

Selected Websites

The Community Tool Box <http://ctb.ku.edu/en/>. The Community Tool Box is a global resource for free information on essential skills for building healthy communities. It offers more than 7000 pages of practical guidance on topics such as leadership, strategic planning, community assessment, advocacy, grant writing, and evaluation. Sections include descriptions of the task, step-by-step guidelines, examples, and training materials.

Developing and Sustaining Community-Based Participatory Research Partnerships: A Skill-Building Curriculum <http://www.cbprcurriculum.info/>. This evidence-based curriculum is intended as a tool for community-institutional partnerships that are using or planning to use a Community-Based Participatory Research (CBPR) approach to improve health. It is intended for use by staff of community-based organizations, staff of public health agencies, and faculty, researchers, and students at all skill levels. Units provide a step-by-step approach, from the development of the CBPR partnership through the dissemination of results and planning for sustainability. The material and information presented in this curriculum are based on the work of the Community-Institutional Partnerships for Prevention Research Group that emerged from the Examining Community Institutional Partnerships for Prevention Research Project.

Health Education Resource Exchange (HERE) in Washington <http://here.doh.wa.gov/>. This clearinghouse of public health education and health promotion projects, materials and resources in the state of Washington is designed to help community health professionals share their experience with colleagues. The website includes sections on community projects, educational materials, health education tools, and best practices.

Knowledge for Health (K4Health) <https://www.k4health.org/node/2>. Funded by USAID and implemented by The Johns Hopkins Bloomberg School of Public Health, the K4Health project's mission is to increase the use and dissemination of evidence-based, accurate, and up-to-date information to improve health service delivery and health outcomes worldwide. The site offers eLearning opportunities, results of needs assessment activities, and toolkits for family planning/reproductive health, HIV/AIDS, and other health topics.

Management Sciences for Health <http://erc.msh.org/>. Since 1971, Management Sciences for Health (MSH), a nonprofit organization, has worked in more than 140 countries and with hundreds of organizations. MSH's resources communicate effective management practices to health professionals around the world. This site, the Manager's Electronic Resource Center, covers topics such as conducting local rapid assessments, working with community members, and developing leaders. The site links to case studies and toolkits from around the world.

National Cancer Institute, Health Behavior Constructs <http://cancercontrol. cancer.gov/BRP/constructs/index.html>. This site provides definitions of major theoretical constructs used in health behavior research and information about the best measures of these constructs. The National Cancer Institute has also published a concise summary of health behavior theories in *Theory at a Glance: A Guide for Health Promotion Practice* with Dr. Barbara K. Rimer and Dr. Karen Glanz as lead authors. It can be accessed from their main site: www.cancer.gov.

The Planned Approach to Community Health <http://wonder.cdc.gov/wonder/ prevguid/p0000064/P0000064.asp>. The Planned Approach to Community Health (PATCH), developed by the Centers for Disease Control and Prevention and its partners, is widely recognized as an effective model for planning, conducting, and evaluating community health promotion and disease prevention programs. It is used by diverse communities in the United States and several nations to address a variety of health concerns such as cardiovascular disease, HIV, injuries, teenage pregnancy, and access to health care. The PATCH Guide is designed to be used by the local coordinator and contains "how to" information on the process, things to consider when adapting the process to a community, and sample overheads and handout materials.

REFERENCES

1. Timmreck TC. *Planning, Program Development, and Evaluation. A Handbook for Health Promotion, Aging and Health Services.* 2nd ed. Boston, MA: Jones and Bartlett Publishers; 2003.
2. Fawcett SB, Francisco VT, Paine-Andrews A, et al. A model memorandum of collaboration: a proposal. [see comment]. *Public Health Reports.* 2000;115(2–3): 174–179.
3. World Health Organization. Framework for countrywide plans of action for health promotion. *Fifth Global Conference for Health Promotion. Health Promotion: Building the Equity Gap.* Mexico; 2000.
4. Soriano FI. *Conducting Needs Assessments. A Multidisciplinary Approach.* Thousand Oaks, CA: Sage Publications; 1995.

5. Witkin BR, Altschuld JW. *Conducting and Planning Needs Assessments. A Practical Guide.* Thousand Oaks, CA: Sage Publications; 1995.
6. Plested BA, Edwards RW, Jumper Thurman P. *Community Readiness: A Handbook for Successful Change.* Fort Collins, CO: Triethnic Center for Prevention Research; 2005.
7. Baker EA, Brennan Ramirez LK, Claus JM, et al. Translating and disseminating research- and practice-based criteria to support evidence-based intervention planning. *J Public Health Manag Pract.* 2008;14(2):124–130.
8. Robinson K, Farmer T, Riley B, et al. Realistic expectations: Investing in organizational capacity building for chronic disease prevention. *Am J Health Promot.* 2007;21(5):430–438.
9. Wallerstein N, Oetzel J, Duran B, et al. What predicts outcomes in community-based participatory research? In: Minkler M, Wallerstein N, eds. *Community-Based Participatory Research for Health: From Process to Outcomes.* San Francisco, CA: Jossey-Bass; 2008.
10. Israel BA, Schulz AJ, Parker EA, et al. Review of community-based research: assessing partnership approaches to improve public health. *Annu Rev Public Health.* 1998;19:173–202.
11. Cargo M, Mercer SL. The value and challenges of participatory research: Strengthening its practice. *Annu Rev Public Health.* 2008;29:325–350.
12. Israel BA, Eng E, Schultz AJ, et al, eds. *Methods in Community-Based Participatory Research for Health.* San Francisco, CA: Jossey-Bass; 2005.
13. Viswanathan M, Ammerman A, Eng E, et al. *Community-Based Participatory Research: Assessing the Evidence.* Rockville, MD: Agency for Healthcare Research and Quality Publication: Evidence Report/Technology Assessment No. 99 (Prepared by RTI—University of North Carolina Evidence-based Practice Center under Contract No. 290–02-0016). AHRQ Publication 04-E022–2; July 2004. 04-E022–2.
14. Cuijpers P, de Graaf I, Bohlmeijer E. Adapting and disseminating effective public health interventions in another country: towards a systematic approach. *Eur J Public Health.* 2005;15(2):166–169.
15. Wang S, Moss JR, Hiller JE. Applicability and transferability of interventions in evidence-based public health. *Health Promot Int.* 2006;21(1):76–83.
16. Lee SJ, Altschul I, Mowbray CT. Using planned adaptation to implement evidence-based programs with new populations. *Am J Commun Psychol.* 2008;41(3–4):290–303.
17. Castro FG, Barrera M, Martinez CR. The cultural adaptation of prevention interventions: Resolving tensions between fidelity and fit. *Prev Sci.* 2004;5(1):41–45.
18. Baker EA, Brownson CA. Defining characteristics of community-based health promotion programs. *J Public Health Manag Pract.* 1998;4(2):1 9.
19. Glanz K, Rimer BK, Viswanath K. *Health Behavior and Health Education. Theory, Research, and Practice.* 4th ed. San Francisco, CA: Jossey-Bass Publishers; 2008.
20. Prochaska JO, DiClemente CC. Stages and processes of self-change of smoking: toward an integrative model of change. *J Consult Clin Psychol.* 1983;51(3):390–395.
21. Prochaska JO. Norcross, JC. *Systems of Psychotherapy: A Transtheoretical Analysis.* 7th ed. Pacific Grove, CA; Brooks/Cole; 2010.
22. Prochaska JO, Velicer WF. The transtheoretical model of health behavior change. *Am J Health Promot.* 1997;12(1):38–48.
23. Israel BA. Social networks and health status: linking theory, research, and practice. *Patient Couns Health Educ.* 1982;4(2):65–79.

24. Israel BA. Social networks and social support: implications for natural helper and community level interventions. *Health Educ Q.* 1985;12(1):65–80.
25. Eng E, Young R. Lay health advisors as community change agents. *Family Commun Health.* 1992;15(1):24–40.
26. Milio N. Priorities and strategies for promoting community-based prevention policies. *J Public Health Manag Pract.* 1998;4(3):14–28.
27. Brennan Ramirez LK, Baker EA, et al. *Promoting Health Equity: A Resource to Help Communities Address Social Determinants of Health.* Atlanta, GA: US Department of Health and Human Services, Centers for Disease Control and Prevention; 2008.
28. Sallis JF, Owen N, Fisher EB. Ecological models of health behavior. In: Glanz K, Rimer BK, Viswanath K, eds. *Health Behavior and Health Education: Theory, Research and Practice.* 4th ed. San Francisco, CA: Jossey-Bass; 2008:464–485.
29. McLeroy KR, Bibeau D, Steckler A, et al. An ecological perspective on health promotion programs. *Health Educ Q.* 1988;15(4):351–377.
30. Operario D, Nemoto T, Ng T, et al. Conducting HIV interventions for Asian Pacific Islander men who have sex with men: challenges and compromises in community collaborative research. *AIDS Educ Prev.* 2005;17(4):334–346.
31. Choi KH, Yep GA, Kumekawa E. HIV prevention among Asian and Pacific Islander American men who have sex with men: A critical review of theoretical models and directions for future research. *AIDS Educ Prev.* 1998;10(3):19–30.
32. Richard L, Potvin L, Kishchuk N, et al. Assessment of the integration of the ecological approach in health promotion programs. *Am J Health Promot.* 1996;10(4): 318–328.
33. Kok G, Gottlieb NH, Commers M, et al. The ecological approach in health promotion programs: a decade later. *Am J Health Promot.* 2008;22(6):437–442.
34. (Entire issue devoted to descriptions of the Planned Approach to Community Health (PATCH)). *J Health Educ.* 23(3):131–192.
35. Goodman RM. Principles and tools for evaluating community-based prevention and health promotion programs. *J Public Health Manage Pract.* 1998;4(2):37–47.
36. Israel BA, Cummings KM, Dignan MB, et al. Evaluation of health education programs: current assessment and future directions. *Health Educ Q.* 1995;22(3):364–389.
37. Bandura A. *Social Foundations of Thought and Action: A Social Cognitive Theory.* Englewood Cliffs, NJ: Prentice Hall; 1986.
38. Glanz K, Bishop DB. The role of behavioral science theory in the development and implementation of public health interventions. *Annu Rev Public Health.* 2010;31:399–418.
39. Simons-Morton BG, Greene WH, Gottlieb NH. *Introduction to Health Education and Health Promotion.* 2nd ed. Prospect Heights, IL: Waveland Press; 1995.
40. Champion VL, Sugg Skinner C. The Health Belief Model. In: Glanz K, Rimer BK, Viswanath K, eds. *Health Behavior and Health Education.* 4th ed. San Francisco, CA: Jossey-Bass; 2008:45–66.
41. Dignan MB, Carr PA. *Program Planning for Health Education and Promotion.* 2nd ed. Philadelphia, PA: Lea & Febiger; 1992.
42. Beresford SA, Thompson B, Feng Z, et al. Seattle 5 a Day worksite program to increase fruit and vegetable consumption. *Prev Med.* 2001;32(3):230–238.
43. Pomerleau J, Lock K, Knai C, et al. Interventions designed to increase adult fruit and vegetable intake can be effective: a systematic review of the literature. *J Nutr.* 2005;135(10):2486–2495.

44. Breckon DJ, Harvey JR, Lancaster RB. *Community Health Education: Settings, Roles, and Skills for the 21st Century*. 4th ed. Rockville, MD: Aspen Publishers; 1998.
45. Green LW, Kreuter MW. *Health Promotion Planning: An Educational and Ecological Approach*. 4th ed. New York, NY: McGraw-Hill; 2005.
46. Bartholomew LK, Parcel GS, Kok G, et al. *Planning Health Promotion Programs: Intervention Mapping*. 2nd ed. San Francisco, CA: Jossey-Bass; 2006.
47. US Dept of Health and Human Services. *Planned Approach to Community Health: Guide for the Local Coordinator*. Atlanta, GA: Centers for Disease Control and Prevention; 1996.
48. Davis JR, Schwartz R, Wheeler F, et al. Intervention methods for chronic disease control. In: Brownson RC, Remington PL, Davis JR, eds. *Chronic Disease Epidemiology and Control*. 2nd ed. Washington, DC: American Public Health Association; 1998: 77–116.
49. Dyal WW. *Program Management. A Guide for Improving Program Decisions*. Atlanta, GA: Centers for Disease Control and Prevention; 1990.
50. U.S. Dept. of Health and Human Services. *Developing Objectives for Health People 2010*. Washington, DC: Office of Disease Prevention and Health Promotion; 1997.
51. King JA, Morris LL, Fitz-Gibbon CT. *How to Assess Program Implementation*. Newbury Park, CA: Sage Publications; 1987.
52. Bracht N, ed. *Health Promotion at the Community Level: New Advances*. 2nd ed. Newbury Park, CA: Sage Publications; 1999.
53. McDermott RJ, Sarvela PD. *Health Education Evaluation and Measurement. A Practitioner's Perspective*. 2nd ed. New York, NY: WCB/McGraw-Hill; 1999.
54. Sleekier A, Orville K, Eng E, et al. Summary of a formative evaluation of PATCH. *J Health Educ*. 1992;23(3):174–178.

10

Evaluating the Program or Policy

You see, but you do not observe.

—Sir Arthur Conan Doyle

Evaluation is an essential part of the evidence-based public health process, answering questions about program needs, the process of implementation, and tracking of outcomes.[1] It can (1) help to plan programs in a way to enhance the likelihood that they will be effective, (2) allow for midcourse corrections and changes, (3) help determine if the program or policy has been effective, and (4) provide information for planning the next program or policy. This chapter reviews some of the key issues to consider in conducting an evaluation and provides linkages to a diverse literature (within and outside public health) for those wishing to go beyond these basics.

BACKGROUND

What Is Evaluation?

Evaluation is the process of analyzing programs and policies and the context within which they occur to determine if changes need to be made in implementation and to assess the intended and unintended consequences of programs and policies; this includes, but is not limited to, determining if they are meeting their goals and objectives. *Evaluation* is "a process that attempts to determine as systematically and objectively as possible the relevance, effectiveness, and impact of activities in light of their objectives."[2] There is variation in the methods used to evaluate programs and perhaps even more variation in the language used to describe each of the various evaluation techniques. There are both quantitative and qualitative evaluation methods and techniques, with the strongest approaches generally including a blending of these.[3,4] A comprehensive review of evaluation

232

is beyond the scope of any single chapter and is the focus of numerous other textbooks.[5-9] Indeed the first textbook on evaluation in public health appeared over four decades ago.[10] This chapter reviews some of the critical issues to consider in conducting an evaluation such as representation of stakeholders in all aspects of the evaluation, types of evaluation, how to decide on the appropriate evaluation methods (e.g., exploratory evaluation, program versus policy evaluation), and considerations when disseminating evaluation findings.

There has been considerable discourse in the literature about the various paradigmatic approaches to evaluation and scientific inquiry. A paradigm is a set of beliefs or a model that helps to guide scientific inquiry. Many of the differences in the paradigms used to guide inquiry within public health are epistemologic (i.e., they reflect different perspectives on the relationship between the inquirer and what can be known) and ontologic (i.e., they reflect different perspectives on the nature of reality and what can be known about it). These paradigms are discussed in detail elsewhere.[11-14] While a complete discussion of these issues is beyond the intent of this chapter, it is essential to recognize that the choices one makes in this regard influence the data collected, the interpretation of the data, and the utilization of evaluation results.[15,16] For example, while most individuals in the field would agree that evaluation in the absence of some stakeholder involvement is generally less useful, there are instances when evaluation is conducted after the program has been completed and data have already been collected. As will be discussed in more depth later in the chapter, this limits the potential for stakeholder involvement in deciding on the types of questions to ask (i.e., what is important to them) and data to be collected. In these instances, the evaluation decisions are influenced by program planning factors such as those regarding timing and available data. Alternately, there are instances where the focus of the evaluation and the type of data collected are decided by the program implementers without the input of a wider group of stakeholders because of the belief that involvement of stakeholders would somehow "contaminate" the evaluation results.

Why Evaluate?

There are many reasons for public health practitioners to evaluate programs and policies. First, practitioners in the public sector must be accountable to national leaders, state policy makers, local governing officials, and citizens for the use of resources.[17] Similarly, those working in the private and nonprofit sectors must be accountable to their constituencies including those providing the funds for programs and policy initiatives. Evaluation also forms the basis for making choices when resources are limited (as they always are), in part by helping to determine the costs and benefits of the various options (for more about this, see Chapter 3). Finally, evaluation is also a source of information for making midcourse corrections,

Table 10-1. Linkages Between Program Planning and Evaluation

Program Planning Activity	Evaluation Data/Sources
Goal	• Outcome data: Assess changes in morbidity, mortality, disability, quality of life —Social indicator data —Census data —National, state, or local survey data
Objectives	• Impact data: Track knowledge, attitude, and behavioral/skill changes —Programmatic surveys —National, state, or local survey data —Qualitative data (observations, interviews, diaries, content analysis)
Action steps	• Process data: Assess how well a program is being delivered —Records of program attendance —Survey of participant satisfaction —Observational data of environment
Program planning	• Formative data: Determine whether a program is feasible and appropriate —Individual or group interviews —Surveys of knowledge or attitudes

improving programs and policies, and serving as the basis for deciding on future programs and policies. It is closely related to the program planning issues and steps described in Chapter 9 (Table 10-1).

In the early stages of planning and evaluation, it is useful to consider a set of factors ("utility standards") that help to frame the reasons for and uses of an evaluation[18] (Table 10-2). In part, these standards frame a set of questions such as the following:

• Who needs to be involved in providing data for the evaluation?
• Who should conduct the evaluation?
• What are the essential questions that need to be answered?
• What should be included in an evaluation report?

The Role of Stakeholders

As discussed in Chapter 5, a stakeholder is anyone who is involved in program operations, is served by the program, or will use the evaluation results.[19] It is important to include representatives of all of these groups in the design of the program or policy as well as in the design, implementation, and interpretation of evaluation results. The inclusion of these lay and professional perspectives will ensure that all voices are considered in the evaluation and that all will benefit from

Table 10-2. Utility Standards for Evaluation

Standard	Description
Stakeholder identification	Persons involved in or affected by the evaluation should be identified so that their needs can be addressed.
Evaluator credibility	The persons conducting the evaluation should be trustworthy and competent in performing the evaluation for findings to achieve maximum credibility and acceptance.
Information scope and selection	Information collected should address pertinent questions regarding the program and be responsive to the needs and interests of clients and other specified stakeholders.
Values identification	The perspectives, procedures, and rationale used to interpret the findings should be carefully described so that the bases for value judgments are clear.
Report clarity	Evaluation reports should clearly describe the program being evaluated, including its context and the purposes, procedures, and findings of the evaluation, so that essential information is provided and easily understood.
Report timeliness and dissemination	Substantial interim findings and evaluation reports should be disseminated to intended users so that they can be used in a timely fashion.
Evaluation impact	Evaluations should be planned, conducted, and reported in ways that encourage follow-through by stakeholders to increase the likelihood of the evaluation being used.

Source: Joint Committee on Standards for Educational Evaluation.[18]

the evaluation. For staff, inclusion in the evaluation process can provide opportunities to develop skills and abilities in evaluation design and interpretation and can ensure that changes suggested in program implementation are consistent with their work experiences. (It is critical to assure staff that program evaluation is not evaluation of *personnel*.[19]) In terms of program participants, inclusion in the evaluation process can increase their investment in the program and ensure that their previous interests and desires are considered when changes are made in programs and policies. Administrators and program funders need to be included to ensure that evaluation activities are conducted with an understanding of where the program or policy fits within the broader organizational or agency mission and to answer questions most urgent to these groups.[19,20] Regardless of who is included, it is essential that the relationships among these stakeholders be based on mutual trust, respect, and open communication.

Before the evaluation begins, all key stakeholders need to agree on the program goals and objectives, along with the purpose of the evaluation. Each stakeholder may harbor a different opinion about the program goals and objectives and the purpose of the evaluation, and these differences should be discussed and resolved before the evaluation plan is developed and implemented[21] (Box 10-1). There are

Box 10-1. A Health Funders Group: What Are We Funding?

A group of philanthropic organizations decided that they would come together to fund a health-related program. After reviewing several proposals, they decided to fund a proposal to provide home visits by nurses to sick infants and children for those families who would not otherwise be able to get these services. The group thought the program proposal would be enhanced if they worked with a group of church-based lay health advisors, and therefore required this collaboration as a condition of funding. The collaboration was considered particularly important because the proposed clients for the program had multiple nonmedical needs (e.g., housing and shelter, food, electricity, clothing). When the outside evaluator was called in, the first step she took was to meet with each of the 10 funders and representatives of the two agencies to determine their expectations. There were 23 different perspectives on the intent of the program, ranging from decreasing infant mortality to enhancing collaboration between agencies and to providing a specific number of certain types of home visits. Following the principles of participatory evaluation,[21] the evaluator presented these numerous perspectives back to the group of health funders in a meeting with agency representatives and worked with the group to narrow in on program goals and on evaluation questions that were most important, useful, and feasible to assess, given the stage of program development and agency collaboration.

several group process techniques that can be helpful in this regard. For example, the Delphi technique, the nominal group technique, and scenario planning (see Chapter 8) all offer opportunities for individual voices to be heard while, at the same time, providing a process for prioritization.

Once the purpose of the evaluation has been agreed on, the next step is to turn stakeholder questions into an evaluation design. The specific roles and responsibilities of each group of stakeholders in creating the questions that guide the evaluation and in developing the methods to collect data may vary. In some evaluation designs, the stakeholders may be notified as decisions are made or have minimal input into evaluation decisions.[15] There are also other evaluation designs (participatory, collaborative, or empowerment evaluation) where stakeholders are seen as co-equal partners in all evaluation decisions, including which questions are to be answered, which data are collected, how data are analyzed, and how results are interpreted. Some of these designs emphasize stakeholder participation as a means of ensuring that the evaluation is responsive to stakeholder needs, while other designs involve stakeholders to increase the control and ownership.[12,15,22] The role of the stakeholders will depend in part on the desires of the stakeholders and the paradigm guiding the evaluation. In all cases, everyone involved should have a clear understanding of their role in the evaluation process.

Before data collection, all stakeholders should also agree on the extent to which the data collected will be kept confidential, not only in terms of protecting the confidentiality of participants in data collection (a nonnegotiable condition for protecting evaluation participants) but also in terms of how information will be shared within the group of stakeholders (all at once or some notified before others). The group should also reach consensus on how and when information will be communicated outside the immediate group of stakeholders and what will be shared.[15]

TYPES OF EVALUATION

There are several types of evaluation, including those related to program formation, context, process, impact, and outcome. Each type has a different purpose and thus is appropriate at different stages in the development of the program or policy. Initial evaluation efforts should focus on population needs and the implementation of program activities, commonly called formative or process evaluation. Impact evaluations and outcome evaluations are only appropriate after the program has been functioning for a sufficient amount of time to see the potential quantitative changes. The exact time will depend on the nature of the program and the changes expected or anticipated. Further, each type of evaluation involves different evaluation designs and data collection methods. Choices of which evaluation types to use are based in part on the interests of the various stakeholders.

Formative Evaluation

The goal of formative evaluation is to determine whether an element of a program or policy (e.g., materials, messages) is feasible, appropriate, and meaningful for the target population.[23] It should be conducted when intervention approaches are being determined, prior to program initiation. Formative evaluation data can be collected through quantitative (questionnaires) or qualitative (individual or group interviews) methods. Information that is useful at this stage is documentation of the context, or setting, within which the health concern is occurring, including an assessment of the social, economic, and physical environment factors.[12,13,19,23] In order to fully assess context, it is important to document the current knowledge and attitudes of potential program participants about various behaviors and their perspectives on proposed programs. For example, suppose a new program for healthy eating is proposed for school-aged children. Formative evaluation questions might include the following:

- What are the attitudes among school officials to the proposed healthy eating program?
- What are current barriers for policies for healthy eating?

- Are there certain schools that have healthier food environments than others?
- What are the attitudes among school-aged children toward healthier food choices?
- What, if anything, has been tried in the past, and what were the results?

Once these data are collected and analyzed by the identified stakeholders, a program plan should be developed. (Chapter 9 describes this process in detail.) The program plan is essential to evaluation. A key component of the program plan is the development of a logic model (an analytic framework) (see Chapter 8 for a description). A logic model lists specific activities and predicts how they will lead to the accomplishment of objectives and how these objectives will enhance the likelihood of accomplishing program goals. A logic model lays out what the program participants will do (attend an educational session on breast cancer screening at their church), what it will lead to (increased knowledge regarding risk factors for breast cancer and specific methods of breast cancer screening), which will in turn have an impact (increase breast cancer screening rates), with the intention that this will therefore produce a long-term outcome (decreased morbidity due to breast cancer). While several authors have conceptualized this process somewhat differently,[15,22,24,25] the overall intent is that the program or policy should be laid out in such a way that it specifies the activities and the program objectives that are expected to affect clearly delineated proximal and distal outcomes. While any logic model is obviously limited in its ability to predict the often important unintended consequences of programs and policies, many argue that, even with this limitation, a logic model is mandatory to evaluate a program effectively. Rossi and colleagues have stated that evaluation in the absence of a logic model results in a "black box" effect in that the evaluation may provide information with regard to the effects but not the processes that produced the effects.[15] Moreover, because so many of the distal outcomes in public health are not evident until long after a program is implemented (e.g., decreases in morbidity due to lung cancer as a result of a tobacco control program), it is essential to ascertain if more proximal outcomes (e.g., decreases in current smoking rates) are being achieved.

Process Evaluation

Process evaluation assesses the way a program is being delivered, rather than the effectiveness of a program.[23] It can function as a form of quality control by assessing what is being provided by a program compared with what is intended. Process evaluation addresses the questions of program implementation:

- To what extent is the program being implemented as planned?
- Are program materials and content appropriate for the population being served?

- How many are attending? Who is attending educational sessions? Who is not attending?
- Are all potential participants participating equally? Is the program reaching the intended audience?
- Does the program have sufficient resources?
- What percent of the program are participants receiving?

These data are important to document changes that have been, and need to be, made to the program to enable the program to be implemented at other sites. Information for process evaluation can be collected through quantitative and qualitative methods, including observations, field notes, interviews, questionnaires, program records, and local newspapers and publications. There are numerous excellent examples of process evaluation.[26–30]

Impact Evaluation

Impact evaluation assesses the extent to which program objectives are being met. Some also refer to this as an assessment of intermediate or proximal outcomes, to acknowledge both the importance of short-term outcomes and that impact evaluation can assess intended as well as unintended consequences.[12] Impact evaluation is probably the most commonly reported type of evaluation in the public health literature.

Impact evaluation requires that all program objectives be clearly specified. A challenge in conducting an impact evaluation is the presence of many program objectives and their variable importance among stakeholders. There are also instances when a national program is implemented at many sites.[31] The national program is likely to require each site to track the attainment of certain objectives and goals. Each site, however, may also have different specific program objectives and activities that they enact to accomplish local and national objectives and achieve the desired changes in outcomes. They may, therefore, be interested in tracking these local program activities and objectives in addition to the national requirements for reporting on program outcomes. Because no evaluation can evaluate all program components, stakeholders should come to an agreement as to which objectives will be measured at what times prior to collecting data.

It may be appropriate to alternate the types of data collected over months or years of a program to meet multiple programmatic and stakeholder needs. For example, suppose one was evaluating the changes in physical activity in a community over a 5-year period. In the initial phases of a program, it may be important to collect baseline data to understand the effects of the environment on physical activity. At each time point, it may be important to collect data on a set of core items (e.g., rates of physical activity) but alternate the data collected for some domains of questions (time 2—data on the role of social support; time 3—data on attitudes toward policies). Moreover, impact evaluation should not occur until participants have completed the program as planned or until policies have been established and implemented for some time. For example, if a program is planned to include five educational sessions, it is not useful to assess impact on objectives after the participants have attended only two sessions. It is also important to include assessments after the program has been completed to determine if the changes made as a result of the program have been sustained over time.

Program objectives assessed by impact evaluation may include changes in knowledge, attitudes, or behavior. For example, changes in knowledge about risk factors associated with breast cancer and/or the benefits of early detection might be tracked through the use of a questionnaire administered before and after an educational campaign or program. Similarly, changes in attitude might be ascertained by assessing a participant's intention to obtain a mammogram both before and after an intervention through the use of a questionnaire.

The Importance of Reliability and Validity.   As described in more depth in Chapter 2, validity is the extent to which a measure accurately captures what it is intended to capture and reliability is the likelihood that the instrument will get the same result time after time.[2] Changes associated with public health programs can be tracked through the use of pre- to post-intervention questionnaires. It is often useful to use items from questionnaires that have already been used to evaluate other programs. Many instruments are available in peer-reviewed articles on the subject of interest (see Chapter 7 on reviewing the scientific literature). If the items are not included in a scientific article, it is possible to contact the researcher and obtain the items or questionnaire directly from them.

Practitioners should consider using measures that have been tested in various surveillance systems such as the Behavioral Risk Factors Surveillance System (BRFSS). Begun in 1984, the BRFSS is the largest telephone health survey in the world.[32] Nelson and colleagues conducted a comprehensive review of reliability and validity studies of the survey questions used in the BRFSS.[33] In this review, measures determined to be of high reliability and high validity were current smoker, blood pressure screening, height, weight, and several demographic characteristics. Measures of both moderate reliability and validity included when last mammography was received, clinical breast examination, sedentary lifestyle, intense leisure-time physical activity, and fruit and vegetable consumption.

Even if the instruments under consideration have been shown to be valid and reliable in one population (e.g., residents of an urban area), it may be important to assess the reliability and validity of measures in the particular population being served by the program (e.g., a rural population). For example, it may be necessary to translate the items from English into other languages in a way that ensures that participants understand the meaning of the questions. This may require more than a simple word-for-word translation (Some words or phrases may be culturally defined and may not have a direct translation.) In addition, the multicultural nature of public health necessitates that the methods used to collect data and the analysis and reporting of the data reflect the needs of diverse populations. It is important to determine that the measures are appropriate for the population that is to be surveyed in terms of content (meeting program objectives), format (including readability and validity), and method of administering the questionnaire (e.g., self-administered versus telephone).[32] Changes in technologies may affect the reliability, validity, and feasibility of various data collection methods. For example, data are often collected by telephone, yet the greater use of answering machines and caller ID has contributed to declines in response rates and has increased the costs of conducting telephone surveys.[34]

Design and Analysis Considerations.   It is also important to consider the evaluation design that is most appropriate to assess the impact of a program or policy. While this is described in Chapter 6, there are a few additional considerations, particularly when conducting community-based programs. One particularly important issue to consider is the unit of assignment to intervention or control versus unit of analysis. Several authors have suggested ways to address these concerns.[35-37] For example, by using the individual as the unit of analysis, it is possible to use relatively fewer communities and collect more data, adjusting for the correlation among individuals within the same unit of assignment (e.g., within communities or within schools) through statistical means.[38] Alternately, one can collect less data across more communities or separate the communities into tracks with some receiving the interventions and others being assigned to a control or delayed treatment group. Others have suggested that the use of control groups may not necessarily be the best approach. Rather, the use of naturalistic inquiry and case studies, which provide in-depth descriptions of single or multiple cases, may be more useful in some evaluations.[12,36,39]

Qualitative data collection, such as individual or group interviews, can also be used to evaluate program impact by documenting changes, exploring the factors related to these changes, and determining the extent to which the intervention, as opposed to other factors, has influenced these changes. Moreover, qualitative data can be particularly helpful in assessing the unintended consequences of programs and policies.[12] Qualitative data must also adhere to standards and criteria of excellence, but these criteria are different than those used for quantitative measures. Lincoln and Cuba[14,40,41] lay out a series of expectations and criteria for ensuring rigor when using qualitative methods. These move from traditional concepts of internal validity to credibility, external validity to transferability, reliability to dependability, and objectivity to conformability. Lastl in examining the impact of a program, some stakeholders may find it important to conduct a cost-benefit or cost-effectiveness analysis. A discussion of these methods and the advantages and disadvantages of each is provided in Chapter 3.

Outcome Evaluation

Outcome evaluation provides long-term feedback on changes in health status, morbidity, mortality, and quality of life that can be attributed to the program. These more distal outcomes are difficult to attribute to a particular program because it takes so long for the effects to be seen and because changes in these outcomes are influenced by factors outside the scope of the program itself. Assessment of a program's influence on these outcomes, therefore, is often thought to require certain types of evaluation designs (experimental and quasi-experimental rather than observational) and long-term follow-up (described in Chapter 6). Some programs, however, may rely on the published literature to extrapolate from proximal to distal outcomes. For example, the link between smoking and lung cancer is well established. Thus, it may be possible to extrapolate from a decrease in smoking rates to the number of lung cancer cases prevented (the concept of population-attributable risk described in Chapter 2).

Data that are collected for purposes of outcome evaluation are more likely to be quantitative than qualitative and include social indicator data collected by the Centers for Disease Control and Prevention (CDC), the World Health Organization (WHO), state health departments, and local surveillance systems such as those sponsored by hospitals or health care systems. An evaluation that has included both impact and outcome data is shown in Box 10-2.[42-45] Qualitative data, however, can be useful in outcome evaluations to enhance understanding of the meaning and interpretation of quantitative findings and increase credibility of the results for many stakeholders.

Some kinds of data will enhance the quality of outcome evaluation. For example, it is helpful to have pre- and post-data available on the outcomes of interest. Comparison or control groups can assist in determining if the changes in desired outcomes are due to the intervention or to other factors. It is also important to have complete data; data collected as part of the program should not be systematically missing from a site or from some segment of the population of interest. In addition, secondary data, or data collected as part of surveillance systems, are most useful if they adequately and completely cover the subgroups of the population that the program or policy is intended to influence. For example, it may be important to have sufficient data to determine if there are differences in effect by race, age, or gender. The data, regardless of its source, should be collected using reliable and

Box 10-2. Evaluating Progress in Tobacco Control in California

In the field of tobacco control, decades of research and thousands of epidemiologic studies comprise the evidence establishing cigarette smoking as the "single most important preventable cause of premature death."[42] Economic studies have shown that increased tobacco taxes are an important tool for decreasing tobacco consumption. To address the issue, California voters passed an earmarked tobacco excise tax in 1988.[43] California raised the excise tax on cigarettes by 25 cents per pack and placed an initial tax of 42 cents on other tobacco products. This effort launched one of the most intensive and aggressive public health interventions ever undertaken. Several data sets were used to evaluate the effects of a tobacco tax (both impact and outcome evaluation). Surveys of youths and adults allowed calculation of rates of smoking initiation and prevalence. Tax records and census statistics provided data on per capita cigarette consumption. The California tobacco excise tax sharply accelerated the drop in both sales of cigarettes and in smoking. Per capita cigarette sales declined 41% between 1988 and 1994. There was a 28% decline in smoking prevalence between 1988 and 1993.[44] The program has also been associated with a reduction in deaths from heart disease in California.[45] This is double the expected decline based on the 1974–1987 trend. Several other states (e.g., Massachusetts, Oregon, Florida) have developed innovative approaches to tobacco control. For example, the effects of tobacco control efforts in Massachusetts appear to be on the same magnitude as those in California (Figure 10-1).

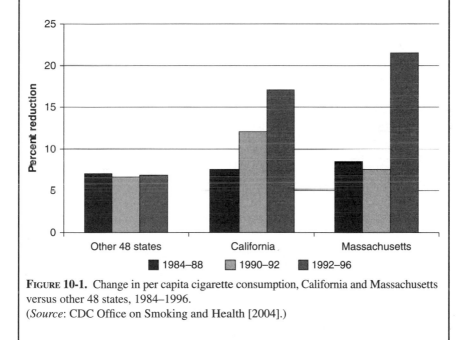

FIGURE 10-1. Change in per capita cigarette consumption, California and Massachusetts versus other 48 states, 1984–1996.
(*Source*: CDC Office on Smoking and Health [2004].)

valid measures and be analyzed using techniques that are appropriate for the questions asked and the types of data being used.[36,46]

Indicators for Impact and Outcome Evaluation

Health indicators are measures of the extent to which targets in health programs are being reached.[47] Therefore, for purposes of evaluation, indicators are not numerical goals in themselves and should not be confused with program objectives and targets, which tend to be quantifiable according to some scale or time. Rather, indicators provide a benchmark—they can help stimulate public health action, aid program managers and policy makers in reformulating existing strategies, and assist in identifying movement toward long-term health goals. Although a large body of literature exists on the uses and usefulness of health indicators within medical care, much less has been published on identifying and applying indicators for impact evaluation at the community level.

Traditionally, indicators have been grouped in broad categories, focusing on sociodemographic characteristics, health status, health risk factors, health care resource consumption, functional status, and quality of life.[48] The CDC developed a consensus set of 18 health status indicators that are useful for outcome evaluation.[49] Most of the CDC consensus indicators are measures of health status or health risk factors (e.g., suicide rate, lung cancer death rate, childhood poverty). They also tend to be widely available at the state, county, and city levels throughout the United States.[50] Zucconi and Carson[51] surveyed all state health departments to gain information on which of these indicators was actually being monitored. Except for work-related deaths, which were tracked in 76% of states, they found that mortality indicators were monitored nearly everywhere. At the county and state levels, these indicators have proved valuable in measuring progress in disease prevention and health promotion.[52] In particular, these indicators can be useful for outcome evaluation if one compares the local data with the national data and/or national goals and objectives, such as *Healthy People 2020,*[53] and determines what might be considered realistic and achievable change within the identified community.

While adequate indicators have been developed for mortality endpoints and for many behavioral risk factors like cigarette smoking or lack of leisure-time activity, shorter-term (intermediate) markers are needed. The rationale for intermediate indicators is founded in the need for evaluators to assess program change in periods of months or years, rather than over longer periods of time. Environmental and policy indicators (unobtrusive measures) may also be useful as an intermediate measure for documenting behavioral changes. Examples of these indicators include the number state laws banning smoking, the number of private worksites banning smoking, the miles of trails in a community, or the availability of low-fat foods in local restaurants (see Chapter 4 for more description of indicators).

DECIDING ON THE APPROPRIATE EVALUATION METHODS

There are many issues to consider in deciding the appropriate methods to use for a particular evaluation, including the type of data to collect (e.g., qualitative versus quantitative data). Qualitative data may include individual and group interviews; diaries of daily or weekly activities; records, newspapers, and other forms of mass media; and photographs and other visual and creative arts (music, poems, etc.). Quantitative data include surveys or questionnaires, surveillance data, and other records. Either form of data may be collected as primary data (designed for purposes of the evaluation at hand) or secondary data (designed for a purpose other than the evaluation at hand but still capable of answering the current evaluation questions to some extent).

These different types of data are often associated with different paradigmatic approaches (i.e., differences regarding what is known and how knowledge is generated) (Table 10-3). Quantitative data are generally collected using a positivist paradigm, or what is often called the "dominant" paradigm. As discussed earlier in this chapter, a paradigm offers guidance because it provides a set of understandings about the nature of reality and the relationship between the knower and what can be known. Within a positivist paradigm, what is known is constant, separate from the method of generating knowledge, the person conducting the inquiry, and the context within which the inquiry is conducted. On the other side of the spectrum, qualitative data are often collected within alternative paradigms that include critical theory and constructionism. While these alternative paradigms vary, they

Table 10-3. Comparison of Quantitative and Qualitative Evaluation Approaches

Type of Evaluation	Type of Data	Method of Collection/Analysis
Quantitative	• Survey questionnaire • Social indicator data • Geographic Information Systems • Environmental assessments	• Telephone, in-person, mail • National (CDC WONDER, Census, BRFSS, WHO) • Secondary review of archival data • Primary data collection or secondary review of data
Qualitative	• Open-ended questions • Individual interviews • Diaries • Group interviews/focus groups • Newspapers/newsletters/printed materials • Photography • Observation/environmental assessments	• Telephone, in-person, mail questionnaire • Telephone, in-person • Self-administered • In-person, telephone conference calls • Primary collection or secondary review of archival data (content analysis) • Primary data collection • Single or multiple observation, structured and unstructured

generally suggest that knowledge is dependent on the context and the interaction between the researcher and the participant in a study. It is important to note, however, that quantitative and qualitative data may be collected and analyzed using any paradigm as the guiding framework for the design of the study. For example, community-based evaluations are often conducted within an alternative paradigm but may use either qualitative or quantitative data or may include both types.

Data Triangulation

Using both quantitative and qualitative data is often referred to as "triangulation" of the data collection and analysis process. Such mixed-method approaches often result in greater validity of inferences, more comprehensive findings, and more insightful understanding.[3] Triangulation generally involves the use of multiple methods of data collection and/or analysis to determine points of commonality or disagreement.[4,54] Triangulation is often beneficial because of the complementary nature of the data. Although quantitative data provide an excellent opportunity to determine how variables are related to other variables for large numbers of people, they provide little in the way of understanding why these relationships exist. Qualitative data, on the other hand, can help provide information to explain quantitative findings, or what has been called "illuminating meaning."[4] The triangulation of qualitative and quantitative data can provide powerful evidence of effectiveness and can also provide insight into the processes of change in organizations and populations.[55] There are many examples of the use of triangulation of qualitative and quantitative data to evaluate health-related programs and policies, including AIDS prevention programs,[56] youth development,[57] occupational health programs and policies,[58] and chronic disease prevention programs in community settings.[59]

Other methods of triangulation have been described. These include "investigator triangulation," in which more than one investigator collects and/or analyzes raw data.[60] When consensus emerges, the results may have higher validity. In "theory triangulation," study findings are corroborated with existing social and/or behavioral science theories.[61]

The Role for Exploratory Evaluation

Exploratory evaluation (aka, evaluability assessment) is a preevaluation activity designed to maximize the chances that any subsequent evaluation will result in useful information.[62] It can be a precursor to either quantitative or qualitative evaluation and is often cost-effective because it can prevent costly evaluation of programs and policies whose logic model is not plausible or where activities and resources are not sufficient or relevant to achieve the objectives.[63]

Although the concept of exploratory evaluation has been around since the mid-1970s when it was first used by the U.S. Department of Health, Education, and Welfare,[64] the method has been underutilized in public health.[63] The use of exploratory evaluation for public health topics has been relatively narrow, including promotion of physical activity,[65] healthy eating,[66] AIDS outreach,[67] and rape prevention.[68]

As summarized by Trevisan[69] and Leviton and colleagues,[63] exploratory evaluation was designed to remedy several common problems in evaluation. First, there have been complaints from policy makers that evaluations are not always useful. Second, an exploratory evaluation can shed light on stakeholder disagreements (about the program goals, logic, how to measure success), which may suggest a program is not ready for evaluation. Next, the underlying logic for a program may not be clear or realistic (i.e., it is not clear how particular interventions will achieve desired results). Third, the cost of an evaluation may be prohibitive. And finally, the relevant decision makers may be unwilling to make changes on the basis of evaluation.

The steps of an exploratory evaluation can be summarized by eight questions that have been adapted from Strosberg and Wholey.[64]

1. What resources, activities, objectives, and causal assumptions make up the program?
2. Do those above the program managers, at the higher levels of the organization, agree with the program manager's description of the program?
3. To what extent does the program have agreed-on measures and data sources?
4. Does the description of the program correspond to what is actually found in the field?
5. Are program activities and resources likely to achieve objectives?
6. Does the program have well-defined uses for information on progress toward its measurable objectives?
7. What portion of the program is ready for evaluation of progress toward agreed-on objectives?
8. What evaluation and management options should organizational leaders consider?

For public health practitioners, exploratory evaluation has many benefits and can lead to more effective and efficient evaluations.[63] For those seeking to learn more about exploratory evaluation, several sources are useful.[62-64]

Evaluation of Dissemination and Implementation Projects

There is growing emphasis on dissemination and implementation (D&I) research, which seeks accelerate the adoption on evidence-based interventions in particular populations and settings.[70] Research on D&I has now taught us several important lessons about how evidence-based programs are spread: (1) D&I does not occur spontaneously, (2) passive approaches to D&I are largely ineffective, and (3) single-source prevention messages are generally less effective than comprehensive approaches.[71] When addressing D&I questions, a modified evaluation framework is needed. A useful model for D&I evaluation is the RE-AIM framework, which takes a staged approach to measure *R*each, *E*fficacy/Effectiveness, *A*doption, *I*mplementation, and *M*aintenance.[72] In RE-AIM, reach refers to the participation rate within the target population and the characteristics of participants versus non-participants. Efficacy/effectiveness relates to the impact of an intervention on specified outcome criteria. Adoption applies at the system level and concerns the percentage and representativeness of organizations that will adopt a given program or policy. Implementation refers to intervention integrity, or the quality and consistency of delivery when the intervention is replicated in real-world settings. And, finally, maintenance describes the long-term change at both individual and system/organizational levels. RE-AIM has been applied across numerous risk factors, diseases, and settings.[73] Its usefulness in evaluating the impact of public health policies has also been documented.[74]

Using Evaluation to Create Change

Another important consideration in the design and implementation of the evaluation is the intent of the evaluation with regard to the creation of knowledge versus the creation of change. Many traditional forms of evaluation act to assess the extent to which a program has met its objectives. Newer methods of evaluation include participants in the evaluation process with the intent of creating changes in the social structure and increasing the capacity of participants to self-evaluate.[11] These later forms of evaluation are often called empowerment evaluation, participatory action research, or community-based participatory research.[11,12,14,21,75,76] Such evaluation methods assess program goals and objectives as they relate to individuals, as well as the context within which individuals live (including economic conditions, education, community capacity, social support, and control).

Change can also come in the form of public health policy (described later). To improve public health outcomes, evidence-based public health policy is developed through a continuous process that uses the best available, quantitative and qualitative evidence.[77] Persuasive use of results of policy evaluations can be critical in the shaping of successful legislative and organizational change.[1]

Policy Evaluation Versus Program Evaluation

While there are many similarities in using evaluation to assess the implementation and effectiveness of programs and health policy, there are some significant differences that should be noted. Just as with program planning, there are several stages in a policy cycle, including formation, design, implementation, and evaluation.[78–80] In considering evaluation within the context of the policy cycle, the first decision is the utilization of evaluation in the agenda setting or policy formation stage and the policy design or formulation stage. This is similar to a community assessment but is likely to differ in terms of consideration of whether the issue warrants a public or government intervention. If there is evidence that policy intervention is warranted, the question becomes whether current policies adequately address the concern or if there is a need to modify existing legislation, create new policy, or enforce existing policy. Issues of cost-effectiveness and public opinion are as likely to have a significant impact on the answers to these questions as are other data collected.

The next phase of the policy cycle is policy implementation.[79] Process evaluation is useful at this stage with a focus on the extent to which the policy is being implemented according to expectations of the various stakeholders. The last stage in the policy cycle is policy accountability.[79] In this stage, impact evaluation and outcome evaluation are appropriate, with a focus on the extent to which the policy has achieved its objectives and goals.

Policy evaluations are critical to understanding the impact of policies on community- and individual-level behavior changes. They should include "upstream" (e.g., presence of zoning policies supportive of physical activity), "midstream" (e.g., the enrollment in walking clubs), and "downstream" (e.g., the rate of physical activity) factors.[81] By far, the most quantitative measures are routinely available for downstream outcomes.[81]

These benchmarks include programmatic as well as structural, social, and institutional objectives and goals. For example, 5 years after implementation of a state law requiring insurance coverage of cancer screenings, several questions might be addressed:

- Do health care providers know about the law?
- Do persons at risk of cancer know about the law?
- Have cancer screening rates changed?
- Are all relevant segments of the population being affected by the law?

There are several challenges in evaluating health policies. One is that the acceptable timing of the evaluation is likely to be determined more by legislative sessions than programmatic needs.[82] Because of the wide variety of objectives and goals, it is important to acknowledge from the outset that evaluation results provide only one piece of the data that are used in decision making regarding maintaining or terminating a health policy. This is in part because the evaluation of public health policy must be considered part of the political process. The results of evaluations of public policy inevitably influence the distribution of power and resources.

Therefore, while it is essential to conduct rigorous evaluations, it must be acknowledged that no evaluation is completely objective, value free, or neutral.[78,80,83]

Resource Considerations

Resources are also important to consider in determining the appropriate evaluation methods. Resources to consider include time, money, personnel, access to information, staff, and participants. It is important to assess stakeholder needs in determining the type of evaluation to conduct. It may be that stakeholders require information in order to maintain program funding or to justify the program to constituents. Alternately, participants may believe that previous programs have not met their needs and may request certain types of data to alleviate these concerns. Similarly, program administrators in a collaborative program may require information as to the benefit of the collaboration or information on how to improve the evaluation to fix managerial problems that are occurring before other process, impact, or outcome measures can be assessed.

The methods of evaluation used should not, however, be constrained by the skill and comfort level of the evaluator. Because there are a broad range of evaluation skills that can be used and few evaluators have all of these skills, there is a temptation to see needs through the evaluator's lens of ability. It is far more useful to define the method of evaluation by the other factors mentioned earlier and the questions asked and then bring together a group of evaluators who have the various skills necessary to conduct the evaluation.[12] In doing so, it is important to consider the ability of the evaluators to work with others who have different technical skills as well as the availability of resources to bring together these multiple types of expertise.

DISSEMINATION: REPORTING AND USING DATA

Once the data are collected and analyzed, it is important to provide the various stakeholders with a full reporting of the information collected and the recommendations for program changes. A formal report should include background information on the evaluation, such as the purpose of the evaluation (including the focus on process, impact, or outcome questions), the various stakeholders involved, a description of the program including program goals and objectives, a description of the methodology used, and the evaluation results and recommendations.[6,19,20] Some important questions to consider when reporting evaluation data are shown in Table 10-4.[84,85]

Utilization of the report and the specific recommendations will depend in part on the extent to which stakeholders have been involved in the process to this point

Table 10-4. Questions to Consider When Reporting Evaluation Information

Question	Audience/Method for Reporting
Who are the audiences (potential consumers) who should be informed?	Key stakeholders (people and agencies) Participants in the program Public health practitioners Public health researchers
How will you inform the community about the results of your program?	Town meetings Meetings of local organizations (civic groups) Newspapers articles Journal articles The Internet
Who will assume responsibility for presenting the results	Public health practitioners Public health researchers Community members
How can this information be used for program improvement?	Needs for new or different personnel Refinement of intervention options Changes in time lines and action steps

Source: Adapted from The Planned Approach to Community Health (PATCH).[84,85]

and the extent to which the various stakeholders have been involved in the data analysis and interpretation. One useful method is to conduct some sort of member validation of the findings prior to presenting a final report.[7,15,19] This is particularly important if the participants have not had other involvement in data analysis and interpretation. Member validation is a process by which the preliminary results and interpretations are presented back to those who provided the evaluation data. These participants are asked to comment on the results and interpretations, and this feedback is used to modify the initial interpretations.

Use of the evaluation report is also influenced by its timeliness and the match between stakeholder needs and the method of reporting the evaluation results.[7,19,25] Often, evaluation results are reported back to the funders and program administrators and are published in academic journals but are not provided to community-based organizations or community members themselves. The ideal method of reporting the findings to each of these groups is likely to differ. For some stakeholders, formal written reports are helpful, while for others, an oral presentation of results or information placed in newsletters or on websites might be more appropriate. It is, therefore, essential that the evaluator considers the needs of all the stakeholders and provides the evaluation results back to the various interest groups in appropriate ways. This includes, but is not limited to, ensuring that the report enables the various stakeholders to use the data for future program or policy initiatives.

SUMMARY

Evaluation is just one step in an evidence-based process of encouraging and creating health-promoting changes among individuals and within communities. As with planning, it is important to provide resources for the evaluation efforts that are appropriate to the scope of the program or policy.

Key Chapter Points

- Because evaluation can influence the distribution of power and resources in communities, it is essential that evaluators strive to include key stakeholders early in the process.
- Information gathered should be shared with all stakeholders in ways that are understandable and useful.
- The types of data used (qualitative, quantitative) should be appropriate to the questions asked. Practitioners are encouraged to seek out other experts from multiple disciplines to assist them with venturing into new data collection approaches.
- It is important to conduct evaluation across the life of a program (formative, process, impact, and outcome) to ensure proper implementation and monitoring.
- Newer techniques such as exploratory evaluation can be a precursor to either quantitative or qualitative evaluation and is often cost-effective.
- Practitioners are encouraged to publish results of their program and policy evaluations and to disseminate their findings widely. This process creates new and sometimes generalizable knowledge that can be highly beneficial to public health professionals and, ultimately, to the communities they serve.

SUGGESTED READINGS AND SELECTED WEBSITES

Suggested Readings

Fink A. Evaluation Fundamentals: Insights Into the Outcomes, Effectiveness, and Quality of Health Programs. 2nd ed. Thousand Oaks, CA: Sage; 2004.

Israel BA, Cummings KM, Dignan MB, et al. Evaluation of health education programs: current assessment and future directions. *Health Educ Q*. 1995;22(3):364–389.

Koepsell TD, Wagner EH, Cheadle AC, et al. Selected methodological issues in evaluating community-based health promotion and disease prevention programs. *Annu Rev Public Health*. 1992;13:31–57.

Leviton L, Kettel Khan L, Rog D, et al. Exploratory evaluation of public health policies, programs and practices. *Annu Rev Public Health*. 2010;31:213–233 .

Patton MQ. Qualitative Evaluation and Research Methods. 3rd ed. Thousand Oaks, CA: Sage; 2002.

Shadish W, Cook T, Campbell D. Experimental and Quasi-Experimental Designs for
Generalized Causal Inference. Boston, MA: Houghton Mifflin; 2002.
Timmreck TC. Planning, Program Development, and Evaluation. A Handbook for Health
Promotion, Aging and Health Services. 2nd ed. Boston, MA: Jones and Bartlett
Publishers; 2003.
Wholey J, Hatry H, Newcomer K, eds. Handbook of Practical Program Evaluation.
2nd ed. San Francisco, CA: Jossey-Bass; 2004.

Selected Websites

American Evaluation Association <http://www.eval.org/Publications/Guiding-
Principles.asp>. The American Evaluation Association is an international professional association of evaluators devoted to the application and exploration
of program evaluation, personnel evaluation, technology, and many other forms of
evaluation.

The CDC Working Group on Evaluation <http://www.cdc.gov/eval/resources.
htm>. The CDC Working Group on Evaluation has developed a comprehensive
list of evaluation documents, tools, and links to other websites. These materials
include documents that describe principles and standards, organizations and foundations that support evaluation, a list of journals and online publications, and
access to step-by-step manuals.

The Community Health Status Indicators (CHSI) Project <http://community
health.hhs.gov/>. The Community Health Status Indicators (CHSI) Project
includes 3141 county health status profiles representing each county in the United
States excluding territories. Each CHSI report includes data on access and utilization of health care services, birth and death measures, *Healthy People 2010*
targets, U.S. birth and death rates, vulnerable populations, risk factors for premature deaths and communicable diseases, and environmental health. The goal of
CHSI is to give local public health agencies another tool for improving their community's health by identifying resources and setting priorities.

The Community Tool Box <http://ctb.ku.edu/en/>. The Community Tool Box
is a global resource for free information on essential skills for building healthy
communities. It offers more than 7000 pages of practical guidance on topics such
as leadership, strategic planning, community assessment, advocacy, grant writing,
and evaluation. Sections include descriptions of the task, step-by-step guidelines,
examples, and training materials.

RE-AIM.org <http://www.re-aim.org/>. With an overall goal of enhancing the
quality, speed, and public health impact of efforts to translate research into practice,
this site provides an explanation of and resources (e.g., planning tools, measures,
self-assessment quizzes, FAQs, comprehensive bibliography) for those wanting to
apply the RE-AIM framework.

The Research Methods Knowledge Base <http://www.socialresearchmethods. net/kb/>. The Research Methods Knowledge Base is a comprehensive web-based textbook that covers the entire research process including formulating research questions, sampling, measurement (surveys, scaling, qualitative, unobtrusive), research design (experimental and quasi-experimental), data analysis, and writing the research paper. It uses an informal, conversational style to engage both the newcomer and the more experienced student of research.

United Nations Development Programme's Evaluation Office <http://www. undp.org/evaluation/index.html>. United Nations Development Programme is the United Nations' global development network, an organization advocating for change and connecting countries to knowledge, experience, and resources to help people build a better life. This site on evaluation includes training tools and a link to their *Handbook on Planning, Monitoring and Evaluating for Development Results, available in English, Spanish and French.* The Evaluation Resource Center allows users to search for evaluations by agency, type of evaluation, region, country, year, and focus area.

REFERENCES

1. Shadish WR. The common threads in program evaluation. *Prev Chronic Dis.* 2006;3(1):A03.
2. Porta M, ed. *A Dictionary of Epidemiology.* 5th ed. New York: Oxford University Press; 2008.
3. Greene J, Benjamin L, Goodyear L. The merits of mixing methods in evaluation. *Evaluation.* 2001;7(1):25–44.
4. Steckler A, McLeroy KR, Goodman RM, et al. Toward integrating qualitative and quantitative methods: An introduction. *Health Educ Q.* 1992;19(1):1–9.
5. Berk R, Rossi P. *Thinking about Program Evaluation 2.* Thousand Oaks, CA:Sage; 1999.
6. Fink A. *Evaluation Fundamentals: Insights into the Outcomes, Effectiveness, and Quality of Health Programs.* 2nd ed. Thousand Oaks, CA: Sage; 2004.
7. Patton MQ. *Qualitative Evaluation and Research Methods.* 3rd ed. Thousand Oaks, CA: Sage; 2002.
8. Timmreck TC. *Planning, Program Development, and Evaluation. A Handbook for Health Promotion, Aging and Health Services.* 2nd ed. Boston, MA: Jones and Bartlett Publishers; 2003.
9. Wholey J, Hatry H, Newcomer K, eds. *Handbook of Practical Program Evaluation.* 2nd ed. San Francisco, CA: Jossey-Bass; 2004.
10. Suchman E. *Evaluative Research: Principles and Practice in Public Service and Social Action Programs.* New York, NY: Russell Sage Foundation; 1967.
11. Fetterman DM, Kaftarian SJ, Wandersman A. *Empowerment Evaluation: Knowledge and Tools for Self-Assessment & Accountability.* Thousand Oaks, CA: Sage Publications; 1996.
12. Israel BA, Cummings KM, Dignan MB, et al. Evaluation of health education programs: current assessment and future directions. *Health Educ Q.* 1995;22(3):364–389.

13. Lincoln Y, Guba E. Paradigmatic controversies, contradictions, and emerging confluences. In: Denzin N, Lincoln Y, eds. *Handbook of Qualitative Research.* 2nd ed. Thousand Oaks, CA: Sage; 2000:163–188.

14. Lincoln YS, Guba EG. *Naturalistic Inquiry.* Beverly Hills, Ca: Sage; 1985.

15. Rossi PH, Lipsey MW, Freeman HE. *Evaluation: A Systematic Approach.* 7th ed. Thousand Oaks, CA: Sage Publications; 2003.

16. Shadish W, Cook T, Campbell D. *Experimental and Quasi-Experimental Designs for Generalized Causal Inference.* Boston, MA: Houghton Mifflin; 2002.

17. Jack L Jr, Mukhtar Q, Martin M, et al. Program evaluation and chronic diseases: methods, approaches, and implications for public health. *Prev Chronic Dis.* 2006; 3(1):A02.

18. Joint Committee on Standards for Educational Evaluation. *Program Evaluation Standards: How to Assess Evaluations of Educational Programs.* 2nd ed. Thousand Oaks, CA: Sage; 1994.

19. Centers for Disease Control and Prevention. Framework for program evaluation in public health. *MMWR.* 1999;48(RR-11):1–40.

20. Herman JL, Morris LL, Fitz-Gibbon C. *Evaluator's Handbook.* Newbury Park, CA: Sage Publications; 1987.

21. Whitmore E. *Understanding and Practicing Participatory Evaluation. New Directions for Evaluation.* San Francisco, CA: Jossey Bass; 1998.

22. Goodman RM. Principles and tools for evaluating community-based prevention and health promotion programs. *J Public Health Manage Pract.* 1998;4(2):37–47.

23. Thompson N, Kegler M, Holtgrave D. Program evaluation. In: Crosby R, DiClemente R, Salazar L, eds. *Research Methods in Health Promotion.* San Francisco, CA: Jossey-Bass; 2006:199–225.

24. Bartholomew LK, Parcel GS, Kok G, et al. *Planning Health Promotion Programs: Intervention Mapping.* 2nd ed. San Francisco, CA: Jossey-Bass; 2006.

25. Patton MQ. *Utilization-Focused Evaluation: The New Century Text.* 3rd ed. Thousand Oaks, CA: Sage Publications; 1997.

26. Baskerville NB, Hogg W, Lemelin J. Process evaluation of a tailored multifaceted approach to changing family physician practice patterns improving preventive care. *J Fam Pract.* 2001;50(3):W242–W249.

27. Berkowitz JM, Huhman M, Heitzler CD, et al. Overview of formative, process, and outcome evaluation methods used in the VERB campaign. *Am J Prev Med.* 2008;34(6 Suppl):S222–S229.

28. Erwin DO, Ivory J, Stayton C, et al. Replication and dissemination of a cancer education model for African American women. *Cancer Control.* 2003;10(5 Suppl): 13–21.

29. Hunt MK, Barbeau EM, Lederman R, et al. Process evaluation results from the Healthy Directions-Small Business study. *Health Educ Behav.* 2007;34(1):90–107.

30. Williams JH, Belle GA, Houston C, et al. Process evaluation methods of a peer-delivered health promotion program for African American women. *Health Promot Pract.* 2001;2(2):135–142.

31. Saxe L, Tighe. The view from Main Street and the view from 40,000 feet: Can a national evaluation understand local communities? In: Telfair J, Leviton LC, Merchant JS, eds. *Evaluating Health and Human Service Programs in Community Settings.* Vol 83. San Francisco, CA: Jossey-Bass; 1999;67–87.

32. Mokdad AH. The Behavioral Risk Factors Surveillance System: past, present, and future. *Annu Rev Public Health.* 2009;30:43–54.

33. Nelson DE, Holtzman D, Bolen J, et al. Reliability and validity of measures from the Behavioral Risk Factor Surveillance System (BRFSS). *Soz Praventivmed.* 2001; 46(1 Suppl):S3–42.
34. Kempf AM, Remington PL. New challenges for telephone survey research in the twenty-first century. *Annu Rev Public Health.* 2007;28:113–126.
35. Braverman MT. *Evaluating Health Promotion Programs.* Vol 43. San Francisco, CA: Jossey-Bass; 1989.
36. Koepsell TD, Wagner EH, Cheadle AC, et al. Selected methodological issues in evaluating community-based health promotion and disease prevention programs. *Annu Rev Public Health.* 1992;13:31–57.
37. Thompson B, Coronado G, Snipes SA, et al. Methodologic advances and ongoing challenges in designing community-based health promotion programs. *Annu Rev Public Health.* 2003;24:315–340.
38. Murray DM. *Design and Analysis of Group-Randomized Trials.* New York, NY: Oxford University Press; 1998.
39. Yin RK. *Case Study Research: Design and Methods.* Thousand Oaks, CA: Sage Publications; 1994.
40. Guba EG, Lincoln YS. The countenances of fourth-generation evaluation: Description, Judgment and negotiation. In: Palumbo D, ed. *The Politics of Program Evaluation.* Newbury Park, CA: Sage Publications; 1987;202–234.
41. Lincoln YS, Guba EG. But is it rigorous? trustworthiness and authenticity in natural-istic evaluation. In: Williams DD, ed. *Naturalisitic Evaluation.* Vol 30. San Fran-cisco, CA: Jossey-Bass; 1986;73–80.
42. US Dept of Health and Human Services. *Reducing the Health Consequences of Smoking—25 Years of Progress: A Report of the Surgeon General.* Vol DHHS publication (CDC) 89–8411. Rockville, MD: US Dept of Health and Human Services, Public Health Service, Centers for Disease Control, Center for Chronic Disease Prevention and Health Promotion, Office on Smoking and Health; 1989.
43. Bal D, Kizer K, Felten P, et al. Reducing tobacco consumption in California: Development of a statewide anti-tobacco use campaign. *JAMA.* 1990;264: 1570–1574.
44. California Department of Health Services. *Toward Tobacco Free California. Mastering the Challenges 1995–1997.* Sacramento, CA: California Department of Health Services; 1996.
45. Fichtenberg CM, Glantz SA. Association of the California Tobacco Control Program with declines in cigarette consumption and mortality from heart disease. *N Engl J Med.* 2000;343(24):1772–1777.
46. Bauman A, Koepsell TD. Epidemiologic issues in community intervention. In: Brownson RC, Pettiti DB, eds. *Applied Epidemiology: Theory to Practice.* New York, NY: Oxford University Press; 2006:164–206.
47. World Health Organization. *Health Program Evaluation. Guiding Principles for Its Application in the Managerial Process for National Development.* Geneva, Switzerland: World Health Organization; 1981. Health for All Series, No.6.
48. Durch JS, Bailey LA, Stoto MA, eds. *Improving Health in the Community: A Role of Performance Monitoring.* Washington, DC: National Academies Press; 1997.
49. Centers for Disease Control. Consensus set of health status indicators for the general assessment of community health status-United States. *MMWR.* 1991;40:449–451.

50. Metzler M, Kanarek N, Highsmith K, et al. Community health status indicators project: the development of a national approach to community health. *Prev Chronic Dis.* 2008;5(3):A94.
51. Zucconi SL, Carson CA. CDC's Consensus Set of Health Status Indicators: monitoring and prioritization by state health departments. *Am J Public Health.* 1994;84:1644–1646.
52. Sutocky JW, Dumbauld S, Abbott GB. Year 2000 health status indicators: a profile of California. *Public Health Rep.* 1996;111:521–526.
53. Fielding J, Kumanyika S. Recommendations for the concepts and form of Healthy People 2020. *Am J Prev Med.* 2009;37(3):255–257.
54. Denzin NK. *The Research Act in Sociology.* London, UK: Butterworth; 1970.
55. Nutbeam D. Evaluating health promotion—progress, problems and solutions. *Health Promot Int.* 1998;13(1):27–44.
56. Dorfman LE, Derish PA, Cohen JB. Hey Girlfriend: an evaluation of AIDS prevention among women in the sex industry. *Health Educ Q.* 1992;19(1):25–40.
57. Shek DT, Siu AM. Evaluation of a positive youth development program in Hong Kong: issues, principles and design. *Int J Adolesc Med Health.* 2006;18(3):329–339.
58. Hugentobler M, Israel BA, Schurman SJ. An action research approach to workplace health: Integrating methods. *Health Educ Q.* 1992;19(1):55–76.
59. Goodman RM, Wheeler FC, Lee PR. Evaluation of the heart to heart project: Lessons from a community-based chronic disease prevention project. *Am J Health Promot.* 1995;9(6):443–455.
60. Guyatt G, Rennie D, eds. *Users' Guides to the Medical Literature. A Manual for Evidence-Based Clinical Practice.* Chicago, IL: American Medical Association Press; 2002.
61. Denzin NK. *Sociological Methods.* New York, NY: McGraw-Hill; 1978.
62. Wholey J. Assessing the feasibility and likely usefulness of evaluation. In: Wholey J, Hatry H, Newcomer K, eds. *Handbook of Practical Program Evaluation.* 2nd ed. San Francisco, CA: Jossey Bass; 2004:33–62.
63. Leviton L, Kettel Khan L, et al. Exploratory evaluation of public health policies, programs and practices. *Annu Rev Public Health.* 2010;30:213–233.
64. Strosberg MA, Wholey JS. Evaluability assessment: from theory to practice in the Department of Health and Human Services. *Public Adm Rev.* 1983;43(1):66–71.
65. Dwyer JJ, Hansen B, Barrera M, et al. Maximizing children's physical activity: an evaluability assessment to plan a community-based, multi-strategy approach in an ethno-racially and socio-economically diverse city. *Health Promot Int.* 2003;18(3):199–208.
66. Durham J, Gillieatt S, Ellies P. An evaluability assessment of a nutrition promotion project for newly arrived refugees. *Health Promot J Austr.* 2007;18(1):43–49.
67. Leviton L, Collins C, Laird B, Kratt P. Teaching evaluation using evaluability assessment. *Evaluation.* 1998;4:389–409.
68. Basile KC, Lang KS, Bartenfeld TA, et al. Report from the CDC: Evaluability assessment of the rape prevention and education program: summary of findings and recommendations. *J Womens Health (Larchmt).* 2005;14(3):201–207.
69. Trevisan M. Evaluability assessment from 1986 to 2006. *Am J Evaluation.* 2007;28:209–303.
70. Rabin BA, Brownson RC, Haire-Joshu D, et al. A glossary for dissemination and implementation research in health. *J Public Health Manag Pract.* 2008;14(2):117–123.

71. Brownson RC, Jones E. Bridging the gap: translating research into policy and practice. *Prev Med.* 2009;49(4):313–315.
72. Glasgow RE, Vogt TM, Boles SM. Evaluating the public health impact of health promotion interventions: the RE-AIM framework. *Am J Public Health.* 1999; 89(9):1322–1327.
73. Dzewaltowski DA, Estabrooks PA, Klesges LM, et al. Behavior change intervention research in community settings: how generalizable are the results? *Health Promot Int.* 2004;19(2):235–245.
74. Jilcott S, Ammerman A, Sommers J, et al. Applying the RE-AIM framework to assess the public health impact of policy change. *Ann Behav Med.* 2007;34(2):105–114.
75. Cargo M, Mercer SL. The value and challenges of participatory research: Strengthening its practice. *Annu Rev Public Health.* 2008;29:325–350.
76. Israel BA, Schulz AJ, Parker EA, et al. Community-based research: a partnership approach to improve public health. *Annu Rev Public Health.* 1998;19:173–202.
77. Brownson RC, Chriqui JF, Stamatakis KA. Understanding evidence-based public health policy. *Am J Public Health.* 2009;99(9):1576–1583.
78. Chelimsky E. The politics of program evaluation. In: Cordray DS, Bloom HS, LIght RJ, eds. *Evaluation Practice in Eeview.* Vol 34. San Francisco, CA: Jossey-Bass; 1987;5–21.
79. Palumbo DJ. Politics and evaluation. In: Palumbo D, ed. *The Politics of Program Evaluation.* Newbury Park, California: Sage Publications; 1987;12–46.
80. Weiss CH. Where politics and evaluation research meet. In: Palumbo DJ, ed. *The Politics of Program Evaluation.* Newbury Park, CA: Sage Publications; 1987;437–472.
81. McKinlay JB. Paradigmatic obstacles to improving the health of populations— implications for health policy. *Salud Publica Mex.* 1998;40(4):369–379.
82. Brownson RC, Royer C, Ewing R, et al. Researchers and policymakers: travelers in parallel universes. *Am J Prev Med.* 2006;30(2):164–172.
83. Savitz DA. *Interpreting Epidemiologic Evidence. Strategies for Study Design and Analysis.* New York, NY: Oxford University Press; 2003.
84. US Department of Health and Human Services. *Planned Approach to Community Health: Guide for the Local Coordinator.* Atlanta, GA: Centers for Disease Control and Prevention; 1996.
85. Cockerill R, Myers T, Allman D. Planning for community-based evaluation. *Am J Eval.* 2000;21(3):351–357.

11

Emerging Issues in Evidence-Based Public Health

> Never let the future disturb you. You will meet it, if you have to, with the
> same weapons of reason which today arm you against the present.
> —Marcus Aurelius

Described in this book are the importance and complexity of the public health problems we face and how these challenges can be addressed through the evidence-based decision-making process. While the evidence base on effective public health interventions has grown considerably in the past few decades, knowledge about how to apply and evaluate the evidence is lacking for many settings and populations. It is essential to keep in mind that as the scientific evidence base grows and new health threats are identified, the process of evidence-based public health (EBPH) needs to take into account changing physical, economic, policy, and sociocultural environments.

Two converging bodies of knowledge hold promise for bridging the gap between discovery of new research findings and application in public health settings. First, the concept of evidence-based public health is growing in prominence due in part to a larger body of intervention research on what works to improve population health (e.g., the *Community Guide* recommendations on effective interventions[1]). Second, effective methods of dissemination and implementation (D&I) are needed to put evidence to work in "real-world" settings. While in its infancy, there is increased attention and growing literature on D&I research.[2,3] This type of research elucidates the processes and factors that lead to widespread use of an evidence-based intervention by a particular population or within a certain setting (e.g., worksite, school). This D&I research has begun to identify a number of important factors to enhance the uptake of evidence-based interventions in both practice (e.g., a state health department) and policy (e.g., a state legislature) settings.[2,4–13]

This chapter briefly describes several emerging issues in public health that influence the body of available evidence and how the evidence is applied across various settings. While these examples are not exhaustive, they are meant to illustrate the myriad of challenges faced by public health practitioners in the coming years and decades.

A GROWING EVIDENCE BASE

Expand the Evidence Base on Intervention Effectiveness

The growing literature on the effectiveness of preventive interventions in clinical and community settings[1,14] does not provide equal coverage of health problems. For example, the evidence base on how to increase immunization levels is much stronger than that on how to prevent poor health outcomes from a natural or man-made disaster. A greater investment of resources to expand the evidence base is therefore essential. Even where we have interventions of proven effectiveness, the populations in which they have been tested often do not include subpopulations with the greatest disease and injury burden. Expanding the base of evidence requires reliance on well-tested conceptual frameworks, especially those that pay close attention to D&I. For example, RE-AIM helps program planners and evaluators to pay explicit attention to *R*each, *E*fficacy/Effectiveness, *A*doption, *I*mplementation, and *M*aintenance.[15,16] Building this evidence base is likely to benefit from greater use of natural experiments, particularly for addressing social and policy determinants of health.[17]

Build the Evidence on External Validity

As described in Chapter 1, there are various forms of evidence. Some forms of evidence inform our knowledge about the etiology and prevention of disease.[18] Other evidence shows the relative effectiveness of specific interventions to address a particular health condition. However, what is often missing is a body of evidence that can help to determine the generalizability of effectiveness of an intervention from one population and setting to another (i.e., the core concepts of external validity) as described in Chapter 2. The issues in external validity often relate to context for an intervention—for example, What factors need to be taken into account when an internally valid program or policy is implemented in a different setting or with a different population subgroup? How does one balance the concepts of fidelity and reinvention? If the adaptation process changes the original intervention to such an extent that the original efficacy data may no longer apply, then the program may be viewed as a new intervention under very different contextual conditions. Green[19] has recommended that the implementation of evidence-based approaches requires careful consideration of the "best processes" needed when generalizing research to alternate populations, places, and times.

Consider Evidence Typologies

In reflecting on what works and what is ineffective, it becomes apparent that trying to put interventions into these two broad categories minimizes the ability of practitioners to discern what is most likely to be effective in their population and context. In addressing this concern, several groups have begun to describe different categories of intervention evidence (Type 2), rather than simply indicating an intervention is or is not "evidence-based" (Table 11-1). These categories of intervention build on work from Canada, the United Kingdom, Australia, the

Table 11-1. Typology for Classifying Interventions by Level of Scientific Evidence

Category	How Established	Considerations for Level of Scientific Evidence	Data Source Examples
Effective: first tier	Peer review via systematic review	Based on study design and execution External validity Potential side benefits or harms Costs and cost-effectiveness	*Community Guide* Cochrane Reviews
Effective: second tier	Peer review	Based on study design and execution External validity Potential side benefits or harms Costs and cost effectiveness	Articles in the scientific literature Research-tested intervention programs Technical reports with peer review
Promising	Intervention evaluation without formal peer review	Summative evidence of effectiveness Formative evaluation data Theory-consistent, plausible, potentially high-reach, low-cost, replicable	State or federal government reports (without peer review) Conference presentations Case studies
Emerging	Ongoing work, practice-based summaries or evaluation works in progress	Formative evaluation data Theory-consistent, plausible, potentially high-reach, low-cost, replicable Face validity	Evaluability assessments[a] Pilot studies NIH RePORTER database Projects funded by health foundations

[a]A "preevaluation" activity that involves an assessment is an assessment that is conducted prior to commencing an evaluation to establish whether a program or policy can be evaluated and what might be the barriers to its evaluation (aka exploratory evaluation).

Netherlands, and the United States on how to recast the strength of evidence, emphasizing the "weight of evidence" and a wider range of considerations beyond efficacy. We define four categories within a typology of scientific evidence for decision-making: effective (first tier), effective (second tier), promising, and emerging. While this continuum provides more variability in categorizing interventions, it has been noted that the criteria for assigning an intervention to one category or another often include research design, with randomized designs being weighted as most beneficial. However, adherence to a strict hierarchy of study designs may reinforce an "inverse evidence law" by which interventions most likely to influence whole populations (e.g., policy change) are least valued in an evidence matrix emphasizing randomized designs.[20,21]

TRACKING PROGRESS

Set Priorities and Measure Progress

Establishing public health and health care priorities in an era of limited resources is a demanding task. The use of the analytic tools discussed in this book can make important contributions to priority setting. Measuring progress toward explicit goals has become an essential feature of goal setting. Global health priorities are set by initiatives such as the Millennium Development Goals,[22] whereas national benchmarks are offered in strategic plans such as *Healthy People 2020*.[23] Progress toward both types of objectives can be tracked in periodic reports as long as (1) the resources required to collect these data are available and (2) data needs are aligned with the interventions being implemented at provincial, state, and local levels. A recent assessment of progress in meeting *Healthy People 2010* targets shows mixed progress with the likelihood of falling short of the majority of targets associated with leading health indicators.[24] Increasingly, these health priorities are focusing on social determinants of health or changes to the physical environment, which often are not tracked in public health surveillance systems.

Improve Surveillance of Policy-Related Variables

Public health surveillance (i.e., the ongoing systematic collection, analysis, and interpretation of outcome-specific health data) is a cornerstone of public health.[25] In the United States, we now have excellent epidemiologic data for estimating which population groups and which regions of the country are affected and how patterns are changing over time with respect to an epidemic. To supplement these data, we need better information on a broad array of environmental and policy factors that determine these patterns. When implemented properly, policy surveillance systems can be an enormous asset for policy development and evaluation. For example, we know that there were nearly 1000 obesity-related bills and resolutions introduced and adopted from 2003 through 2005 across the 50 states and the District of Columbia.[26] These data allow us to compare progress among states, determine the types of bills that are being introduced and passed (e.g., school nutrition standards, safe routes to school programs), and begin to track progress over time.

PARTNERSHIPS AND ENGAGEMENT

Address the Tension between Participatory Decision Making and EBPH

As noted in Chapter 1, participatory approaches are designed to actively involve community-based organizations, government agencies, and community members in research and intervention projects.[27-29] These collaborative approaches are promising because they move beyond the "parachute" approach to public health practice and research (where community members are simply the objects of study) to one where a wide variety of stakeholders are actively involved in the process. Yet, there is a potential for tension between participatory approaches and evidence-based decision making. For example, a well-conducted community assessment might lead to a specific set of health-related priorities and intervention approaches (e.g., diabetes, arthritis, suicide, sexually transmitted diseases). There may be community support for addressing some of these issues but not others. Moreover, while several of these may have common determinants (e.g., physical activity), there may be funding available for a particular disease (e.g., diabetes) and not for others. It is important to develop structures for discussing these issues and weighing the best ways to move forward. Some communities may decide to apply for funds with one group and have another group continue to seek funding for other priority areas. Alternately, the group might support funding in one area, recognizing that addressing common determinants will assist in the prevention of a variety of health issues. Last, the assessment might find that there are underlying root causes of these issues, such as inadequate transportation to resources and support services in a rural community. The community might incorporate policy development and/or environmental changes to develop these infrastructures in a way that they remain in the community beyond the grant funding.

Enhance Transdisciplinary Work across Sectors and Systems

As illustrated at numerous points in this book, effective approaches to prevention will require attention from many sectors, including government, private industry, and academe. This relates to the growing scholarly work on team science, which is often accomplished through transdisciplinary research. Transdisciplinary research provides valuable opportunities for practice-research collaboration to improve the health and well-being of both individuals and communities.[30,31] Tobacco control efforts have been successful in facilitating cooperation among disciplines such as advertising, policy, business, medical science, and behavioral science. Activities within these multidisciplinary tobacco networks try to fill the gaps between scientific discovery and research translation by engaging a wide range of stakeholders.[32–34] A transdisciplinary approach has also shown some evidence of effectiveness in obesity prevention in Canada.[35,36] As networks to promote public health develop, it will be important to engage new disciplines and organizations. It is particularly important to engage "nontraditional" partners (i.e., those whose mission is not directly focused on health) such as business and industry, local and state departments of transportation, city planners, and local/state media.

CAPACITY AND LEADERSHIP

Engage Leadership

As noted elsewhere in this book, leadership is essential to promote adoption of evidence-based decision making as a core part of public health practice.[37] This includes an expectation that decisions will be made on the basis of the best science, needs of the target population, and what will work locally. In some cases, additional funding may be required, but in many circumstances, not having the will to change (rather than dollars) is the major impediment. Use of evidence-based decision making can be incorporated as part of performance reviews for key public health personnel and as part of explicit goals and objectives for all program directors.

Expand Training Opportunities

More practitioner-focused training is needed on the rationale for EBPH, how to select interventions, how to adapt them to particular circumstances, and how to monitor their implementation. The CDC Taskforce on Public Health Workforce Development has recommended that the essential public health services[38] be used as a framework to build the basic, cross-cutting and technical competencies required to address public health problems. As outlined in Chapter 1, we would supplement this recommendation by inclusion of EBPH-related competencies.[18,39] Some training programs show evidence of effectiveness.[40,41] The most common format uses didactic sessions, computer labs, and scenario-based exercises, taught by a faculty team with expertise in EBPH. The reach of these training programs can be increased by emphasizing a train-the-trainer approach.[42] Other formats have been used, including Internet-based self-study,[43,44] CD-ROMs,[45] distance and distributed learning networks, and targeted technical assistance. Training programs may have greater impact when delivered by "change agents" who are perceived as experts yet share common characteristics and goals with trainees.[46] A commitment from leadership and staff to lifelong learning is also an essential ingredient for success.[47] Because many of the health issues that require urgent attention in local communities will require the involvement of other organizations (e.g., nonprofit groups, hospitals, employers), their participation in training efforts is essential.

Enhance Accountability for Public Expenditures

Public health agencies should be good stewards of society's resources. Thus, economic evaluation must play a larger role in public health. Although there are challenges in using economic evaluation in public health, there is growing consensus on the appropriate methods and a growing evidence base.[48,49] Public health agencies should use the economic evaluation evidence base, in combination with evidence of effectiveness, to guide their allocation of resources. Grants made by public health agencies to outside organizations should contain language explicitly requiring use of such evidence, when it exists, to justify expenditure of funds. While the science base for many topics is still evolving, it is irresponsible not to use existing evidence in the design and implementation of proven public health interventions. Evaluations of such efforts can thus contribute to a better understanding of what works in different settings. Simultaneously, the adoption of EBPH by the public health system as a whole and its impact on the community's health should be tracked. A central criterion in the accreditation of public health departments, soon to be implemented,[50] must be the use of best evidence in every effort to improve health and health equity.

SPECIAL POPULATIONS AND SECTORS

Understand How to Better Use Evidence-Based Approaches to Address Disparities

To what degree do specific evidence-based approaches reduce disparities while improving overall current and/or future health? For many interventions, there is no clear answer to this question. Despite the national goals aimed at eliminating health disparities, recent data show large and growing differences in disease burden and health outcomes between high- and low-income groups.[51] Most of the existing intervention research has been conducted among higher-income populations. and programs focusing on elimination of health disparities have often been short-lived.[52] Yet, in both developed and developing countries, poverty is strongly correlated with poor health outcomes.[53] When sufficient evidence exists, systematic reviews should focus specifically on interventions that show promise in eliminating health disparities.[54–56] Policy interventions hold the potential to influence health determinants more broadly and could significantly reduce the growing disparities across a wide range of health problems.[57]

Make Evidence More Accessible for Policy Audiences

Evidence becomes more relevant to policy makers when it involves a local example and when the effects are framed in terms of its direct impact on one's local community, family, or constituents.[58] In the policy arena, decision makers indicate that relevance to current debates is a critical factor in determining which research will be used and which proposals will be considered. Research on contextual issues and the importance of narrative communication that presents data in the form of story and helps to personalize issues is beginning to emerge.[59]

Learn from Global Efforts

Nearly every public health issue has a global footprint, because diseases do not know borders and shared solutions are needed. This can readily be seen if one lines up the goals of the World Health Organization with national health plans. There are many areas that are likely to lead to advances in EBPH. These could include (1) adapting methods of public health surveillance from one country to another,[60] (2) understanding how to adapt an effective intervention in one geographic region to the context of another geographic region,[61] (3) implementing innovative methods of training practitioners in EBPH,[42] and (4) identifying effective methods for delivery of health care services in one country that could be applied to another.[62] Importantly, public challenges in less developed countries are compounded by poverty and hunger, diminished public infrastructure, and the epidemiologic transition to behaviors that pose risks more typically found in higher income countries.[63]

SUMMARY

Public health history teaches us that a long "latency period" often exists between the scientific understanding of a viable disease control method and its widespread application on a population basis.[64] For example, the Papanicolaou (Pap) test was perfected in 1943 but was not widely used until the early 1970s. Not until 1993 were programs available in all states to provide Pap testing to low-income women. Prevention was the major contributor to the health gains of the past century, yet it is vastly underfunded.[65] The power of scientific evidence combined with community action is illustrated when examining the public health achievements over the past century.[66] This offers hope for the future. By expanding the evidence base for public health, and applying the evidence already in hand, we can shorten the latency period and will then begin to fully achieve the promise of prevention.

SUGGESTED READINGS AND SELECTED WEBSITES

Suggested Readings

Cuijpers P, de Graaf I, Bohlmeijer E. Adapting and disseminating effective public health interventions in another country: towards a systematic approach. *Eur J Public Health.* 2005;15(2):166–169.

Fielding J, Kumanyika S. Recommendations for the concepts and form of Healthy People 2020. *Am J Prev Med.* 2009;37(3):255–257.

Green LW. From research to "best practices" in other settings and populations. *Am J Health Behav.* 2001;25(3):165–178.

McGinnis JM. Does proof matter? Why strong evidence sometimes yields weak action. *Am J Health Promot.* 2001;15(5):391–396.

Nutbeam D. How does evidence influence public health policy? Tackling health inequalities in England. *Health Promot J Aust.* 2003;14:154–158.

Petticrew M, Roberts H. Systematic reviews—do they "work" in informing decision-making around health inequalities? *Health Econ Policy Law.* 2008;3(Pt 2):197–211.

Selected Websites

The Global Health Council <https://www.globalhealth.org/>. The Global Health Council is the world's largest membership alliance dedicated to saving lives by improving health throughout the world. Its diverse membership is comprised of health care professionals and organizations that include nongovernment organizations, foundations, corporations, government agencies, and academic institutions. This web site provides policy briefs, research briefs, fact sheets, and roundtable discussions on many topics.

Kaiser Family Foundation <http://www.kff.org/>. The Kaiser Family Foundation (not associated with Kaiser Permanente or Kaiser Industries) is a nonprofit, private operating foundation that focuses on the major health care issues facing the United States, as well as the U.S. role in global health policy. It compiles and presents public data and also develops its own research. Intended audiences are policymakers, the media, and the general public, and data are easily accessible.

Links provide comparable data for U.S. states (www.statehealthfacts.org) and for countries (www.globalhealthfacts.org).

National Conference of State Legislators <http://www.ncsl.org/>. The National Conference of State Legislatures (NCSL) is a bipartisan organization that serves the legislators and staffs of the nation's 50 states and its commonwealths and territories. NCSL provides research, technical assistance, and opportunities for policymakers to exchange ideas on the most pressing state issues. The NCSL site provides information about each state's governing bodies as well as bill summaries, reports, and databases on numerous public health policy topics.

RE-AIM.org <http://www.re-aim.org/>. With an overall goal of enhancing the quality, speed, and public health impact of efforts to translate research into practice, this site provides an explanation of and resources (e.g., planning tools, measures, self-assessment quizzes, FAQs, comprehensive bibliography) for those wanting to apply the RE-AIM framework.

Research-Tested Intervention Programs (RTIPS) <http://rtips.cancer.gov/rtips/index.do>. At this site, the National Cancer Institute translates research-tested intervention programs. Program materials are available to order or download, and the site provides details of an intervention such as the time required, suitable settings, and the required resources.

Using What Works: Adapting Evidence-Based Programs to Fit Your Needs <http://cancercontrol.cancer.gov/use_what_works/start.htm>. The National Cancer Institute provides a train-the-trainer course designed to teach health promoters how to adapt evidence-based programs to their local communities. Materials describe how to conduct a needs assessment and how to find, adapt, and evaluate evidence-based programs.

World Health Organization <http://www.who.int/en/>. The World Health Organization (WHO) is the directing and coordinating authority for health within the United Nations system. It is responsible for providing leadership on global health matters, shaping the health research agenda, setting norms and standards, articulating evidence-based policy options, providing technical support to countries, and monitoring and assessing health trends. From this site, one can access *The World Health Report*, WHO's leading publication that provides an expert assessment on global health with a focus on a specific subject each year.

REFERENCES

1. Zaza S, Briss PA, Harris KW, eds. *The Guide to Community Preventive Services: What Works to Promote Health?* New York, NY: Oxford University Press; 2005.
2. Kerner J, Rimer B, Emmons K. Introduction to the special section on dissemination: dissemination research and research dissemination: how can we close the gap? *Health Psychol.* 2005;24(5):443–446.

3. Rabin BA, Brownson RC, Haire-Joshu D, et al. A glossary for dissemination and implementation research in health. *J Public Health Manag Pract.* 2008;14(2):117–123.

4. Brownson RC, Ballew P, Dieffenderfer B, et al. Evidence-based interventions to promote physical activity: what contributes to dissemination by state health departments. *Am J Prev Med.* 2007;33(1 Suppl):S66–73; quiz S74–68.

5. Brownson RC, Chriqui JF, Stamatakis KA. Understanding evidence-based public health policy. *Am J Public Health.* 2009;99(9):1576–1583.

6. Brownson RC, Royer C, Ewing R, McBride TD. Researchers and policymakers: travelers in parallel universes. *Am J Prev Med.* 2006;30(2):164–172.

7. Innvaer S, Vist G, Trommald M, Oxman A. Health policy-makers' perceptions of their use of evidence: a systematic review. *J Health Serv Res Policy.* 2002;7(4):239–244.

8. Kerner JF. Integrating research, practice, and policy: what we see depends on where we stand. *J Public Health Manag Pract.* 2008;14(2):193–198.

9. Rabin BA, Brownson RC, Kerner JF, Glasgow RE. Methodologic challenges in disseminating evidence-based interventions to promote physical activity. *Am J Prev Med.* 2006;31(4 Suppl):S24–34.

10. Rutten A, Luschen G, von Lengerke T, et al. Determinants of health policy impact: comparative results of a European policymaker study. *Soz Praventivmed.* 2003;48(6):379–391.

11. Weiss CH. Research for policy's sake: the enlightenment function of social research. *Policy Analysis.* 1977;3:531–547.

12. Weissert CS, Weissert WG. State legislative staff influence in health policy making. *J Health Polit Policy Law.* 2000;25(6):1121–1148.

13. White M, McDonnell S. Public health surveillance in low-and middle-income countries. In: Teutsch S, Churchill R, eds. *Principles and Practice of Public Health Surveillance.* 2nd ed. New York: Oxford University Press; 2000:287–315.

14. Agency for Healthcare Research and Quality. Guide to Clinical Preventive Services, 3rd ed, Periodic Updates. Accessed October 11, 2005. http://www.ahrq.gov/clinic/gcpspu.htm

15. Glasgow RE, Vogt TM, Boles SM. Evaluating the public health impact of health promotion interventions: the RE-AIM framework. *Am J Public Health.* 1999;89(9):1322–1327.

16. Jilcott S, Ammerman A, Sommers J, et al. Applying the RE-AIM framework to assess the public health impact of policy change. *Ann Behav Med.* 2007;34(2):105–114.

17. Petticrew M, Cummins S, Ferrell C, et al. Natural experiments: an underused tool for public health? *Public Health.* 2005;119(9):751–757.

18. Brownson RC, Baker EA, Leet TL, Gillespie KN. *Evidence-Based Public Health.* New York, NY: Oxford University Press; 2003.

19. Green LW. From research to "best practices" in other settings and populations. *Am J Health Behav.* 2001;25(3):165–178.

20. Nutbeam D. How does evidence influence public health policy? tackling health inequalities in England. *Health Promot J Aust.* 2003;14:154–158.

21. Ogilvie D, Egan M, Hamilton V, et al. Systematic reviews of health effects of social interventions: 2. Best available evidence: how low should you go? *J Epidemiol Commun Health.* 2005;59(10):886–892.

22. World Health Organization. *Health in the Millennium Development Goals.* Geneva, Switzerland: World Health Organization; 2004.

23. Fielding J, Kumanyika S. Recommendations for the concepts and form of Healthy People 2020. *Am J Prev Med.* 2009;37(3):255–257.

24. Sondik EJ, Huang DT, Klein RJ, et al. Progress toward the Healthy People 2010 goals and objectives. *Annu Rev Public Health.* 2010;31:271–281.
25. Thacker SB, Berkelman RL. Public health surveillance in the United States. *Epidemiol Rev.* 1988;10:164–190.
26. Boehmer TK, Brownson RC, Haire-Joshu D, et al. Patterns of childhood obesity prevention legislation in the United States. *Prev Chronic Dis.* 2007;4(3):A56.
27. Green LW, George MA, Daniel M, et al. *Review and Recommendations for the Development of Participatory Research in Health Promotion in Canada.* Vancouver, British Columbia: The Royal Society of Canada; 1995.
28. Israel BA, Schulz AJ, Parker EA, et al. Review of community-based research: assessing partnership approaches to improve public health. *Annu Rev Public Health.* 1998;19:173–202.
29. Cargo M, Mercer SL. The value and challenges of participatory research: Strengthening its practice. *Annu Rev Public Health.* 2008;29:325–350.
30. Harper GW, Neubauer LC, Bangi AK, et al. Transdisciplinary research and evaluation for community health initiatives. *Health Promot Pract.* 2008;9(4): 328–337.
31. Stokols D. Toward a science of transdisciplinary action research. *Am J Commun Psychol.* 2006;38(1–2):63–77.
32. Kobus K, Mermelstein R. Bridging basic and clinical science with policy studies: the Partners with Transdisciplinary Tobacco Use Research Centers experience. *Nicotine Tob Res.* 2009;11(5):467–474.
33. Kobus K, Mermelstein R, Ponkshe P. Communications strategies to broaden the reach of tobacco use research: examples from the Transdisciplinary Tobacco Use Research Centers. *Nicotine Tob Res.* 2007;9(Suppl 4):S571–582.
34. Morgan GD, Kobus K, Gerlach KK, et al. Facilitating transdisciplinary research: the experience of the transdisciplinary tobacco use research centers. *Nicotine Tob Res.* 2003;5(Suppl 1):S11–19.
35. Byrne S, Wake M, Blumberg D, et al. Identifying priority areas for longitudinal research in childhood obesity: Delphi technique survey. *Int J Pediatr Obes.* 2008;3(2):120–122.
36. Russell-Mayhew S, Scott C, Stewart M. The Canadian Obesity Network and interprofessional practice: members' views. *J Interprof Care.* 2008;22(2):149–165.
37. Scutchfield FD, Knight EA, Kelly AV, et al. Local public health agency capacity and its relationship to public health system performance. *J Public Health Manag Pract.* 2004;10(3):204–215.
38. Centers for Disease Control and Prevention. *CDC Taskforce on Public Health Workforce Development.* Atlanta, GA: CDC; 1999.
39. Brownson R, Ballew P, Kittur N, et al. Developing competencies for training practitioners in evidence-based cancer control. *J Cancer Educ.* 2009;24(3):186–93.
40. Dreisinger M, Leet TL, Baker EA, et al. Improving the public health workforce: evaluation of a training course to enhance evidence-based decision making. *J Public Health Manag Pract.* 2008;14(2):138–143.
41. Maylahn C, Bohn C, Hammer M, et al. Strengthening epidemiologic competencies among local health professionals in New York: teaching evidence-based public health. *Public Health Rep.* 2008;123(Suppl 1):35–43.
42. Brownson RC, Diem G, Grabauskas V, et al. Training practitioners in evidence-based chronic disease prevention for global health. *Promot Educ.* 2007;14(3):159–163.

43. Linkov F, LaPorte R, Lovalekar M, et al. Web quality control for lectures: Supercourse and Amazon.com. *Croat Med J.* 2005;46(6):875–878.
44. Maxwell ML, Adily A, Ward JE. Promoting evidence-based practice in population health at the local level: a case study in workforce capacity development. *Aust Health Rev.* 2007;31(3):422–429.
45. Brownson RC, Ballew P, Brown KL, et al. The effect of disseminating evidence-based interventions that promote physical activity to health departments. *Am J Public Health.* 2007;97(10):1900–1907.
46. Proctor EK. Leverage points for the implementation of evidence-based practice. *Brief Treat Crisis Interv.* 2004;4(3):227–242.
47. Chambers LW. The new public health: do local public health agencies need a booster (or organizational "fix") to combat the diseases of disarray? *Can J Public Health.* 1992;83(5):326–328.
48. Neumann P. *Using Cost-Effectiveness Analysis to Improve Health Care.* New York, NY: Oxford University Press; 2005.
49. Weatherly H, Drummond M, Claxton K, et al. Methods for assessing the cost-effectiveness of public health interventions: key challenges and recommendations. *Health Policy.* 2009;93(2–3):85–92.
50. Tilson HH. Public health accreditation: progress on national accountability. *Annu Rev Public Health.* 2008;29:xv–xxii.
51. Ezzati M, Friedman AB, Kulkarni SC, et al. The reversal of fortunes: trends in county mortality and cross-county mortality disparities in the United States. *PLoS Med.* 2008;5(4):e66.
52. Shaya FT, Gu A, Saunders E. Addressing cardiovascular disparities through community interventions. *Ethn Dis.* 2006;16(1):138–144.
53. Subramanian SV, Belli P, Kawachi I. The macroeconomic determinants of health. *Annu Rev Public Health.* 2002;23:287–302.
54. Masi CM, Blackman DJ, Peek ME. Interventions to enhance breast cancer screening, diagnosis, and treatment among racial and ethnic minority women. *Med Care Res Rev.* 2007;64(5 Suppl):195S–242S.
55. Peek ME, Cargill A, Huang ES. Diabetes health disparities: a systematic review of health care interventions. *Med Care Res Rev.* 2007;64(5 Suppl):101S–156S.
56. Petticrew M, Roberts H. Systematic reviews—do they "work" in informing decision-making around health inequalities? *Health Econ Policy Law.* 2008;3(Pt 2):197–211.
57. Brownson RC, Haire-Joshu D, Luke DA. Shaping the context of health: a review of environmental and policy approaches in the prevention of chronic diseases. *Annu Rev Public Health.* 2006;27:341–370.
58. Jones E, Kreuter M, Pritchett S, et al. State health policy makers: what's the message and who's listening? *Health Promot Pract.* 2006;7(3):280–286.
59. Stamatakis K, McBride T, Brownson R. Communicating prevention messages to policy makers: The role of stories in promoting physical activity. *J Phys Act Health.* 2010;7 Suppl 1:S99–107.
60. Schmid T, Zabina H, McQueen D, et al. The first telephone-based health survey in Moscow: building a model for behavioral risk factor surveillance in Russia. *Soz Praventivmed.* 2005;50(1):60–62.
61. Cuijpers P, de Graaf I, Bohlmeijer E. Adapting and disseminating effective public health interventions in another country: towards a systematic approach. *Eur J Public Health.* 2005;15(2):166–169.

62. Clancy CM, Cronin K. Evidence-based decision making: global evidence, local decisions. *Health Aff (Millwood).* 2005;24(1):151–162.
63. Institute for Alternative Futures. *Survey on Key Levers of Change to Prevent and Control Chronic Disease: Preliminary Summary.* Copenhagen, Denmark: WHO NCD Strategy Development and Oxford Vision 2020; November 28, 2003.
64. Brownson RC, Bright FS. Chronic disease control in public health practice: looking back and moving forward. *Public Health Rep.* 2004;119(3):230–238.
65. McGinnis JM. Does proof matter? why strong evidence sometimes yields weak action. *Am J Health Promot.* 2001;15(5):391–396.
66. Centers for Disease Control and Prevention. Ten great public health achievements—United States, 1900–1999. *MMWR Morb Mortal Wkly Rep.* 1999;48(12):241–243.

Glossary

Action planning: Planning for a specific program or policy with specific, time-dependent outcomes.

Adjusted rates: Rate in which the crude (unadjusted) rate has been standardized to some external reference population (e.g., an age-adjusted rate of lung cancer). An adjusted rate is often useful when comparing rates over time or for populations (e.g., by age, gender, race) in different geographic areas.

Advocacy: Set of skills that can be used to create a shift in public opinion and mobilize the necessary resources and forces to support an issue. Advocacy blends science and politics in a social-justice value orientation with the goal of making the system work better, particularly for individuals and populations with the least resources.

Analytic epidemiology: Study designed to examine associations, commonly putative or hypothesized causal relationships. An analytic study is usually concerned with identifying or measuring the effects of risk factors or is concerned with the health effects of specific exposures.

Analytic framework: (causal framework, logic model) Diagram that depicts the inter relationships among population characteristics, intervention components, shorter-term intervention outcomes, and longer-term public health outcomes. Its purpose is to map out the linkages on which to base conclusions about intervention effectiveness. Similar frameworks are also used in program planning to assist in designing, implementing, and evaluating effective interventions.

Basic priority rating (BPR): A method of prioritizing health issues based on the size of the problem, the seriousness of the problem, the effectiveness of intervention, and its propriety, economics, acceptability, resources, and legality (known as PEARL).

Case-control study: Method of study in which persons with the disease (or other condition) of interest are compared with a suitable control group of persons without the disease.

273

The relationship of an attribute to the disease is examined by comparing the diseased and nondiseased with regard to how frequently the attribute is present. Risk is estimated by the odds ratio.

Category-specific rates: Rates that characterize patterns of disease by person, place, or time for a defined population.

Causality: Relationship of causes to the effects they produce. A cause is termed "necessary" when it must always precede an effect. This effect need not be the sole result of the one cause. A cause is termed "sufficient" when it inevitably initiates or produces an effect. Any given causal factor may be necessary, sufficient, neither, or both.

Causal framework: See Analytic framework, logic model.

Changeability: Likelihood that a risk factor or behavior can be altered by a public health program or policy.

Coalition: Group of individuals and/or organizations that join together for a common purpose.

Cohort study: Method of study in which subsets of a defined population can be identified by those who are, have been, or in the future may be exposed or not exposed, or exposed in different degrees, to a factor or factors hypothesized to influence the probability of occurrence of a given disease or other outcome. The main feature of a cohort study is observation of large numbers over a long period (commonly years) with comparison of incidence rates in groups that differ in exposure levels. Risk is estimated by the relative risk.

Community: Group of people with diverse characteristics who are linked by social ties, share common perspectives, and engage in joint action in geographical locations or settings.

Confounding bias: An error that distorts the estimated effect of an exposure on an outcome, caused by the presence of an extraneous factor associated with both the exposure and the outcome.

Consensus conference: Mechanism commonly used to review epidemiologic evidence in which expert panels convene to develop recommendations, usually within a period of a few days.

Context or setting: Surroundings within which a health issue occurs, including assessment of the social, cultural, economic, political, and physical environment.

Cost-benefit analysis: Economic analysis that converts effects into the same monetary terms as the costs and compares them, yielding a measure of net benefits or a cost-benefit ratio. Lower cost-benefit ratios and higher net benefits are desirable.

Cost-effectiveness analysis: An economic analysis in which the total costs of an intervention are measured in monetary terms and then compared with the health outcomes (such as lives saved or cases detected) achieved by the intervention to yield a cost-effectiveness ratio. Lower ratios are preferred.

Cost-minimization analysis: Economic analysis in which the costs of different programs with equivalent benefits are compared, to determine the least costly alternative. The requirement of equal benefits among the programs compared severely limits its usefulness.

Cost-utility analysis: Economic analysis that converts benefits into a preference-based measure of health-related quality of life and compares this to the costs of the program to determine a cost-utility ratio, such as cost per additional quality-adjusted life-year. Lower ratios are preferred. Cost-utility analysis is sometimes considered a subset of cost-effectiveness analysis.

Cross-sectional studies: Method of study in which the presence or absence of a disease and the presence or absence of other variables are determined in each member of the study population or in a representative sample at one particular time.

Crude (unadjusted) rate: Rate that represents the actual frequency of disease in a defined population for a specified period.

Decision analysis: Technique used under conditions of uncertainty for systematically representing and examining all the relevant information for a decision and the uncertainty around that information. The available choices are plotted on a decision tree. At each branch, or decision node, each outcome and its probability of occurrence are listed.

Delphi method: Iterative circulation to a panel of experts of questions and responses that are progressively refined in light of responses to each round of questions; preferably, participants' identities should not be revealed to each other. The aim is to reduce the number of viable options or solutions, perhaps to arrive at a consensus judgment on an issue or problem, or a set of issues or problems, without allowing anyone to dominate the process. The method was originally developed at the RAND Corporation.

Descriptive epidemiology: Study of the occurrence of disease or other health-related characteristics in human populations. General observations are often made concerning the relationship of disease to basic characteristics such as age, sex, race, social class, geographic location, or time. The major characteristics in descriptive epidemiology can be classified under the headings of person, place, and time.

Determinant of health: Factor associated with or which influences a health outcome. Determinants include social, cultural, environmental, economic, behavioral, biological, and other factors.

Direct costs: All costs necessary to directly conduct an intervention or program. Include supplies, overhead, and labor costs, often measured by the number of full-time equivalent employees (FTEs) and their wages and fringe benefits.

Discounting: Conversion of amounts (usually currency) received over different periods to a common value in the current period, with the goal of determining the current payments that would be equal in value to distant payments.

Dissemination: Process of communicating either the procedures or the lessons learned from a study or program evaluation to relevant audiences in a timely, unbiased, and consistent fashion.

Distal outcomes: Long-term changes in morbidity and mortality.

Ecological framework: Model relating individual, interpersonal, organizational, community (including social and economic factors), and health policy factors to individual behavior change and their direct effect on health.

Economic evaluation: Analysis of the costs and benefits of a program or intervention, using existing or prospective data to determine the additional cost per additional unit of benefit.

Environmental assessment: Analysis of the political, economic, social, and technological contexts as part of the strategic planning process.

Epidemiology: Study of the health and illness of populations and the application of findings to improve community health.

Evaluation: Process that attempts to systematically and objectively determine the relevance, effectiveness, and impact of activities in the light of their objectives.

Evaluation designs: The qualitative and quantitative methods used to evaluate a program that may include both experimental and quasi-experimental studies.

Evidence-based medicine: Conscientious, explicit, and judicious use of current best evidence in making decisions about the care of individual patients. The practice of evidence-based medicine means integrating individual clinical expertise with the best available external clinical evidence from systematic research.

Evidence-based public health: Process of integrating science-based interventions with community preferences to improve the health of populations.

Experimental study design: Study in which the investigator has full control over the allocations and/or timing of the interventions. The ability to allocate individuals or groups randomly is a common requirement of an experimental study.

Expert panel: Group of individuals who provide scientific peer review of the quality of the science and scientific interpretations that underlie public health recommendations, regulations, and policy decisions.

External validity: Study is externally valid, or generalizable, if it can produce unbiased inferences regarding a target population (beyond the subjects in the study). This aspect of validity is only meaningful with regard to a specified external target population.

Formative evaluation: Type of evaluation conducted in the early stages of an intervention to determine whether an element of a program or policy (e.g., materials, messages) is feasible, appropriate, and meaningful for the target population.

"Fugitive" literature ("grey" literature): Government reports, book chapters, the proceedings of conferences, and published dissertations that are therefore difficult to retrieve.

Guide to Clinical Preventive Services: Set of guidelines, published by the U.S. Preventive Services Task Force, that document the effectiveness of a variety of clinic-based interventions in public health through systematic review and evaluation of scientific evidence.

Guide to Community Preventive Services: Systematic Reviews and Evidence-Based Recommendations (the Community Guide): Set of guidelines, published by the Task Force on Community Preventive Services and supported by the Centers for Disease Control and Prevention (CDC), that summarize what is known about the effectiveness and cost-effectiveness of population-based interventions designed to promote health and prevent disease, injury, disability, and premature death, as well as to reduce exposure to environmental hazards.

Guidelines: Standardized set of information based on scientific evidence of the effectiveness and efficiency of the best practices for addressing health problems commonly encountered in public health or clinical practice. Where such evidence is lacking, guidelines are sometimes based on the consensus opinions of experts.

Health Belief Model: Value expectancy theory stating that individuals will take action to ward off, screen for, or control an ill-health condition if they regard themselves as susceptible to the condition, believe it to have potentially serious consequences, believe that a course of action available to them would be beneficial in reducing either their susceptibility to or the severity of the condition, and believe that the anticipated barriers to (or costs of) taking the action are outweighed by its benefits.

Health disparities: Inequalities in health indicators (such as infant mortality rates and life expectancy) that are observed among subpopulations. Health disparities often correlate with socioeconomic status.

Health impact assessment: Type of analysis requiring screening, scoping, appraisal, reporting, and monitoring to measure the effect of a nonhealth intervention on the health of a community.

Health indicator: Variable, susceptible to direct measurement, that reflects the state of health of persons in a community. Examples include infant mortality rates, incidence rates based on notifiable cases of disease, and disability days.

Impact evaluation: Assessment of whether intermediate objectives of an intervention have been achieved. Indicators may include changes in knowledge, attitudes, behavior, or risk-factor prevalence.

Incidence: Number of new cases of a disease.

Incidence rate: Occurrence of new cases of disease in a specific time period over the person-time for the population; reflects the true rate of disease occurrence.

Indirect costs: Expenses that are not directly linked to an intervention but are incurred by providers, participants, or other parties. In cost-utility analysis, these include time and travel costs to participants, averted treatment costs (future treatment costs that will be saved as a result of the intervention), and costs of treating side effects.

Information bias: Systematic error in measuring exposures or outcomes that affects the accuracy of information between study groups.

Intermediate measure ("upstream" measure): Short-term outcome most directly associated with an intervention, often measured in terms of knowledge, attitudes, or behavior change.

Internal validity: Degree to which the inference drawn from a study is warranted when account is taken of the study methods, the representativeness of the study sample, and the nature of the population from which it is drawn. Index and comparison groups are selected and compared in such a manner that the observed differences between them on the dependent variables under study may, apart from sampling error, be attributed only to the hypothesized effect under investigation.

Logic model: See Analytic framework, causal model.

Management: Process of constructing, implementing, and monitoring organized responses to a health problem or a series of interrelated health problems.

MATCH (the Multilevel Approach to Community Health): Conceptual and practical intervention planning model. MATCH consists of five phases: health goals selection, intervention planning, development, implementation, and evaluation.

Media advocacy: Advocacy that involves strategic use of the mass media in reaching policy, program, or educational goals.

Member validation: Process by which the preliminary results and interpretations are presented back to those who provided the evaluation data.

Meta-analysis: Systematic, quantitative method for combining information from multiple studies in order to derive a meaningful answer to a specific question.

Multiple linear regression: Mathematical modeling technique that finds the best linear model that relates given data on a dependent variable y to one or several independent variables x_1, x_2, etc. Other common regression models in epidemiology are the logistic and proportional hazards models.

Natural experiment: Study or evaluation design that generally takes the form of an observational study in which the researcher cannot control or withhold the allocation of an intervention to particular areas or communities but where natural or predetermined variation in allocation occurs. A common natural experiment would study the effects of the enactment of a policy on health status.

Needs assessment: Systematic procedure that makes use of epidemiologic, sociodemographic, and qualitative methods to determine the nature and extent of health problems, experienced by a specified population, and their environmental, social, economic, and behavioral determinants. The aim is to identify unmet health care needs and preventive opportunities.

Nominal group technique: Structured, small-group process designed to achieve consensus. Individuals respond to questions and then are asked to prioritize ideas as they are presented.

Objectivity: Ability to be unaffected by personal biases, politics, history, or other external factors.

Observational study design: Study that does not involve any intervention, experimental or otherwise. Such a study may be one in which nature is allowed to take its course, with changes in one characteristic being studied in relation to development of disease or other health condition. Examples of observational studies include the cohort study or the case-control study.

Odds ratio: Ratio of the odds of an event in the exposed group to the odds of an event in the control (unexposed) group. Commonly used in the case-control method to estimate the relative risk. The prevalence odds ratio is often calculated for cross-sectional data.

Original research article: Paper written by the author(s) who conducted the research.

Outcome evaluation: Long-term measure of effects such as changes in morbidity, mortality, and/or quality of life.

Paradigm: Pattern of thought or conceptualization; an overall way of regarding phenomena within which scientists normally work.

Participatory approaches: Collaborative, community-based research method, designed to actively involve community members in research and intervention projects

PATCH (the Planned Approach to Community Health): Community health planning model that relies heavily on local data to set priorities, design interventions, and evaluate progress. The goal of PATCH is to increase the capacity of communities to plan, implement, and evaluate comprehensive, community-based interventions.

Peer review: Process of reviewing research proposals, manuscripts submitted for publication, and abstracts submitted for presentation at scientific meetings, whereby they are judged for scientific and technical merit by other scientists in the same field.

Person-time: Sum of the amount of time that each at-risk person in a given population is free from disease (often measured in person-years)

PERT: The Program Evaluation and Review Technique involves a graphically displayed timeline for the tasks necessary in the development and implementation of public health programs.

Policy: Laws, regulations, and formal and informal rules and understandings that are adopted on a collective basis to guide individual and collective behavior.

Pooled analysis: Use of data from multiple studies where the data are analyzed at the level of the individual participant with the goal of obtaining a quantitative estimate of effect.

Population attributable risk (PAR): Incidence of a disease in a population that is associated with or attributable to exposure to the risk factor.

Population-based process: Administrative strategy that seeks to maximize expected health and well-being across an entire community or population, rather than maximizing outputs and outcomes within specific programs and organizations.

PRECEDE-PROCEED: Systematic planning framework developed to enhance the quality of health education interventions. The acronym PRECEDE stands for Predisposing, Reinforcing, and Enabling Constructs in Educational Diagnosis and Evaluation. The model is based on the premise that, just as medical diagnosis precedes a treatment plan, so should educational diagnosis precede an intervention plan. The acronym PROCEED stands for Policy, Regulatory, and Organizational Constructs in Educational and Environmental Development. This part of the model is based on recognition of the need for health promotion interventions that go beyond traditional educational approaches to changing unhealthy behaviors.

Precision: Quality of being sharply defined or stated. In statistics, precision is defined as the inverse of the variance of a measurement or an estimate.

Prevalence rate: Number of existing cases of disease among surviving members of the population.

Preventable burden (preventability; prevented fraction): Proportion of an adverse health outcome that potentially can be eliminated as a result of a prevention strategy.

Primary data: New evidence collected for a particular study or program through methods such as community surveys, interviews, and focus groups. The process of primary data collection usually occurs over a relatively long period of time.

Process evaluation: Analysis of inputs and implementation experiences to track changes as a result of a program or policy. This occurs at the earliest stages of public health intervention and often is helpful in determining midcourse corrections.

Program: Organized public health action, such as direct service interventions, community mobilization efforts, policy development and implementation, outbreak investigations, health communication campaigns, health promotion programs, and applied research initiatives.

Program objectives: Statements of short-term, measurable, specific activities having a specific time limit or timeline for completion. Program objectives must be measurable and are designed to reach goals.

Public health surveillance: The ongoing systematic collection and timely analysis, interpretation, and communication of health information for the purpose of disease prevention and control.

Publication bias: Bias in the published literature where the publication of research depends on the nature and direction of the study results. Studies in which an intervention is not found to be effective are sometimes not published or submitted for publication. Therefore, systematic reviews that fail to include unpublished studies may overestimate the true effect of an intervention or a risk factor.

Quality-adjusted life-years (QALYs): Frequently used outcome measure in cost-utility analysis that incorporates the quality or desirability of a health state with the duration of survival.

Each year of life is weighted on a scale from 0 (death) to 1 (perfect health), with weights derived from patient or population surveys.

Quality of the evidence: Quality refers to the appropriateness and integrity of the information obtained. High-quality data are reliable, valid, and informative for their intended use.

Qualitative data: Nonnumerical observations, using approved methods such as participant observation, group interviews, or focus groups. Qualitative data can enrich understanding of complex problems and help to explain why things happen.

Quantitative data: Data that are expressed in numerical quantities, such as continuous measurements or counts.

Quasi-experimental designs: Study in which the investigator lacks full control over the allocation and/or timing of intervention but nonetheless conducts the study as if it were an experiment, allocating subjects to groups. Inability to allocate subjects randomly is a common situation that may be best studied as a quasi-experiment.

Randomized controlled trials: Experiment in which subjects in a population are randomly allocated to two groups, usually called study and control groups, to receive or not receive an experimental preventive or therapeutic procedure, maneuver, or intervention. The scientifically rigorous nature of RCTs increases the internal validity while limiting the external validity, and the use of RCTs is often determined by the availability of resources as well as the research question at hand.

Rate: Rate is a measure of the frequency of occurrence of a phenomenon (e.g., a disease or risk factor) for a defined population during a specified period.

RE-AIM: Framework for consistent reporting of research results that takes account of Reach to the target population; Effectiveness or Efficacy; Adoption by target settings or institutions; Implementation of consistency of delivery of intervention; and Maintenance of intervention effects in individuals and settings over time.

Registries: Regularly updated listings of information containing all identified disease or health problem cases. Active registries seek data and use follow-up to obtain more reliable and complete information. Passive registries accept and merge reports but do not update or confirm information.

Relative risk (rate ratio, risk ratio): Ratio of the rate of disease or death among the exposed to the rate among the unexposed; synonymous with rate ratio or risk ratio.

Relative standard error: Standard error (i.e., the standard deviation of an estimate) as a percentage of the measure itself. A relative standard error of 50% means the standard error is half the size of the rate.

Reliability: Degree of stability exhibited when a measurement is repeated under identical conditions. Reliability refers to the degree to which the results obtained by a measurement procedure can be replicated. Lack of reliability may arise from divergences between observers or instruments or instability of the attribute being measured.

Reportable diseases: Selected diseases for which data are collected, as mandated by law and/or regulation at national, state, and local levels.

Resource-based decision making: In the resource-based planning cycle, the spiral of increased resources and increased demand for resources helps to drive the cost of health care services continually higher, even as the health status for some populations decline. This is one among several theories of why health care costs increase.

Review articles: Summary of what is known on a particular topic through review of original research articles.

Risk assessment: Qualitative and quantitative estimation of the likelihood of adverse effects that may result from exposure to specified health hazards or from the absence of beneficial influences. Includes four steps: hazard identification, risk characterization, exposure assessment, and risk estimation.

Scenario planning: In this small-group method, future-oriented scenarios are developed, based on how an event or a system will look at some target time horizon. In some cases, scenario planning has been used when other, more quantitative, forecasting methods fail to anticipate a changing environment.

Scientific literature: Theoretical and research publications in scientific journals, reference books, textbooks, government reports, policy statements, and other materials about the theory, practice, and results of scientific inquiry.

Secondary data: Evidence routinely collected by others, usually at a local, state, or national level. The availability of secondary data from government, university, and nonprofit agencies saves time and money.

Selection bias: Bias (error) due to systematic differences in characteristics between those who take part in the study and those who do not.

Sensitivity· Ability of a screening test to correctly identify presence of a disease.

Sensitivity analysis: Evaluation to assess how robust the results of a study or systematic review are to changes in how it was done. Assumptions about the data are systematically varied and the analysis repeated to determine the stability of the results.

Small area analysis: Investigation containing fewer than twenty cases of the disease of interest; often requires special considerations and statistical tests to deal with the low incidence of events.

Specificity: Ability of a screening test to correctly identify absence of a disease

Stakeholder: Individual or organization with an interest in an intervention, health policy, or health outcome.

Strategic planning: Process of identifying objectives and essential actions (preventive and therapeutic) believed sufficient to control a health problem.

Survey: Systematic (but not experimental) method of data collection that often consists of questionnaires or interviews Survey data differ from surveillance data in that they are not ongoing but rather sporadic.

Systematic review: Review of a clearly formulated question that uses systematic and explicit methods to identify, select, and critically appraise relevant research and to collect and analyze data from the studies that are included in the review, the goal of which is an unbiased assessment of a particular topic Statistical methods (meta-analysis) may or may not be used to analyze and summarize the results of the included studies.

Time-series analyses: Quasi-experimental research design in which measurements are made at several different times, thereby allowing trends to be detected.

TOWS analysis: TOWS analysis takes into account the external Threats and Opportunities that face an organization in light of the Weaknesses and Strengths within the organization.

Transferability: Degree to which the results of a study or systematic review can be extrapolated to other circumstances, in particular to routine health care situations.

Transtheoretical model: Theory of health behavior change. It suggests that people move through one of five stages (precontemplation, contemplation, preparation, action, maintenance) and that health behavior change is an evolving process that can be more effectively achieved if the intervention processes match the stage of readiness to change behavior.

Triangulation: Triangulation generally involves the use of multiple methods of data collection and/or analysis to determine points of commonality or disagreement. It often involves a combination of qualitative and quantitative data.

Type 1 evidence: Analytic data showing the importance of a particular health condition and its link with some preventable risk factor. For example, a large body of epidemiologic evidence shows that smoking causes lung cancer.

Type 2 evidence: Data that focus on the relative effectiveness of specific interventions to address a particular health condition. For example, a growing body of evidence shows that several interventions are effective in preventing the uptake (initiation) of smoking in youth.

Type 3 evidence: Data that document the context under which an intervention is appropriate.

Unit of analysis: Unit of assignment in an intervention study. Most commonly, the unit will be an individual person but, in some studies, people will be assigned in groups to one or another of the interventions. This is done either to avoid contamination or for convenience, and the units might be schools, hospitals, or communities.

Vital statistics: Data compiled by state health agencies concerning births, deaths, marriages, divorces, and abortions.

REFERENCES

Some definitions are adapted from the following sources:

Brownson RC, Baker EA, Leet TL, Gillespie KN. *Evidence-Based Public Health.* New York: Oxford University Press; 2003.

Centers for Disease Control and Prevention. Framework for program evaluation in public health. Morbidity and Mortality Weekly Report 1999;48(RR-11):1–40.

Ginter PM, Swayne LM, Duncan WJ. *Strategic Management of Health Care Organizations.* Fourth ed. Malden, MA: Blackwell Publishers Inc.; 2002.

Glanz K, Rimer BK, Viswanath K. *Health Behavior and Health Education. Theory, Research, and Practice.* Fourth ed. San Francisco: Jossey-Bass Publishers; 2008.

Green LW, Kreuter MW. *Health Promotion Planning: An Educational and Ecological Approach.* 4th ed. New York, NY: McGraw Hill; 2005.

Haddix AC, Teutsch SM, Corso PS. *Prevention Effectiveness. A Guide to Decision Analysis and Economic Evaluation.* 2nd ed. New York: Oxford University Press; 2002.

Kohatsu ND, Robinson JG, Torner JC. Evidence-based public health: an evolving concept. *Am J Prev Med.* Dec 2004;27(5):417–421.

Last JM. *A Dictionary of Public Health.* New York: Oxford University Press; 2007.

Porta M, ed. *A Dictionary of Epidemiology.* Fifth Edition ed. New York: Oxford University Press; 2008.

Novick LF, Morrow CB, Mays GP, eds. Public Health Administration. Principles for Population-Based Management. Second Edition. Sudbury, MA: Jones and Bartlett Publishers; 2008.

Petticrew M, Cummins S, Ferrell C, et al. Natural experiments: an underused tool for public health? *Public Health.* Sep 2005;119(9):751–757.

Sackett DL, Straus SE, Richardson WS, Rosenberg W, Haynes RB. Evidence-Based Medicine. How to Practice and Teach EBM. 2nd ed. Edinburgh: Churchill Livingston, 2000.

Witkin BR, Altschuld JW. Conducting and Planning Needs Assessments. A Practical Guide. Thousand Oaks, CA: Sage Publications, 1995.

Index

Accountability for public expenditures, 265
Accreditation, 265
Action, public health
   related issues when considering, 47–53
Action planning
   background, 207–210
   defined, 206
   stepwise approach to successful, 219–226
Action plans
   characteristics, 206
   developing, 206–207
Action (stage of change), 216
Acquired immunodeficiency syndrome
   (AIDS), 53–54
Adjusting rates, 143–144
Adult learning, 18
Advocates, public health, 128
Agency for Healthcare Research and Quality
   (AHRQ), 175
Alcohol consumption, and breast cancer, 68
Alcohol-related traffic fatalities, 91
American Evaluation Association, 253
American Public Health Association
   (APHA), 26
Analytic frameworks, 194–199. *See also*
   Logic models

constructing, 198
developing and using, 194–199
   considering the broad environment,
      198–199
   effects of primary prevention, 195
   effects of point-of-decision prompts, 196
Analytic tools, 92–93
   for assessing risk and intervention
      effectiveness, 62–70
   background, 61
   for comparing options and weighing benefits
      vs. costs, 70–84
   to enhance evidence-based public health
      uptake, 14–17
Analysis Grid for Elements Linked to Obesity
   (ANGELO) model, 182
Annual Review of Public Health, 175
Applicability, 209–210
   rating of the attributes, 209
AssessNow, 113
Association of Public Health
   Observatories, 94

Back to Sleep campaign, 150
Barriers to quality health care, 103
Basic Priority Rating (BPR), 185–186, 188

Behavior change, health-related
    beliefs important in, 216–217
Beliefs important in health behavior change,
    216–217
Benefits, 78. *See also* Cost-benefit analysis
    determining, 78–80
    perceived, 215
"Best practices," 92
Best Practices for Comprehensive Tobacco
    Control Programs, 91
Biological plausibility, 41, 42
Birth Defects Prevention Act, 146–147
Blood alcohol concentration (BAC) laws, 91
Breast cancer
    alcohol consumption and, 68
    environmental agents, and, 37
    incidence and mortality, 139–140
        among Missouri women, 140–141
        select European countries, 140
        trends in, 52
Breast cancer control, initial issue statements
    for, 123
Breast cancer screening guidelines
    chronology and statements from the
        development of, 49
    establishing, 49
Behavioral Risk Factor Surveillance System
    (BRFSS), 130
    intermediate measures, 136–137
Budget planning worksheet, generic, 224

Canadian Task Force on Preventive Health Care
    (CTF), 26, 94
Cancer. *See also* Breast cancer
    disease burden, 49–50
    lung, trachea, and bronchus, 143, 144
Cancer Control P.L.A.N.E.T., 26
Cancer Surveillance, Epidemiology and End
    Results (SEER), 146
Capacity and leadership, 264–265
    engage leadership, 264
    enhance accountability for public
        expenditures, 265
    expand training opportunities, 264–265
Cardiovascular health programs, searching for
    evidence on effectiveness of, 165
Case-control studies, 151–153
Category-specific rates, 139–140

Causal frameworks. *See* Analytic frameworks
CDC BRFSS, 130–131, 136–137, 147, 154
CDC Community Health Resources, 26–27
CDC Social Determinants of Health Maps, 113
CDC WONDER, 131, 135
CDC Working Group on Evaluation, 200, 253
CEA Registry: Center for the Evaluation of
    Value and Risk in Health, 94
Center for Rural Health, 103
Centers for Disease Control (CDC), 135,
    138, 242
Centers for Disease Control and Prevention
    Working Group on Evaluation, 200, 253
Change, stages of, 216
Clinical guidelines, 6. *See also* Practice
    guidelines
Clinically preventable burden (CPB), 182, 183
Clinical settings, guidelines for interventions in,
    89–90
Coalitions,
    defined, 103
    characteristics of effective, 104–105
    continuum of integration, 104
    stages of development, 104
Cochrane Collaboration, 90, 94, 159, 176
Cohort studies, 151
Community assessment, 21
    background, 102
    dissemination of findings, 111–112
    role of stakeholders in, 102-103
    why conduct, 102
Community audits, 108–109
Community-based participatory research
    (CBPR), 208–209
Community coalitions. *See* Coalitions
Community factors,
    action planning, 211–212
    assessment of, 106, 107–108
Community forums/ listening sessions, 110
Community Guide. *See* Guide to Community
    Preventive Services
Community Health Improvement Resources,
    113–114
Community Health Status Indicators (CHSI)
    Project, 131, 253
Community level, prioritizing public health
    issues at, 184–188
Community readiness, 207–208

Community settings, guidelines for
    interventions in, 90–91, 218
Community Tool Box, 114, 227, 253
Conferences, 174
Conducting a Community Assessment, 114
Confounding bias, 44
Consensus conferences, 86–88
Consistency (evidence), 40, 41
Consumers, 128
Contemplation (stage of change), 216
Coronary heart disease (CHD)
    modifiable risk factors for, 51
Cost-benefit analysis (CBA), 73–74, 79. *See
    also* Economic evaluation
    comparing costs to benefits, 80–82
    determining benefits, 78–80
    interpreting and using the results, 83–84
Cost-effectiveness analysis (CEA), 73–74, 79
Cost-effectiveness (CE), 182, 183
Costs, 76. *See also* Funds
    determining, 76–78
    perceived, 215
    types of, 76–77
Cost-utility analysis (CUA), 73–74, 80, 83
County Health Rankings, 155
Cross-sectional studies, 22, 153
Cues to action, 215

Data
    analysis, 110–111
    collection, 106–110
    consolidation of, 66
    reporting and utilizing, 250–251
    triangulation, 246
    types/sources of, 65
        qualitative, 109–110
        quantitative, 108–109
Data abstraction, conducting, 66
Database(s), bibliographic, 22
    computer-stored, 163
    selecting a, 161
Data collection
    and analysis, 245–246
    methods of, 245
Decision analysis, 71–73
    steps in, 72
Decision making in public health
    evidence-based, 35

barriers and solutions for use of, 24–25
    characteristics, 12–14
    domains that influence, 5
    tension between participatory, and, 263
    factors influencing, 47–48
    participatory, 263
Decision tree, analyzing, 71–72
Delphi method(s), 191–192
    flowchart of, 193
Descriptive studies, 22
Design and implementation research, 247–248
Developing and Sustaining Community-Based
    Participatry Research Partnerships: A
    Skill-Building Curriculum, 227
Diabetes, Type 2
    costs of screening for, 81
Dietary change, 217
Discounting, 82
Disease Control Priorities Project (DCPP),
    54–55, 200
Disease frequency, estimating, 134–136
    for smaller populations, 137–138
Disease prevention, 199. *See also* Prevention;
    specific topics
    contrasting approaches to
Diseases. *See also specific diseases*
    perceived severity, 216
    reportable, 146
Dissemination and implementation research, 259
Documents for review, 167. *See also* Journal
    articles; Publications; Scientific literature
Dose-response relationship, 41, 42

Ecological framework(s), 105–106, 210–213
    levels of intervention, 210–212
    objectives and intervention approaches across
        levels of, 211
Economic evaluation, 16, 61, 73, 265. *See also*
    Cost-benefit analysis
    challenges and opportunities in using, 84–86
    conceptual framework for, 75–76
    ensuring effective implementation, 86
    possible outcomes of, 74–75
    types of, 73–74
Economic evaluation ratio, 76
Electromagnetic fields (EMFs), extremely low
    frequency
    and childhood cancer, 41

Emerging issues, 259–260
Environmental analysis, questions to consider
    in, 120
Epidemiology, 121, 134
    analytic, 134, 148–153
    descriptive, 134
Epidemiology Supercourse, 155
Equipment needed, 222
Etiology, 179
European Health for All Database, 131
Evaluation, 23, 252
    creation of change, 248
    defined, 232
    dissemination and implimentation projects,
        247–248
    exploratory, 246–247
    linkages between program planning and, 234
    nature of, 232–233
    principles, 14
    progress in tobacco control, 243
    reasons for, 233–234
    types/methods of, 237–245
        deciding on the appropriate, 245–250
        resource considerations, 248
        policy vs. program, 248–250
        quantitative and qualitative, 245–246
Evaluability assessment. See Exploratory
    evaluation
Evaluation information, questions to consider
    when reporting, 251
Evidence, vii
    accessible for policy makers, 266
    assessing for quality and limits of, 35–37
    challenges related to, 8–9
    consolidation of, 66
    cultural and geographic differences, 9
    defined, 6
    examining a body of scientific, 37–39
    forms of, 6
    finding, 38
    in public health practice, increasing the use
        of, 17–23
    intervention effectiveness, expanding the base
        on 260
    translating it into recommendations and
        action, 86–92
    triangulating, 9
    types of, 7

typologies, 261–262
    understanding the context for, 7–8
    user groups for, vii–ix
Evidence-based behavioral practice, 26, 176
Evidence-based medicine, 10
    citations for, 11
    similarities to and differences from
        Evidence-based public health, 10–12
Evidence-based public health, 3–5, 35–37. See
    also Decision making in public health,
    evidence-based
    addressing health disparities, 265–266
    advances in, 266
    audiences for, 9–10
    competencies, 17–20
    learning from global efforts, 266
    rationale for, 18–19
    sequential framework for enhancing, 18, 21–23
    similarities to and differences from
        evidence-based medicine, 10–12
    tools and approaches to enhance, 14–17
Excess disease, 133
Exercise. See Physical activity
Experimental evidence, 41, 42
Experimental study designs, 148–149
Expert panels, 86–88
Exposure to risk factors, 151, 153

Facilities needed, 222
5-a-Day for Better Health program, 217
Fidelity, 209
Funds, 222. See also Costs

Global Health Council, 267
"Golden diamond," 185
Google Scholar, 176
Group decision making, advantages and
    disadvantages of, 191
Group process, advantages to, 198
Group processes for enhancing creativity,
    190–194
Groupthink, 191
Guidelines. See Clinical guidelines; Practice
    guidelines
Guide to Clinical Preventive Services, 94, 182
Guide to Community Preventive Services, 27,
    90–91, 94–95, 200. See also
    Community Guide

Health Belief Model (HBM), 215–216
Health-care professionals, 128
Health Data, Advocacy, Training, Assistance (DATA) Program, 114
Health disparities
  evidence-based approaches to address, 265–266
Health Education Resource Exchange (HERE), 227
Health Evidence Network (HEN), 55
Health Funders Group, 236
Health Impact Assessment, 16
  Centers for Disease Control and Prevention Health Places, 95
Health Risk Appraisal (HRA), 183–184
Healthy People, 55, 201
Healthy People 2020, 53, 262
Healthy People 2010 Toolkit, 188
Henle-Koch Postulates, 40
"High-risk" strategy, 126
HIV prevention among Asian and Pacific Islander American men, 213

Immunization rates, U.S. adults, by race, 125
Impact evaluation, 239–240
  considerations, design and analysis, 241–242
  importance of reliability and validity, 240–241
  indicators for, 244
Implementation guides, 45
Influenza vaccination among elderly
  intitial issue statements for, 127
Incidence rates, standard error of, 138
Indirect costs, 76–78
Individual factors,
  assessment of, 105, 107–108
Infant mortality in Texas, reducing, 129
Information bias, 44
Investigator triangulation, 246
Internet, use of, 147, 166
Interpersonal factors,
  action planning, 210–211
  assessment of, 106, 107–108
Intervention approaches based on best possible evidence, 12
Interventions. *See also specific topics*
  adapt to community, 208–210
  developing and prioritizing options. *See* Program options

typology for classifying, 261
expand the evidence base on, 260
implementing, 23
steps in designing a successful public health, 219
Interviews, 109
Ischemic heart disease deaths, European countries, 124
Issue(s)
  characterizing it by person, place, and time, 139–144
  dividing it into its component parts, 120–129
  quantifying, 21–22
Issue statement(s), 117–118
  background regarding, 118–120
  components, 121–127
    background/ epidemiologic data, 121–125
    questions about the program or policy, 125–126
    potential solutions, 126
    potential outcomes, 126–127
  developing an initial, 21
  steps in, 122
  importance of stakeholder input, 127–129
  reviewing the, 161

Johns Hopkins Center for Global Health, 27
Journal articles, 159. *See also* Documents for review
  publication, 38–39
  tags used to index, 163

Kaiser Family Foundation, 267–269
Kansas Information for Communities (KIC), 155
Key informant interviews, 173–174, 175
Key words, identifying, 164, 165
Knowledge for Health (K4Health), 227

Latency period, 266–267
Leadership, engagement 264
Life expectancy, 77–78. *See also* Quality adjusted life years
Literature review(s), 22, 63–64, 174–175. *See also* Scientific literature, search of the
  inclusion and exclusion criteria used in, 64–65
  summarizing and applying, 168

Logic models. *See also* Analytic frameworks
    program to improve oral health, 197
    role in program planning, 213–214
Long Island Breast Cancer Study Project
    (LIBCSP), 37–38
Lung cancer
    incidence, 51–52
    mortality rates, 52, 142, 143
        age-adjusted, 144

Maintenance (stage of change), 216
Management Sciences for Health (MSH), 228
Managerial decisions, making the correct,
    219–220
Materials needed, 222
Measures, intermediate
    using, 136–137
MEDLINE, 162, 164. *See also* PubMed
    tags used to index articles in, 163
Member validation, 251
Meta-analysis, 67–69, 159
Missouri Information for Community
    Assessment (MICA), 155
Millennium Development Goals, 180, 201, 262
Mortality rates, 145–146
    standard error of, 138
Multidisciplinary problem solving, xii, 142
Multilevel Approach to Community Health
    (MATCH), 218

National Academy of Sciences: Institute of
    Medicine, 176
National Cancer Institute,
    Health Behavior Constructs, 228
    Using What Works: Adapting Evidence-Based
        Programs to Fit Your Needs, 268
National Center for Health Statistics
    (NCHS), 154
National Conference of State Legislators, 268
National health goals, priority setting
    via, 52–53
National Health Interview Survey (NHIS), 147
National Health Service (NHS) Centre for
    Reviews and Dissemination, 95
National Institutes of Health (NIH), 87
National Registry of Evidence-based Programs
    and Practices (NREEP), 27
National standards for local needs, 87

Needs assessment, 118. *See also* Community
    Assessment
Nominal group technique (NGT), 192

Obesity, prioritizing environmental interventions
    to prevent, 182
Observatoins, 109–110
Observational study designs, 151–153
Office of the Surgeon General, 55
Oral health program, logic model, 197
Organizational factors
    action planning, 211
    community assessment, 106, 107–108
Outcome evaluation, 242–244
    considering potential outcomes, 126–127
    indicators for, 244

Panels, expert, 86–88
Papanicolaou (Pap) test, 266–267
Paradigms, 233
Participatory approaches, 16, 263
Partnerships and engagement, 263–264
Partnership for Prevention, 27, 131
Partners In Information Access for Public
        Health Professionals, 55, 131, 176, 201
PEARL (propriety, economics, acceptability,
        resources, and legality), 185–186
Peer review, 38
Personnel needed, 222
Photovoice, 110
Physical activity
    and coronary heart disease, 51
    effects of point-of-decision prompts on, 196
    evidence matrix for literature on, 169–172
    promoting in youth, 13
Pilot testing the intervention, 225–226
Planned Approach to Community Health
    (PATCH), 218, 228
Planning frameworks, 213, 218.*See also* Action
        planning
    common principles across, 218
Policies, public health. *See* Programs and
        policies
Policy evaluation, 248–250. *See also* Evaluation
Policy factors,
    assessment of, 106, 107–108
Policy implementation, 248
Policy makers, evidence and, viii

Policy surveillance, 262–263
Politicians, 128
Pooled analysis, 69
Pooling, 45–46
Population-based interventions, 90
Population burden, estimating, 48–51
Population strategy, 126
Positivist paradigm, 245
Practice guidelines, 88–91, 126. *See also*
    Clinical guidelines
    defined, 88
Practitioners, public health. *See also* Health-care
    professionals
    evidence and, viii
PRECEDE-PROCEED model, 218
Precontemplation (stage of change), 216
Preparation (stage of change), 216
Preventable burden, 50, 182
Prevented fraction (PF), estimating, 50–51
Prevention. *See also* Disease prevention
    effects of primary, 195
Preventive services, clinical
    prioritizing, 182–184
Print media/written documents, 109
Prioritizing clinical preventive services,
    182–184. *See also* Program options
    ranking of, 183
Priority Missouri Information for Community
    Assessment (MICA), 186
Priority ranks and indicators for Maryland,
    consensus set of, 185
Priority setting. *See also* Basic Priority Rating
    via national health goals, 52–53
    worksheet for, 188
    measure progress and, 262
Problem identification, 62
Problem definition, 119
Process evaluation, 238–239
Productivity losses, averted, 78
Professional, 174
Program development
    and implementation, planning cycle
        for, 207
    innovation and creativity in, 189–190
        creativity in developing alternatives, 190
        group processes for enhancing creativity,
            190–194
Program/direct costs, 76. *See also* Costs

Program evaluation, 248–250. *See also*
    Evaluation
Program evaluation and review technique
    (PERT), 217–218
Program objectives
    examples of, and linkages to action
        strategies, 221
    setting, 220–221
Program options, prioritizing
    analytic methods for, 181–189
        clinical preventive services, 182–184
        community level, 184–188
    background regarding, 179–181
    considerations in, 187
    developing and, 22–23, 178–179
Program planning, and evaluation, 234
Program planning approaches, systematic, 13
Programs and policies, public health
    disseminating results of, 14
    evaluating, 23
Progress
    tracking, 262–263
        set priorities and measure, 262
Publication bias, 38–39
Publications. *See also* Documents for review;
    Scientific literature
    types of, 159–160
PubMed, 176. *See also* MEDLINE

Qualitative data collection, 109–110
Qualitative evaluation, 245–246
Quality-adjusted life years (QALYs),
    79–85, 182
Quasi-experimental study designs, 149–151
    comparison of, 152

RE-AIM, 248, 260
    website, 253, 268
Registries, 146–147
Reliability, 240–241
Research. *See also* specific topics
    assessing causality in, 40
    criteria for, 40–42
Research articles, 159
Research Portfolio Online Reporting Tool
    (RePORTER), 176
Researchers on population health issues,
    evidence and, vii

Research methodology
    addressing methodological issues, 85
    level of analysis, 64–65
    type of analysis, 65
Research Methods Knowledge Base, 55, 254
Research (study) design issues
    external validity, 44–46
    internal validity, 43–44
Research (study) designs, 64. *See also* Research
    experimental, 148–149
    hierarchy of, 43–44, 72, 89–90
    observational, 151–153
    quasi-experimental, 149–151
Research-Tested Intervention Programs
        (RTIPS), 268
Resources, evaluation consideration, 250
Resource needs, assessing, 222
Review articles, 159–160
Reviews, systematic, 15, 61, 62
    checklist for evaluationg the methodological
        quality of, 63
    challenges and opportunities in using, 84–86
    methods for conducting, 62–70
Risk
    perceived, 215
    population attributable, 50,
Risk assessment, 69. *See also* Epidemiology,
        analytic
Risk factors. *See also specific topics*
    exposure to, 151

Scenario planning, 194
Scientific evidence. *See* Evidence
Scientific literature, 158. *See also* Documents
        for review
    background regarding, 158–161
    levels of reading the, 159
    search of the, 161–168, 174–175.*See also*
        Literature review(s)
    conducting a, 164–167
    flowchart for organizing a, 162
    purpose, 161
    seeking sources outside the searchable,
        168, 173–174
    "fugitive" or "grey" literature, 173
    types of publications, 159–160
Seattle 5-a-Day, 217
Selection bias, 44

Self-efficacy, 215–216
Sensitivity analysis, 72, 82–83
    ways to conduct, 82–83
Smoking rates, Asian countries, by gender, 124
Solutions, potential, 126
Special populations and sectors, 265–266
SPOT guidelines, 45
Staff, identifying and training, 86, 222–225
Stages of change, 216–217
    intervention for promoting fruit and vegetable
        consumption, 217
Stakeholders,
    developing an initial issue
        statement, 127–129
    evidence and, viii
    input in developing helaht policy options, 23
    major health policy considerations
        among, 128
    role in community assessment, 102–104
    role in evaluation, 234–237
State standards for local needs, 86
Strategic planning, key aspects of, 119–120
Strength (evidence), 40, 41
Study designs. *See* Research (study) designs
Study execution, 43
Substance Abuse and Mental Health Services
        Administration, 27
Sudden infant death syndrome (SIDS), 150
Suicide rates
    by person, place, and time, 139
Surveillance, public health, 15
    improvement, 262–263
Surveillance systems, public health, 108,
        144–145, 144–147
Surveys, 108, 147
Susceptibility, perceived, 215

Task Force on Community Preventive Services,
        90. *See also* Guide to Community
        Preventive Services
Temporality (evidence), 41–42
Termination (stage of change), 216
Texas Health Data, 155
Theory(ies)
    defined, 214
    individual-level, 215–219
    role in creating programs and policies,
        213–217

Theory of Reasoned Action/Theory of Planned Behavior, 215
Theory triangulation, 246
Time and travel costs, 77, 222
Time line for implementing intervention, 223
Timetables, developing the, 221–222
Time trends, assessing, 51–52
Tobacco control, evaluating progress, 243
Threats, Opportunities, Weaknesses and Strengths (TOWS) analysis, 119–120
  components, 120
Toxic shock syndrome, 36
Training
  opportunities to expand, 264–265
  staff, 86, 222–225
Transdisciplinary research, 264
Transferability, 210
  Rating of the attributes, 209
Transtheoretical Model, 216–217
Travel, and travel costs, 77, 222
Treatment costs, 77–78
  averted, 78
Triangulation of data collection and analysis process, 246. *See also* Investigator triangulation, Theory triangulation

UCLA Center for Health Policy Research, 114
UCLA Health Impact Assessment
  Clearinghouse Learning and Information Center, 27, 95

UCSF School of Medicine: Virtual Library in Epidemiology, 55
United Nations Development Programme, 254
Using What Works: Adapting Evidence-Based Programs to Fit Your Needs, 268
U.S. Preventive Services Task Force (USPSTF), 27, 66, 88
  hierarchy of research designs, 89
U.S. Public Health Service, 44
U.S. Census, 108, 135

Validity, 240–241
  internal, 43–44
  external, 44–46
    build the evidence on, 260
    quality rating criteria, 46
Value expectancy theory, 215–216
Vital statistics, 145–146

World Health Report, 56, 268
World Health Organization (WHO), 55–56, 266, 268
WHO Health Impact Assessment, 28, 95
WHO Statistical Information System (WHOSIS), 131
Wisconsin Clearinghouse for Prevention Resources, 114
WONDER, 131, 135
Workplan, developing the, 221–222